FOURTH EDITION

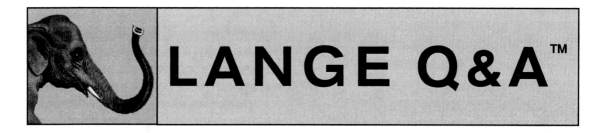

LANGE Q&A™

USMLE STEP 3

Donald A. Briscoe, MD
Associate Program Director
Family Medicine Residency Program
CHRISTUS St. Joseph Hospital
Houston, Texas

McGraw-Hill
Medical Publishing Division

New York Chicago San Francisco Lisbon London Madrid Mexico City Milan
New Delhi San Juan Seoul Singapore Sydney Toronto

Lange Q&A™: USMLE Step 3, Fourth Edition

1 2 3 4 5 6 7 8 9 0   QPD/QPD   0 9 8 7 6 5

ISBN: 0-07-144579-X

Notice

Medicine is an ever-changing science. As new research and clinical experience broaden our knowledge, changes in treatment and drug therapy are required. The authors and the publisher of this work have checked with sources believed to be reliable in their efforts to provide information that is complete and generally in accord with the standards accepted at the time of publication. However, in view of the possibility of human error or changes in medical sciences, neither the authors nor the publisher nor any other party who has been involved in the preparation or publication of this work warrants that the information contained herein is in every respect accurate or complete, and they disclaim all responsibility for any errors or omissions or for the results obtained from use of the information contained in this work. Readers are encouraged to confirm the information contained herein with other sources. For example and in particular, readers are advised to check the product information sheet included in the package of each drug they plan to administer to be certain that the information contained in this work is accurate and that changes have not been made in the recommended dose or in the contraindications for administration. This recommendation is of particular importance in connection with new or infrequently used drugs.

This book was set in Palatino by International Typesetting and Composition.
The editor was Catherine A. Johnson.
The production supervisor was Phil Galea.
Project management was provided by International Typesetting and Composition.
The cover designer was Aimee Nordin.
Quebecor World Dubuque was printer and binder.

This book is printed on acid-free paper.

Library of Congress Cataloging-in-Publication Data

Lange Q & A. USMLE Step 3 / [edited by] Donald A. Briscoe.—4th ed.
    p. ; cm.
  Rev. ed. of: Appleton & Lange's review for the USMLE Step 3 / [edited by] Samuel L. Jacobs. 3rd ed. c2001.
  Includes index.
  ISBN 0-07-144579-X
  1. Medicine—Examinations, questions, etc. 2. Physicians—Licenses—United States—Examinations—Study guides. I. Title: Lange Q and A. USMLE Step 3. II. Title: USMLE Step 3. III. Briscoe, Donald A. IV. Appleton & Lange's review for the USMLE Step 3.
  [DNLM: 1. Medicine—Examination Questions. W 18.2 L2742 2005]
R834.5.A662 2005
610'.76—dc22
                                                                2005041516

Contents

Color insert appears between pages 110 and 111.

Contributors

Douglas Adler, MD
Assistant Professor
University of Texas Medical School at Houston
Houston, Texas
Internal Medicine—Gastroenterology

S. Sohail Ahmed, MD
Assistant Professor
Boston University School of Medicine
Boston, Massachusetts
Internal Medicine—Rheumatology

Cesar Arias, MD
Resident
University of Texas Medical School at Houston
Houston, Texas
Internal Medicine

Sean Blitzstein, MD
Clinical Assistant Professor of Psychiatry
University of Illinois at Chicago
Chicago, Illinois
Psychiatry

Kristina Bogar, DO
Chief Resident, Family Practice
CHRISTUS St. Joseph Hospital
Houston, Texas
Internal Medicine, Pediatrics

Donald A. Briscoe, MD
Associate Program Director
Family Medicine Residency Program
CHRISTUS St. Joseph Hospital
Houston, Texas
Preventive Medicine, Internal Medicine

Joan Bull, MD
Professor
University of Texas Medical School at Houston
Houston, Texas
Internal Medicine—Oncology

Edison Catalano, MD
Professor and Chief
Robert Wood Johnson Medical School at Camden
Camden, New Jersey
Pathology

Abigail Caudle, MD
Chief Resident
University of North Carolina School of Medicine
Chapel Hill, North Carolina
Surgery

Evelyn Chan, MD
Assistant Professor
University of Texas Medical School at Houston
Houston, Texas
Internal Medicine—Medical Ethics

Christian Chisholm, MD
Assistant Professor
University of Virginia School of Medicine
Charlottesville, Virginia
Obstetrics and Gynecology

Mohamed Elfar, MD
Resident, Surgery
CHRISTUS St. Joseph Hospital
Houston, Texas
Surgery

Miguel Escobar, MD
Assistant Professor
University of Texas Medical School at Houston
Houston, Texas
Internal Medicine—Hematology

Elise Everett, MD
Clinical Instructor
University of Virginia School of Medicine
Charlottesville, Virginia
Obstetrics and Gynecology

Christopher Greeley, MD
Assistant Professor
Vanderbilt University School of Medicine
Nashville, Tennessee
Pediatrics

Vanessa Gregg, MD
Resident
University of Virginia School of Medicine
Charlottesville, Virginia
Obstetrics and Gynecology

Eric Haas, MD
Colorectal Surgical Associates
Department of Surgery
CHRISTUS St. Joseph Hospital
Houston, Texas
Surgery

Mark Hughes, MD
Assistant Professor
The Johns Hopkins School of Medicine
Baltimore, Maryland
Internal Medicine—Medical Ethics

Kathie Hullfish, MD
Associate Professor
University of Virginia School of Medicine
Charlottesville, Virginia
Obstetrics and Gynecology

William Irvin, MD
Associate Professor
University of Virginia School of Medicine
Charlottesville, Virginia
Obstetrics and Gynecology

David Johnson, PhD
Associate Professor
Duquesne University Mylan School of Pharmacy
Pittsburgh, Philadelphia
Internal Medicine—Pharmacology

Philip C. Johnson, MD
Professor
University of Texas Medical School at Houston
Houston, Texas
Internal Medicine—Infectious Disease

Judianne Kellaway, MD
Associate Professor
University of Texas Medical School at Houston
Houston, Texas
Ophthalmology

Uday Khosla, MD
Private Practice
Houston, Texas
Internal Medicine—Nephrology

Hong Jin Kim, MD
Assistant Professor
University of North Carolina School of Medicine
Chapel Hill, North Carolina
Surgery

Steven Mays, MD
Assistant Professor
University of Texas Medical School at Houston
Houston, Texas
Internal Medicine—Dermatology

Amal Melhem, MD
Resident
University of Texas Medical School at Houston
Houston, Texas
Internal Medicine

Philip Orlander, MD
Professor
University of Texas Medical School at Houston
Houston, Texas
Internal Medicine—Endocrinology

Alberto Puig, MD, PhD
Assistant Professor
University of Texas Medical School at Houston
Houston, Texas
Internal Medicine—General Medicine

Husam Saad-Eddin, MD
Resident, Family Practice
CHRISTUS St. Joseph Hospital
Houston, Texas
Preventive Medicine, Internal Medicine

Margaret Walkup, MD
Resident
University of North Carolina School of Medicine
Chapel Hill, North Carolina
Surgery

Christopher Williams, MD
Assistant Professor
University of Virginia School of Medicine
Charlottesville, Virginia
Obstetrics and Gynecology

Introduction

This book is designed for those preparing for the United States Medical Licensing Examination (USMLE) Step 3. It provides a comprehensive review source with over 850 "exam-type" multiple choice questions covering the clinical sciences. Detailed explanations are provided for each question, with attempts to explain both why the correct answer is correct and, when appropriate, why the incorrect answers are incorrect. In addition, the last section of this book provides integrated, multispecialty practice tests, both to provide self-assessment and to simulate the multiple choice parts of the Step 3 examination.

The United States Medical Licensing Examination, Step 3

Purpose of the Examination

The purpose of Step 3 is to determine if a physician possesses and can apply the medical knowledge and understanding of clinical science considered essential for the unsupervised practice of medicine, with emphasis placed on patient management in ambulatory care settings. The inclusion of Step 3 in the USMLE sequence of examinations ensures that attention is devoted to the importance of assessing the knowledge and skills of physicians who are assuming independent responsibility for providing general medical care to patients.

Examination Format

Step 3 consists of multiple choice items and computer-based simulations, distributed according to the content blueprint. The examination material is prepared by committees broadly representing the medical profession. The committees comprise recognized experts in their fields, both academic and nonacademic practitioners, as well as members of state medical licensing boards.

Step 3 is a 2-day examination. You must complete each day within 8 hours. The examination has approximately 480 multiple choice items divided into blocks of 35 to 50 items. There will be 45–60 minutes of time allowed for the completion of each block, depending on the number of items in the block. There are also approximately 9 computer-based simulations, with one case in each block, which you will complete on the second day of the exam. You will have up to 25 minutes to complete each block.

Forty-five minutes is allotted for break time each day. The break time can be divided in any way that you choose. You may take a short break between blocks or a longer break for a meal. If you complete a block early, you may use any remaining time for breaks. You may not use any excess time to complete other blocks of the test. If you take too much break time, your time to complete the last block in the testing session will be reduced. If you run out of time while working on a block, you will not be able to move to any new screens. Some versions of the software used will close the session while others will allow you to answer the question that you are viewing. In the latter case, your overall session time is still running and the amount of time that you have remaining for breaks or to complete the session will be reduced.

Step 3 is organized along two principal dimensions: clinical encounter frame and physician task. Encounter frames are the circumstances surrounding physicians' clinical encounters with patients. These include encounters with patients seen for the first time for nonemergency issues, known patients seen for continued care, and patients seen for life-threatening emergency situations. These encounters may occur in clinics, offices, skilled nursing facilities, hospitals, emergency rooms, or on the phone.

Each test item also represents one of six physician tasks. These are obtaining history and performing a physical examination, using laboratory and diagnostic studies, formulating a most likely diagnosis, evaluating the severity of the patient's problems, applying scientific contents and mechanisms of disease, and managing the patient. Patient management includes issues of health maintenance, clinical intervention, therapeutics, and legal/ethical issues.

The 2005 USMLE Bulletin of Information specifies that the clinical encounter frames will be broken down as follows: 20–30% initial care; 50–60% continued care; and 15–25% emergency care. The physician tasks will be broken down as follows: 8–12% obtaining history and performing physical examination; 8–12% using laboratory and diagnostic studies; 8–12% formulating most likely diagnosis; 8–12% evaluating severity of patient's problems; 8–12% applying scientific concepts and mechanisms of disease; and 45–55% managing the patient. All of these percentages are subject to change. The most up-to-date information is available at the USMLE web site (*www.usmle.org*).

During the allowed time for an individual block, the questions may be answered in any order, reviewed, and changed. After exiting a block, no further review of items or change of answers within that block is possible. Policies regarding review of test items may be changed without notice. The most current policies regarding review are posted on the USMLE web site at *www.USMLE.org*. The computer interface includes, among other features, clickable icons for marking questions for review, automated review of marked and incomplete items, and a clock indicating the amount of time remaining. A tutorial on using the computer interface is available at the USMLE web site. A 15-minute optional tutorial will be available for your use on the day of your examination.

Step 3 cases are intended to reflect the diversity of health care populations with respect to age, cultural group, and occupation. The patient population mix is intended to be representative of data collected from various national databases that study health care in the United States.

Clinical Settings

The multiple choice items are organized into blocks that correspond to the clinical settings in which you will encounter the patients. Each setting is described at the beginning of its block. These descriptions are shown here as they would appear during the examination.

Setting I: Office/Health Center

You see patients in two locations: at your office suite, which is adjacent to a hospital, and at a community-based health center. Your office practice is a primary care generalist group. Most of the patients you see are from your own practice and are appearing for regularly scheduled return visits. Occasionally you will encounter a patient whose primary care is managed by one of your associates. Reference may be made to the patient's medical records. Known patients may be managed by the telephone. You may have to respond to questions about information appearing in the public media, which will require interpretation of the medical literature. The laboratory and radiology departments have a full range of services available.

Setting II: Inpatient Facilities

You have general admitting privileges to the hospital, including the children's and women's services. On occasion you will see patients in the critical care unit. Postoperative patients are usually seen in their rooms, unless the recovery room is specified. You may also be called to see patients in the psychiatric unit. There is a short-stay unit where you may see patients undergoing same-day operations or being held for observation. Also, you may visit patients in the adjacent nursing home/extended care facility and the detoxification unit.

Setting III: Emergency Department

Most patients in this setting are new to you, but occasionally you arrange to meet there with a known patient who has telephoned you. Generally, patients encountered here are seeking urgent care. Also available to you are a full range of social services, including rape crisis intervention, family support, and security assistance backed up by local police.

Step 3 Test Item Formats

Multiple Choice Items

Multiple choice items are presented in several formats within each test block. Each of the formats requires selection of the one best choice. The general instructions for answering items are as follows:

Read each question carefully and in the order in which it is presented. Then select the one best response option of the choices offered. More than one option may be partially correct. You must select ONE BEST answer by clicking your mouse on the appropriate answer button or pressing the letter on the keyboard.

Single Items

This is the traditional, most frequently used multiple choice format. It usually consists of a patient in a clinical setting and a reason for the visit. The item vignette is followed by four or five response options lettered A, B, C, D, and E. You are required to select the best answer to the question. Other options may be partially correct, but there is only ONE BEST answer.

Process for single items:

- Read the patient description of each item carefully.
- Try to formulate an answer and then look for it in the list of options.
- Alternatively, read each option carefully and eliminate those that you think are incorrect.
- Of the remaining options, select the one that you believe is most correct.
- If unsure about an answer, it is better to guess, as unanswered questions are counted as incorrect.

Directions for this format and an example item follow:

Example item 1

1. A 45-year old Black man comes to the office for the first time because he says, "I had blood in my urine this morning." He reports no other symptoms. On physical examination, his blood pressure is elevated and his kidneys are palpable bilaterally. The information in his history that is most pertinent to his current condition is

(A) chronic use of analgesics
(B) cigarette smoking
(C) a family history of renal disease
(D) occupational exposure to carbon tetrachloride
(E) recent sore throats

The correct answer is (**C**).

Multiple Item Sets

A single patient-centered vignette may be associated with two or three consecutive questions about the information presented. Each question is linked to the vignette, but is testing a different point. Items are designed to be answered independently of each other. You are required to select the one best choice for each question. Other options may be partially correct, but there is only ONE BEST answer. The process of answering these items is the same as for single items.

Example Items 2–4

A 38-year-old White woman, who is a part-time teacher and mother of three children, comes to the office for evaluation of hypertension. You have been her physician since the birth of her first child 8 years ago. One week ago, an elevated blood pressure was detected during a regularly scheduled examination for entrance into graduate school. Vital signs today are:

Temp.: 98.6°F
Pulse: 100 bpm
Resp.: 22 per minute
BP: 164/100 mmHg (right arm, supine)

2. The most likely finding on physical examination is

(A) an abdominal bruit
(B) cardiac enlargement
(C) decreased femoral pulses
(D) thyroid enlargement
(E) normal retinas

The correct answer is (**E**).

3. The most appropriate next step is to order

(A) complete blood count
(B) serum electrolytes and creatinine
(C) serum glucose

(D) serum thyroxine

(E) urine culture

The correct answer is (**B**).

4. To assess this patient's risk factors for atherogenesis, the most appropriate test is determination of

(A) plasma renin activity

(B) serum cholesterol

(C) serum triglycerides

(D) urinary aldosterone excretion

(E) urinary metanephrine excretion

The correct answer is (**B**).

Cases

A single-patient or family-centered vignette may ask as few as two and as many as three questions, each related to the initial opening vignette. Information is added as the case unfolds. *It is extremely important to answer the questions in the order presented.* Time often passes within a case and your orientation to an item early in a case may be altered by the additional information presented later in the case. If you do skip items, be sure to answer earlier questions with only the information presented to that point in the case. Each item is intended to be answered independently. You are required to select the ONE BEST choice to each question.

Example Items 5–7

A 24-year-old man comes to the office because of intermittent chest pain that began a few weeks ago. You have been his physician for the past 2 years and he has been in otherwise good health. He says that he is not having pain currently. A review of his medical record shows that his serum cholesterol concentration was normal at a preemployment physical examination 1 year ago. You have not seen him since that visit and he says that he has had no other complaints or problems in the interim. He reminds you that he smokes a pack of cigarettes a day. When you question him further, he says that he does not use any alcohol or illicit drugs. Although the details are vague, he describes the chest pain as a substernal tightness that is not related to exertion.

5. The finding on physical examination that would be most consistent with costochondritis as the cause of his chest pain is

(A) crepitance over the second and third ribs anteriorly

(B) deep tenderness to hand pressure on the sternum

(C) localized point tenderness in the parasternal area

(D) pain on deep inspiration

(E) normal physical examination

The correct answer is (**C**).

6. In light of the patient's original denial of drug use, the most appropriate next step to confirm a diagnosis of cocaine use is to

(A) ask the lab if serum is available for a toxicologic screening on his previous blood sample

(B) call his family to obtain corroborative history

(C) obtain a plasma catecholamine concentration

(D) obtain a urine sample for a routine urinalysis but also request a toxicologic screen

(E) present your findings to the patient and confront him with the suspected diagnosis

The correct answer is (**E**).

7. Cocaine use is confirmed. The patient admits a possible temporal relationship between his cocaine use and his chest pain. He expresses concern about long-term health risks. He should be advised that

(A) Cocaine-induced myocardial ischemia can be treated with beta-blockers.

(B) Death can occur from cocaine-induced myocardial infarction or arrhythmia.

(C) The presence of neuropsychiatric sequelae from drug use indicates those at risk for sudden death associated with cocaine use.

(D) Q wave myocardial infarction occurs only with smoked "crack" or intravenous cocaine use.

(E) Underlying coronary artery disease is the principal risk for sudden death associated with cocaine use.

The correct answer is (**B**).

Primum Computer-Based Case Simulations (CCS)

Primum CCS allows you to provide care for a simulated patient. You decide which diagnostic information to obtain and how to treat and monitor the patient's progress. In Primum CCS, you may request information from the history and physical examination; order labs, diagnostic studies, procedures, or consultations; and start medications or other therapies. As time passes, the patient's condition changes based on the underlying problem and the interventions that you order. You must monitor the results of the tests that you order and the interventions that you make. When you confirm that there is nothing further that you want to do, you may advance simulated time in order to reevaluate the patient's condition. You cannot go back in time but you can change your orders to reflect your updated management plan. The patient's chart contains an order sheet and reports resulting from your orders. You can review the vital signs, progress notes, patient updates, and test results. You may care for and move the patient among the office, home, emergency department, intensive care unit, and hospital ward.

The CCS scoring process compares your patient management strategy with policies obtained from experts. Actions resembling a range of optimal strategies will produce a higher score. Dangerous and unnecessary actions will detract from your score. You must balance thoroughness, efficiency, avoidance of risk, and timeliness in responding to the clinical situation.

Practice time with the CCS software is not available on the day of the test. You must review the CCS orientation material and practice the sample cases well in advance of your testing day in order to have an understanding of how the CCS system works. Sample cases are provided to Step 3 applicants on the USMLE CD and are available at the USMLE website.

Specific Information of the Step 3 Examination

The USMLE is sponsored by the Federation of State Medical Boards (FSMB) and the National Board of Medical Examiners (NBME). Rules for the USMLE program are established by a composite committee that includes representatives of the FSMB, NBME, Educational Commission for Foreign Medical Graduates (ECFMG), and the American public. Information is published in an annual Bulletin of Information, which is available for download at the USMLE website (*www.usmle.org*). You must be familiar with and will be subject to the policies and procedures of the Bulletin of Information for the year in which you take your examination. Changes in the USMLE program may occur after the release of the bulletin. If changes occur, information will be posted on the USMLE website.

The registration entity for the Step 3 examination is the FSMB. You must contact the FSMB for information on how to apply for the USMLE, application materials, information on the status of your application or scheduling permit, or information on obtaining a replacement scheduling permit (in the event that it is lost). The FSMB may be contacted at:

FSMB
Department of Examination Services
P.O. Box 619850
Dallas, TX 75261-9850
Website: *www.fsmb.org*
Email: *usmle@fsmb.org*

To be eligible for Step 3, prior to submitting your application, you must

- Meet the Step 3 requirements set by the medical licensing authority to which you are applying.
- Obtain the MD degree (or its equivalent) or the DO degree.
- Pass Step 1, Step 2 CK and, if required based on the rules, Step 2 CS.
- Obtain certification by the ECFMG or successfully complete a "Fifth Pathway" program if you are a graduate of a medical school outside of the United States or Canada.

Application procedures for Step 3 vary among jurisdictions. You should begin inquiries at least

3 months in advance of the dates on which you expect to take the test.

The Step 3 examination is given at Prometric Test Centers in the United States and its territories. Prometric is a division of Thomson Learning, Inc. Once your application has been approved, an eligibility period is assigned. A scheduling permit will be issued to you with instructions for making an appointment at a Prometric Test Center. The eligibility period starts immediately and extends for approximately 90 calendar days, so you should contact Prometric immediately after receiving your scheduling permit to schedule your test dates. If you are unable to take the test during your eligibility period, contact the FSMB to inquire about a 3-month eligibility period extension (a fee is charged for this and restrictions may apply). If you fail to take your examination within your eligibility period and wish to take it in the future, you will need to submit a new application and fee(s).

Physical Conditions

On the day(s) of your test, you should arrive at the Prometric center 30 minutes before your scheduled testing time. If you arrive late, you may not be admitted. If you arrive more than 30 minutes after your scheduled time, you will not be admitted.

When you arrive at the test center, you must present your scheduling permit and an acceptable form of identification. These include: passport, driver's license with photograph, national identity card, other government-issued identification, and ECFMG-issued identification card. If you do not have your scheduling permit and identification, you will not be admitted to the test.

Test center staff monitors all testing sessions. You must follow their instructions throughout the examination. They are not authorized to answer questions regarding examination content, software, or scoring.

On the day of the examination, you are not allowed to bring any personal belongings into the testing area. If you bring any personal belongings to the test center, you must store them in a designated locker or cubicle outside of the testing room. You will be provided with laminated writing surfaces, dry erase markers, and an eraser, which must be returned after the test. Making notes of any kind, except on the materials provided, is not permitted. You may not leave your testing station for breaks unless the break screen is visible on your computer monitor. During testing breaks, you may use a telephone or other communication device, but only for purposes not related to test content. You may not remove any materials (written, printed, recorded, and so forth) from the test center. Complete rules of conduct are available in the Bulletin of Information.

Organization of this Book

This book is organized to cover each of the clinical science areas that you will encounter on the Step 3 examination. Each chapter lists questions first, followed by the answers and explanations, and a bibliography for further study. The question formats here have been chosen to conform to the style that you will encounter on the examination. This is done to familiarize you before you sit for the examination.

As is done for the actual examination, the practice test items are arranged in blocks of 50, for which 1 hour should be allotted, and organized by one of the three clinical settings described above. The amount of time allowed is proportional to the amount of time that will be available for each block of questions during the actual examination.

Answers, Explanations, and Bibliography

In each of the sections of the book, the question sections are followed by a section containing the answers, explanations, and references to the questions. This section tells you the answer to each question, provides an explanation and review of both why the answer is correct and why the other answers are incorrect, and tells you where you can find more information on the subject. We encourage you to use this section as a basis for further study and understanding.

If you choose the correct answer to a question, you can then read the explanation for reinforcement and to add to your knowledge of the subject matter. If you choose the wrong answer to a question, you can read the explanation for a discussion of the material in question. You can also look up the reference cited for a more in-depth discussion.

How to Use this Book

There are two logical ways to get the most value from this book. We will call them Plan A and Plan B.

In Plan A, you go straight to the practice tests and complete them according to the instructions. After taking the tests and checking your answers, the number of questions that you answered incorrectly will be a good indicator of your initial knowledge state and the types of questions that you answered incorrectly will help point you in the right direction for further preparation and review. At this point, you can use the individual specialty chapters of the book to help you improve any areas of relative weakness.

In Plan B, you go through the clinical chapters first. Once you've completed this process, then you take the practice tests, check your answers and see how well prepared you are at this point. If you still have an area of significant weakness, it should be apparent in time for you to take remedial action.

In Plan A, by taking the practice test first, you get quick feedback regarding your initial areas of strength and weakness. You may find that you know all of the material very well, indicating that perhaps only a cursory review is necessary. This may be good to know early on in your exam preparation. On the other hand, you may find that you have some specific areas of weakness (such as pediatrics and psychiatry) and could then focus on these areas in your preparation—not only with this book but also with textbooks of pediatrics and psychiatry.

However, it is unlikely that you will not do some preparation prior to taking the USMLE Step 3 (especially since you have this book). Therefore, it may be more realistic to take the practice test after you have reviewed the specialty sections—as in Plan B. This will probably give you a more realistic test-type situation, as few of us may sit down for a test without studying first. In this case, you will have done some reviewing (from superficial to in-depth) and your practice test will reflect this studying time. If, after reviewing the specialty sections and taking the practice test, your scores indicate some weaknesses, you can then go back for further review of the subject sections and supplement your preparations with appropriate texts.

Now take a deep breath, relax, and good luck!

Acknowledgments

While one name may go on the cover of this book, this was far from a one person job. I would first like to thank all of the contributors to this book. This project gave me the chance to work with some old friends and with some new ones. I appreciate everyone's excellent contributions and dedication. I also would like to acknowledge the work of the contributors to the previous editions of the book, published as *Appleton & Lange's Review for the USMLE Step 3*. We made significant changes in this edition, but it was built on the foundations of the previous title. I truly appreciate the assistance of Catherine Johnson and the professional staff at McGraw-Hill for leading me through this endeavor.

I also appreciate the assistance of everyone at CHRISTUS St. Joseph Hospital. My colleagues in the Family Practice Residency—Dan Kalb, Neeta Gautam, Juan Garcia, Olufunke Odetunde, Kent Lee, and Anush Pillai—who gave me some room to work and provided helpful comments and suggestions throughout. I thank the residents with whom I have the privilege of working and from whom I learn something new everyday. To Shaylor Thomas, Tracy Salinas, the clinical and administrative staffs of the FPC and CMG, thank you for all that you do for the residency and the patients. A special thank you goes to Eugene Toy, who gave me a first writing opportunity and introduced me to those responsible for this book.

This would not have been possible without the support of my family. To Heather, Cal, Casey, and my parents, I give my thanks and love. To Lisa Peden, Eileen Lafleur, and all of our family in Maryland and Texas, thanks for all of your help during this busy time.

Finally, on behalf of everyone involved with this project, I dedicate this book to those for whom it is intended—residents in the midst of their medical training. Step 3 is just one more hurdle to clear as you go. We wish you the best of luck on your examinations and in your careers.

Donald A. Briscoe, MD

	REFERENCE RANGE	SI REFERENCE INTERVALS
BLOOD, PLASMA, SERUM		
* Alanine aminotransferase (ALT), serum	10–40 U/L	10–40 U/L
* Alkaline phosphatase, serum	Male: 30–100 U/L	Male: 30–100 U/L
	Female: 45–115 U/L	Female: 45–115 U/L
Amylase, serum	25–125 U/L	25–125 U/L
* Aspartate aminotransferase (AST), serum	15–40 U/L	15–40 U/L
* Bilirubin, serum (adult), total // direct	0.1–1.0 mg/dL // 0.0–0.3 mg/dL	2–17 µmol/L // 0–5 µmol/L
Calcium, serum (total)	8.4–10.2 mg/dL	2.1–2.8 mmol/L
* Cholesterol, serum		
Total	150–240 mg/dL	3.9–6.2 mmol/L
HDL	30–70 mg/dL	0.8–1.8 mmol/L
LDL	<160 mg/dL	<4.2 mmol/L
Cortisol, serum	8:00 AM: 5–23 µg/dL // 4:00 PM: 3–15 µg/dL	138–635 nmol/L // 82–413 nmol/L
	8:00 PM: # 50% of 8:00 AM	Fraction of 8:00 AM: # 0.50
Creatine kinase, serum	Male: 25–90 U/L	25–90 U/L
	Female: 10–70 U/L	10–70 U/L
* Creatinine, serum	0.6–1.2 mg/dL	53–106 µmol/L
Electrolytes, serum		
* Sodium (Na^+)	135–146 mEq/L	135–146 mmol/L
* Potassium (K^+)	3.5–5.0 mEq/L	3.5–5.0 mmol/L
* Chloride (Cl^-)	95–105 mEq/L	95–105 mmol/L
* Bicarbonate (HCO_3^-)	22–28 mEq/L	22–28 mmol/L
Ferritin, serum	Male: 15–200 ng/mL	15–200 µg/L
	Female: 12–150 ng/mL	12–150 µg/L
Follicle-stimulating hormone, serum/plasma	Male: 4–25 mIU/mL	4–25 U/L
	Female: premenopause 4–30 mIU/mL	4–30 U/L
	midcycle peak 10–90 mIU/mL	10–90 U/L
	postmenopause 40–250 mIU/mL	40–250 U/L
Gases, arterial blood (room air)		
PO_2	75–100 mmHg	10.0–14.0 kPa
PCO_2	35–45 mmHg	4.4–5.9 kPa
pH	7.35–7.45	[H^+] 36–44 nmol/L
* Glucose, serum	Fasting: 70–110 mg/dL	3.8–6.1 mmol/L
	2-h postprandial: <120 mg/dL	<6.6 mmol/L
Immunoglobulins, serum		
IgA	76–390 mg/dL	0.76–3.90 g/L
IgE	0–380 IU/mL	0–380 kIU/L
IgG	650–1500 mg/dL	6.5–15 g/L
IgM	40–345 mg/dL	0.4–3.45 g/L
Iron	50–170 µg/dL	9–30 µmol/L
Lactate dehydrogenase, serum	45–90 U/L	45–90 U/L
Luteinizing hormone, serum/plasma	Male: 6–23 mIU/mL	6–23 U/L
	Female: follicular phase 5–30 mIU/mL	5–30 U/L
	midcycle 75–150 mIU/mL	75–150 U/L
	postmenopause 30–200 mIU/mL	30–200 U/L
Osmolality, serum	275–295 mOsmol/kg H_2O	275–295 mOsmol/kg H_2O
Phosphorus (inorganic), serum	3.0–4.5 mg/dL	1.0–1.5 mmol/L
Proteins, serum		
Total (recumbent)	6.0–7.8 g/dL	60–78 g/L
Albumin	3.5–5.5 g/dL	35–55 g/L
Globulin	2.3–3.5 g/dL	23–35 g/L
Thyroid-stimulating hormone (TSH), serum	0.5–5.0 µU/mL	0.5–5.0 mU/L
Thyroxine (T_4), serum	5–12 µg/dL .	64–155 nmol/L
Triglycerides	35–160 mg/dL	0.4–1.81 mmol/L
Triiodothyronine (T_3) resin uptake	25–35%	0.25–0.35
* Urea nitrogen, serum (BUN)	7–18 mg/dL	1.2–3.0 mmol/L
Uric acid, serum	3.0–8.2 mg/dL	0.18–0.48 mmol/L
CEREBROSPINAL FLUID		
Cell count	0–5 cells/mm³	0–5 × 10⁶/L
Chloride	118–132 mEq/L	118–132 mmo
Gamma globulin	3–12% total proteins	0.03–0.12
Glucose	40–70 mg/dL	2.2–3.9 mmol/L

(Continued)

	REFERENCE RANGE	SI REFERENCE INTERVALS
Pressure	70–180 mm H_2O	70–180 mm H_2O
Proteins, total	<40 mg/dL	<0.40 g/L
HEMATOLOGIC		
Bleeding time (template)	2–7 minutes	2–7 minutes
CD4 cell count	>500/mm³	
Erythrocyte count	Male: 4.3–5.9 million/mm³	$4.3–5.9 \times 10^{12}$/L
	Female: 3.5–5.5 million/mm³	$3.5–5.5 \times 10^{12}$/L
Erythrocyte sedimentation rate (Westergren)	Male: 0–15 mm/h	0–15 mm/h
	Female: 0–20 mm/h	0–20 mm/h
Hematocrit	Male: 41–53%	0.41–0.53
	Female: 36–46%	0.36–0.46
Hemoglobin blood	Male: 13.5–17.5 g/dL	2.09–2.71 mmol/L
	Female: 12.0–16.0 g/dL	1.86–2.48 mmol/L
Hemoglobin A_{1c}	≤6%	≤0.06%
Leukocyte count and differential		
Leukocyte count	4500–11,000/mm³	$4.5–11.0 \times 10^9$/L
Neutrophils, segmented	54–62%	0.54–0.62
Neutrophils, band	3–5%	0.03–0.05
Eosinophils	1–3%	0.01–0.03
Basophils	0–0.75%	0.0–00.75
Lymphocytes	25–33%	0.25–0.33
Monocytes	3–7%	0.03–0.07
Mean corpuscular hemoglobin (MCH)	25–35 pg/cell	0.39–0.54 fmol/cell
Mean corpuscular hemoglobin concentration (MCHC)	31–36% Hb/cell	4.81–5.58 mmol Hb/L
Mean corpuscular volume (MCV)	80–100 µm³	80–100 fl
Partial thromboplastin time (activated)	<28 s	<28 s
Platelet count	150,000–400,000/mm³	$150–400 \times 10^9$/L
Prothrombin time	<12 seconds	<12 seconds
Reticulocyte count	0.5–1.5% of red cells	0.005–0.015
Volume		
Plasma	Male: 25–43 mL/kg	0.025–0.043 L/kg
	Female: 28–45 mL/kg	0.028–0.045 L/kg
Red cell	Male: 20–36 mL/kg	0.020–0.036 L/kg
	Female: 19–31 mL/kg	0.019–0.031 L/kg
URINE		
Calcium	100–300 mg/24 h	2.5–7.5 mmol/24 h
Creatinine clearance	Male: 97–137 mL/min	
	Female: 88–128 mL/min	
Osmolality	50–1400 mOsmol/kg H_2O	
Oxalate	8–40 µg/mL	90–445 µmol/L
Proteins, total	<150 mg/24 h	<0.15 g/24 h

An astrisk (*) indicates a laboratory value included in the biochemical profile.

CHAPTER 1

Internal Medicine
Questions

Questions 1 through 3

A 45-year-old male comes to your office for his first annual checkup in the last 10 years. On first impression, he appears overweight but is otherwise healthy and has no specific complaints. He has a brother with diabetes and a sister with high blood pressure. Both of his parents are deceased and his father died of a stroke at age 73. He is a long standing heavy smoker and only drinks alcohol on special occasions. On physical examination, his blood pressure is 156/90 in the left arm and 154/88 in the right arm. The rest of the examination is unremarkable. He is concerned about his health and does not want to end up on medication, like his siblings.

1. Regarding your initial recommendations, which of the following would be most appropriate?

    (A) You should take no action and ask him to return to clinic in 1 year for a repeat blood pressure check.

    (B) You should immediately start him on an oral antihypertensive medication and ask him to return to clinic in 1 week.

    (C) You should advise him to stop smoking, start a strict diet and exercise routine with the goal of losing weight, and return to clinic in 6 months.

    (D) You should consider starting a workup for potential causes of secondary hypertension.

    (E) You should screen him for diabetes and evaluate him for other cardiovascular risk factors before proceeding any further.

2. In the initial evaluation of a patient such as this, which of the following should be routinely recommended?

    (A) a urine microalbumin/creatinine ratio

    (B) an echocardiogram

    (C) thyroid function tests

    (D) renal function tests (serum creatinine and blood urea nitrogen [BUN])

    (E) an exercise stress test

3. Your patient returns to clinic a few weeks later for a follow-up appointment. Despite having lost 3 lb and increasing his activity to walking 2 mi three times per week, his blood pressure remains elevated at 148/92. His initial evaluation revealed a fasting blood sugar of 156 and a hemoglobin A1C of 7.5. Along with starting hypoglycemic medications to control his diabetes, you recommend that he take an antihypertensive medication. Which of the following classes of antihypertensive medications would you start this patient on?

    (A) an angiotensin-converting enzyme (ACE) inhibitor

    (B) a beta-blocker

    (C) a central acting alpha-blocker

    (D) a calcium channel blocker

    (E) a diuretic

Questions 4 and 5

A 52-year-old male construction worker is seen in the emergency department at a local hospital with complaints of persistent cough for the past 4 months. He has been relatively healthy until a few months ago, when he lost his mother and developed severe depression which left him socially and professionally paralyzed. He has stopped doing any exercise or outdoor activity and spends most of his time at home eating, sleeping, and watching TV. In addition, he has noticed a 20-lb weight gain over this period but attributes it to his lack of exercise and increased food intake. His cough is worse at night, or any time when he lies down to sleep, and he notices a burning sensation in his throat associated with it. It is not associated with fever or chills, and his wife complains that he is constantly clearing his throat after meals. He smoked a few cigarettes per day as a young man in the Navy but quit more than 30 years ago. He denies recent travel or incarceration and has no recollection of any sick contacts. On examination, he is afebrile and appears mildly obese. His lung examination is clear. His oropharynx is red and mucosal membranes are dry and not inflamed.

4. Which of the following statements describes the likely cause of his chronic cough?

    (A) The patient likely suffers from a common cold due to a viral infection and will improve with symptomatic medications.

    (B) The patient most likely suffers from chronic bronchitis exacerbated by a bacterial infection.

    (C) The patient has developed gastroesophageal reflux disease (GERD).

    (D) The patient has developed late onset occult asthma.

    (E) The patient has a "nervous" cough due to severe depression.

5. Which of the following therapies would be most beneficial in alleviating this patient's symptoms?

    (A) an inhaled, short-acting beta-2 agonist

    (B) a proton pump inhibitor (PPI)

    (C) an antitussive-expectorant syrup

    (D) weight loss and exercise

    (E) prolonged course of antibiotics

6. You are asked to interview a young couple who wish to conceive a child. Their first and only son was born with a rare, autosomal recessive glycogen storage disorder known as Pompe's disease. Both parents are healthy and unaffected by this disease, but the father believes that he has heard of a distant cousin who also has this disease. They are concerned about the possibility that their next child will also be born with the affliction. In giving them advice about their chances of having a healthy child, you should:

    (A) Tell them not to worry about it; their next child will surely be healthy.

    (B) Tell them that their next child has a 25% chance of being born with the disease.

    (C) Tell them that there is a 50:50 chance that their next child will be affected.

    (D) Tell them that it is impossible to predict the likelihood that their next child will have the disease.

    (E) Advise them not to have any more children because they all will certainly be affected.

Questions 7 and 8

A 53-year-old female has made an appointment to see you concerning the recent onset of menopause. Her last menstrual period was 8 months ago and, over the last year, she had noticed that her periods were becoming lighter and less frequent. In addition, she has developed frequent hot flashes, and her mood has become very labile. She wishes to know what your advice is regarding hormone replacement therapy. She has heard recent reports in the news concerning an increase risk of developing cardiovascular complications, especially heart attacks and strokes. Although she is in great health, her father died at age 50 of a massive heart attack. Her mother is alive and well, and there is no history of breast cancer among the females in her family.

7. Regarding postmenopausal hormone replacement therapy (HRT), which of the following statements would be correct?

   (A) Known benefits from HRT in postmenopausal women include a reduction in the incidence of osteoporosis and bone fractures (particularly hip fractures).

   (B) Known benefits from HRT in postmenopausal women include a cardioprotective effect, which reduces the incidence of coronary artery disease (CAD) and myocardial infarction (MI).

   (C) HRT increases the incidence of endometrial cancer in all patients.

   (D) Although HRT reduces vasomotor instability and hot flashes after menopause, this effect is short-lived and there is no effect in mood stability.

   (E) Despite recent press reports, any woman at risk for osteoporosis should take HRT, regardless of cardiovascular risk factors.

8. Which of the following would be the strongest argument to avoid HRT in this patient?

   (A) HRT is unlikely to relieve her hot flashes.

   (B) She has a positive family history of CAD.

   (C) She is at high risk for developing breast cancer.

   (D) She is at high risk for developing venous thromboembolism.

   (E) She probably would develop breast tenderness and bloating.

9. A young college student is brought to your office by his fiancé for evaluation of weight loss. He tells you that, over the past few months, he seems to be unable to gain any weight despite having a ferocious appetite and that he is steadily losing weight. He has also noticed increased thirst and urination. Over the past few nights he has awakened several times to go to the bathroom. You suspect that he may have developed diabetes. Which of the following is a diagnostic criterion for diabetes mellitus (DM)?

   (A) a fasting plasma glucose level of >140 mg/dL

   (B) a nonfasting plasma glucose level of >126 mg/dL

   (C) a fasting (overnight fast) plasma glucose level of >126 mg/dL

   (D) a blood glucose level of 180 mg/dL, 2 h after completing a glucose tolerance test with a 75-g oral glucose load.

   (E) a serum glycosylated hemoglobin (A1C) level higher than 5%

Questions 10 and 11

A 67-year-old male with a history of type II diabetes and hypertension is hospitalized with complaints of retrosternal chest pain that radiates to the left arm and jaw. In the emergency department, an electrocardiogram (ECG) showed S-T segment depressions in the inferior and lateral leads. He has been given the diagnosis of *acute coronary syndrome* and admitted to the coronary care unit for further evaluation and treatment. Admission laboratory values reveal a total cholesterol of 270, a low-density lipoprotein (LDL) of 190, and a high-density lipoprotein (HDL) of 28. He is currently smoking a pack of cigarettes per day and lives a sedentary life. He is clearly overweight and his blood pressure, despite medication, remains elevated at 150/88. His last hemoglobin A1C less than a month ago was 9.8%.

10. After being discharged from the hospital, which of the following cholesterol lowering regimens should be recommended to this patient?

   (A) Low fat diet and exercise four times per week should reduce his cholesterol profile to acceptable levels.

   (B) Starting a statin (3-hydroxy-3-methylglutaryl coenzyme A [HMG-CoA] reductase inhibitor) in addition to smoking cessation, diet, and exercise may reduce his risk of developing further cardiovascular complications.

   (C) Starting niacin and recommending smoking cessation classes should be the first line therapy in order to increase his HDL and reduce his risk for further cardiovascular complications.

   (D) There is no role for cholesterol lowering medications in secondary prevention of cardiovascular disease.

   (E) The role of cholesterol lowering drugs in reducing the risk for CAD is not well established and routine recommendation of such therapy after acute coronary syndrome should be avoided.

11. In addition to diet, exercise, and smoking cessation, which of the following would have the largest impact in reducing his cholesterol?

   (A) controlling his blood pressure

   (B) increasing his consumption of alcoholic beverages to three to four glasses of wine per day

   (C) improving his sleeping habits

   (D) adding thyroid hormone to his medications

   (E) controlling his diabetes

Questions 12 through 14

A 48-year-old female with a history of mild congestive heart failure (CHF) treated with furosemide presents to the ER for evaluation of 24 h of epigastric pain, nausea, and vomiting after eating a large meal in a restaurant. Previously, the patient had experienced intermittent right upper quadrant pain after eating. On examination, the patient has a temperature of 98.5°F and a pulse of 100. Her examination is remarkable for epigastric tenderness to palpation, normal bowel sounds, and no rebound tenderness or guarding.

Lab studies are as follows:

Leukocyte count	4800/mm^3
Alanine aminotransferase	258 U/L
Aspartate aminotransferase	287 U/L
Alkaline phosphatase, serum	350 U/L
Bilirubin (total)	2.0 mg/dL
Bilirubin (indirect)	0.4 mg/dL
Amylase	2865 U/L
Lipase	3453 U/L

12. Which of the following is the most likely diagnosis?

   (A) acute gastroenteritis

   (B) acute gallstone pancreatitis

   (C) drug induced pancreatitis

   (D) acute cholecystitis

   (E) acute cholangitis

13. The most appropriate next test to order would be:

   (A) abdominal x-ray

   (B) abdominal computed tomographic (CT) scan

   (C) abdominal ultrasound

   (D) magnetic resonance imaging (MRI) of the abdomen

   (E) stool cultures and assessment for ova and parasites

14. The patient is made NPO and vigorously hydrated. After 3 days, the amylase and lipase normalize, but the bilirubin rises to 4.2 mg/dL. An endoscopic retrograde cholangiopancreatography (ERCP) is performed, and the following cholangiogram is obtained (see Fig. 1-1). The best treatment option at this time is:

   (A) papillary dilation and stone extraction

   (B) papillotomy (aka. sphincterotomy) and stone extraction

   (C) placement of a transpapillary stent in the biliary tree

(D) placement of a transpapillary stent in the pancreatic duct

(E) no further manipulations are required

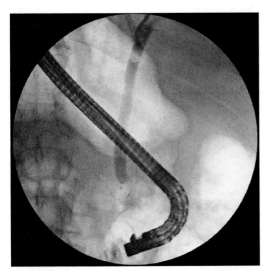

FIG. 1-1 (*Courtesy of Douglas G. Adler, MD.*)

15. The biological half-life of a drug is generally related to which of the following?

(A) the time for a drug to be absorbed into the blood

(B) the time for a drug to take effect following administration

(C) the time for the body burden of a drug to be reduced by 50%

(D) the serum concentration of a drug that is 50% of the toxic level

(E) a value that is half the duration of action of a drug

16. Which of the following organs/systems is especially sensitive to toxic interactions between acetaminophen and alcohol?

(A) kidney

(B) stomach

(C) liver

(D) inner ear

(E) peripheral nervous system

Questions 17 through 19

A 42-year-old man without prior significant medical history comes to your office for evaluation of chronic diarrhea of 12 months duration, although the patient states he has had loose stools for many years. During this time he has lost 25 lb. The diarrhea is large volume, occasionally greasy, and non-bloody. In addition, the patient has mild abdominal pain for much of the day. He has been smoking a pack of cigarettes a day for 20 years and drinks approximately five beers per day. His physical examination reveals a thin male with temporal wasting and generalized muscle loss. He has glossitis and angular cheilosis. He has excoriations on his elbows and knees and scattered papulovesicular lesions in these regions as well.

17. Which of the following is the most likely diagnosis for this patient?

(A) chronic pancreatitis

(B) Crohn's disease

(C) celiac Sprue

(D) Whipple's disease

(E) ulcerative colitis

18. The best test to confirm the suspected diagnosis is:

(A) abdominal CT scan with contrast

(B) small bowel x-ray

(C) esophagogastroduodenoscopy with small bowel biopsy

(D) colonoscopy with colonic biopsy

(E) 72-h fecal fat quantification

19. The most serious long-term complication this patient could face is:

(A) pancreatic cancer

(B) small bowel cancer

(C) gastric cancer

(D) colon cancer

(E) rectal cancer

Questions 20 through 22

A 24-year-old male medical student is admitted to the hospital for the evaluation of a 3-month history of bloody stools. The patient has approximately six blood stained or blood streaked stools per day, associated with relatively little, if any, pain. He has not had any weight loss, and he has been able to attend classes without interruption. He denies any fecal incontinence. He has no prior medical history. Review of systems is remarkable only for occasional fevers and the fact that the patient quit smoking approximately 8 months ago. A colonoscopy is performed and reveals a granular, friable colonic mucosal surface with loss of normal vascular pattern from the anal verge to the hepatic flexure of the colon. Biopsies reveal prominent neutrophils in the epithelium and cryptitis with focal crypt abscesses, and no dysplasia. The patient is diagnosed with ulcerative colitis.

20. Which of the following is the best initial treatment for this patient?

    (A) colectomy
    (B) oral prednisone
    (C) oral metronidazole
    (D) cortisone enemas
    (E) intravenous cyclosporine

21. While on the inpatient service, the patient is noted to have a serum alkaline phosphatase of 380 U/L and a bilirubin of 2.4 mg/dL. An ERCP is performed, and the following cholangiogram is obtained (see Fig. 1-2). In addition to ulcerative colitis, the patient likely has what other illness?

    (A) primary biliary cirrhosis
    (B) Wilson's disease
    (C) alpha-1 antitrypsin deficiency
    (D) hereditary hemochromatosis
    (E) primary sclerosing cholangitis (PSC)

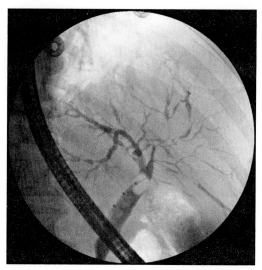

FIG. 1-2 (*Courtesy of Douglas G. Adler, MD.*)

22. In addition to an increased lifetime risk of colon cancer, the patient is also at increased risk for which of the following tumors?

    (A) hepatocellular carcinoma
    (B) hepatoblastoma
    (C) desmoid tumors
    (D) small bowel lymphoma
    (E) cholangiocarcinoma

Questions 23 and 24

A 61-year-old man comes to your office for a checkup. He currently feels well and has no focal complaints. He has a past medical history significant for well-controlled hypertension, and his gallbladder was removed 3 years ago in the setting of acute cholecystitis. He does not smoke and drinks one to two alcoholic beverages per day. Family history is remarkable for colon cancer in his mother at age 45 and a brother at age 49. He has a sister who developed endometrial cancer at age 53. He has never undergone colon cancer screening and is interested in pursuing this.

23. Which colorectal cancer screening test would be best for this patient?

    (A) virtual colonoscopy (aka CT colography)
    (B) barium enema alone
    (C) barium enema with flexible sigmoidoscopy

(D) fecal occult blood testing three times

(E) colonoscopy

24. The patient's family history is strongly suggestive of which of the following:

(A) familial adenomatous polyposis syndrome (FAP)

(B) hereditary nonpolyposis colorectal cancer syndrome (HNPCC)

(C) Peutz-Jeghers syndrome

(D) Cronkhite-Canada syndrome

(E) Turcot's syndrome

Questions 25 through 27

A 50-year-old female presents to your office for evaluation of solid food dysphagia without weight loss. Symptoms have been present for 6 months and are progressive. The patient has had two episodes of near impaction, but copious water ingestion and repeated swallows allowed the food bolus to pass. She has never had to present to the emergency room for disimpaction. She drinks five to six beers per day, loves spicy foods, and smokes a pack of cigarettes daily with a total lifetime history of 30 pack-years. She has had intermittent heartburn symptoms for years and has not sought treatment. She takes hydrochlorothiazide for hypertension. Review of symptoms reveals chronic cough. Physical examination is unremarkable. Upper endoscopy reveals a distal esophageal stricture with inflammatory changes. Esophageal biopsies reveal benign mucosa with chronic inflammation. Gastric biopsies are unremarkable. *Helicobacter pylori* testing is negative.

25. What is the most likely etiology of the patient's stricture?

(A) alcohol ingestion

(B) tobacco use

(C) gastroesophageal reflux

(D) hydrochlorothiazide

(E) spicy food ingestion

26. What is the next best step in therapy for this patient?

(A) esophageal dilation

(B) histamine receptor antagonist therapy

(C) PPI therapy

(D) esophageal dilation with histamine receptor antagonist therapy

(E) esophageal dilation with PPI inhibitor therapy

27. The patient is at increased risk for which of the following illnesses?

(A) esophageal squamous cell cancer

(B) esophageal adenocarcinoma

(C) gastric cancer

(D) gastric lymphoma

(E) duodenal adenocarcinoma

Questions 28 through 32

A 65-year-old man presents to your office for evaluation of abdominal pain. The patient states that he has epigastric pain that radiates to his back. The pain is worse with eating and improves with fasting. The pain has been present for 6 months and is gradually worsening. The patient has lost 15 lb but feels his oral intake has been adequate. He complains of greasy stools and frequent thirst and urination. Examination reveals a thin male with temporal wasting and moderate abdominal pain with palpation. The patient consumes approximately 10–15 beers per day and smokes a pack of cigarettes per day for the past 20 years.

28. What would be the best initial test to do in this patient?

(A) spot fecal fat collection

(B) 72-h fecal fat collection

(C) CT scan of the abdomen

(D) ERCP

(E) upper endoscopy

29. On further questioning, the patient reports that he recently had a motor vehicle accident at night because he felt he could not see clearly. The most likely cause of this symptom is:

(A) vitamin B_{12} deficiency

(B) vitamin C deficiency

(C) vitamin D deficiency

(D) vitamin A deficiency

(E) vitamin K deficiency

30. On further evaluation, the patient is found to be diabetic. He has an elevated hemoglobin A1C and fasting hyperglycemia. The patient is sent for diabetic teaching sessions and begun on insulin therapy, but is unable to achieve euglycemia. He experiences frequent bouts of symptomatic hypoglycemia requiring emergency room visits. What is the most likely cause for these episodes?

    (A) insulin overdose
    (B) impaired glucagon production
    (C) inadequate oral intake
    (D) vitamin K deficiency
    (E) vitamin B_{12} deficiency

31. The patient's weight loss would be best treated by which of the following regimens?

    (A) pancreatic enzyme replacement therapy
    (B) liquid caloric supplementation by mouth
    (C) liquid caloric supplementation via gastrostomy tube
    (D) total parenteral nutrition (TPN)
    (E) partial parenteral nutrition (PPN)

32. The patient's abdominal pain worsens and his weight loss progresses despite therapy, and you suspect that he may have a malignancy. If a malignancy was present, which tumor marker would be most likely to be elevated in this patient?

    (A) carcinoembryonic antigen (CEA)
    (B) prostate-specific antigen (PSA)
    (C) cancerantigen (CA)-125
    (D) α-fetoprotein (AFP)
    (E) CA-19-9

Questions 33 and 34

A 60-year-old woman arrives at your office for a routine physical examination. During the course of her examination she asks you about osteoporosis. She is concerned about her risk for osteoporosis, as her mother suffered from multiple vertebral compression fractures at the age of 60. Your patient reports that she still smokes cigarettes ("although I know they are bad for me") and has one alcoholic beverage a week. She reports having had menopause 5 years ago. She is proud of the fact that she regularly exercises at the local fitness center. She has been taking 1500 mg of calcium with 800 IU of vitamin D every day. You suspect that she is at risk for osteoporosis.

33. Which of the following tests is best to detect and monitor osteoporosis?

    (A) plain film radiography
    (B) dual-photon absorptiometry
    (C) single-photon absorptiometry
    (D) dual-energy x-ray absorptiometry (DEXA)
    (E) quantitative CT scan

34. After performing the appropriate imaging study, you determine that your patient has osteoporosis. Of the following choices, which is a risk factor most likely contributing to her osteoporosis?

    (A) active lifestyle
    (B) late menopause
    (C) cigarette smoking
    (D) frequency of alcohol intake
    (E) her intake of calcium and vitamin D

Questions 35 through 37

A 28-year-old male, well known to your clinic, presents for management of swelling, pain, and tenderness that has developed in his left ankle and right knee. It has persisted for 1 month. Your patient reports that he developed severe diarrhea after a picnic 1 month prior to the onset of his arthritis. During the interval between the diarrhea and onset of arthritis, he developed a "pink eye" that lasted for 4 days. He denies any symptoms of back pain or stiffness. You remember that he was treated with ceftriaxone and doxycycline for gonorrhea 2 years ago, which he acquired from sexual activity with multiple partners. Since that time, he has been in a monogamous relationship with his wife and has not had any genitourinary symptoms. He promises that he has been faithful to his wife and has not engaged in unprotected sexual activity outside his marriage. His physical examination is notable for a swollen left ankle, swollen right knee, and the absence of penile discharge or any skin lesions.

35. Which of the following is the most likely diagnosis?

(A) pseudogout
(B) gout
(C) reactive arthritis
(D) resistant gonococcal arthritis
(E) ankylosing spondylitis

36. What would be the appropriate management for this patient's arthritis?

(A) Screen him for the suspected disease with HLA-B27 testing.
(B) Treat with daily indomethacin (150–200 mg daily).
(C) Start him on empiric antibiotics.
(D) Start treatment with prednisone 10 mg daily.
(E) Assume that the patient is not being honest and perform the appropriate urogenital testing to confirm gonorrhea.

37. The patient's symptoms do not respond to your initial therapeutic management. You suspect that his condition is refractory to treatment. Which of the following should you consider at this time?

(A) He may have human immunodeficiency virus (HIV) infection and should be tested.
(B) His condition will require high doses of prednisone (60 mg daily) for adequate control.
(C) His joints are obviously not infected and should be directly injected with corticosteroids.
(D) He must have a disseminated bacterial infection that will require IV antibiotics.
(E) He is resistant to indomethacin, so the dose should be doubled to 400 mg daily.

38. What is the mechanism of action of the uricosuric agent probenecid?

(A) inhibition of xanthine oxidase
(B) inhibition of cyclooxygenase
(C) facilitation of urea metabolism
(D) inhibition of renal urate reabsorption
(E) facilitation of hepatic urate reabsorption

39. An acute attack of gout is most effectively treated by which of the following agents?

(A) probenecid
(B) allopurinol
(C) indomethacin
(D) sulfinpyrazone
(E) aspirin

40. Which of the following produces the greatest increase in bone mineral density in patients with osteoporosis?

(A) estrogen
(B) calcitonin
(C) alendronate
(D) teriparatide
(E) raloxifene

41. A concerned mother brings in her 18-month-old infant girl. The baby's developmental milestones have been normal. The mother states that there is a "funny glint" in her baby's eyes. She also states that sometimes the infant's eyes look crossed. Which of these supports the diagnosis of a serious life threatening disease?

(A) Baby reaches for small objects.
(B) Baby fusses when each eye is covered.
(C) Bright red reflex in one eye, a white reflex in the other.
(D) Baby rubs both eyes.
(E) Baby holds objects close to inspect them.

Questions 42 through 44

A 23-year-old female graduate student with acne and asthma presents to you with a chief complaint of headaches. She has noted a gradual increase in the intensity and frequency of the headaches to the point where they are interfering with her daily activities and studies. Your examination shows an obese young lady with papilledema. The remainder of your physical examination is normal.

42. Which of the following is the most appropriate management at this time?

    (A) order an erythrocyte sedimentation rate
    (B) order a glucose tolerance test
    (C) urine pregnancy test
    (D) obtain a lumbar puncture to measure opening pressure
    (E) obtain an MRI of the brain and orbits, with and without contrast

43. The test ordered above was negative. Which of the following is your most appropriate next step?

    (A) instruct the patient on a weight loss program and follow-up in 3 months
    (B) begin diuretic therapy
    (C) start the patient on sumatriptan for migraine headaches
    (D) perform a lumbar puncture to measure opening pressure
    (E) obtain an MRI of the brain and orbits, with and without contrast

44. Which of the following is most commonly associated with this condition?

    (A) obesity
    (B) steroid use during asthma attacks
    (C) tetracycline treatment for acne
    (D) oral contraceptives
    (E) pregnancy

Questions 45 and 46

A 64-year-old Hispanic female with type II diabetes mellitus and hypertension for 15 years comes to your office after not seeing a physician for 5 years. The hemoglobin A1C is 9. She reports that her vision has been deteriorating but new glasses from the optometrist have helped.

45. Which of the following findings during your examination would represent the highest risk for blindness in this patient?

    (A) microaneurysms
    (B) neovascularization at the optic nerve
    (C) arteriovenous nicking
    (D) cotton wool spots or focal infarcts
    (E) hard exudates or lipid deposits

46. Your examination findings include all of the above. These form the diagnosis of:

    (A) nonproliferative diabetic retinopathy
    (B) proliferative retinopathy
    (C) central serous chorioretinopathy
    (D) microangiopathy of the retina
    (E) hypertensive retinopathy

Questions 47 through 49

A 54-year-old Asian female with no significant medical history presents with frontal headache, eye pain, nausea, and vomiting. Her abdominal examination shows mild diffuse tenderness but no rebound or guarding. Her mucous membranes are dry. Her vision is blurry in both eyes, her eyes are injected but her extraocular muscles are intact.

47. Which of the following is most likely to provide a diagnosis?

    (A) abdominal ultrasound
    (B) emergency exploratory laparoscopy
    (C) MRI of the brain
    (D) arterial blood gas
    (E) ocular tonometry

48. What other finding is this patient most likely to have?

    (A) cloudy corneas
    (B) anemia
    (C) anorexia
    (D) dizziness or vertigo
    (E) polyuria and polydipsia

49. Which of the following is the most likely diagnosis?

    (A) diabetic ketoacidosis
    (B) appendicitis
    (C) angle closure glaucoma
    (D) perforated colon due to inflammatory bowel disease
    (E) cerebellar malignancy

50. Primidone has effects that are similar to phenobarbital because:

(A) It is in the same chemical class as phenobarbital.

(B) Both drugs have the same mechanism of action.

(C) Primidone is metabolized to phenobarbital.

(D) Both drugs are antipsychotics.

(E) Both primidone and phenobarbital block glutamate receptors.

51. Which of the following is utilized primarily as a supplement to maintain general anesthesia?

(A) halothane
(B) enflurane
(C) nitrous oxide
(D) cyclopropane
(E) D-tubocurarine

52. Which of the following statements about the hypnotic effects of the benzodiazepines is true?

(A) Only flurazepam has true sedative-hypnotic properties.

(B) They have no effect on rapid-eye movement (REM) patterns.

(C) They are all absorbed rapidly and thus can be taken at bedtime.

(D) The accumulation of metabolites enhances the hypnotic activity and duration of activity of some benzodiazepines.

(E) They do not produce withdrawal syndromes.

53. Which antidepressant drug has the least anticholinergic side effect?

(A) imipramine
(B) fluoxetine
(C) nortriptyline
(D) amitriptyline
(E) doxepin

54. Which of the following is effective for prophylaxis in treating manic depression?

(A) fluoxetine
(B) lithium
(C) amitriptyline
(D) tranylcypromine
(E) haloperidol

55. The drug-metabolizing capability of the liver may be inhibited by:

(A) cimetidine
(B) phenobarbital
(C) ethyl alcohol
(D) methylcholanthrene
(E) penicillin

56. Which of the following is indicated in the treatment of moderate to severe Alzheimer's disease?

(A) tacrine (Cognex)
(B) donepezil (Aricept)
(C) rivastigmine (Exelon)
(D) memantine (Namenda)
(E) galantamine (Reminyl)

57. Which of the following drugs can be used to treat anxiety without sedation as a side effect?

(A) diazepam
(B) amitriptyline
(C) doxepin
(D) oxazepam
(E) buspirone

58. The use of which of the following is contraindicated in patients taking sildenafil (Viagra)?

(A) nitroglycerin
(B) metoprolol
(C) verapamil
(D) captopril
(E) clonidine

59. Bupivacaine is a local anesthetic agent that is much more potent and whose duration of action is considerably longer than procaine. Possible reasons for this difference include:

(A) higher partition coefficient for bupivacaine than for procaine

(B) covalent binding to the receptor site

(C) lower protein binding of bupivacaine than procaine

(D) decreased rate of metabolism of procaine compared to bupivacaine

(E) bupivacaine constricts blood vessels

Questions 60 through 63

A 68-year-old White male, with a history of hypertension, an 80 pack year history of tobacco use and emphysema, is brought into the emergency room because of 4 days of progressive confusion and lethargy. His wife notes that he takes amlodipine for his hypertension. He does not use over-the-counter medications, alcohol, or drugs. Furthermore, she indicates that he has unintentionally lost approximately 30 lb in the last 6 months. His physical examination shows that he is afebrile with a blood pressure of 142/85, heart rate of 92 (no orthostatic changes), and a room-air oxygen saturation of 91%. He is 70 kg. The patient appears cachectic. He is arousable but lethargic and unable to follow any commands. His mucous membranes are moist, heart rate regular without murmurs or a S3/S4 gallop, and extremities without any edema. His pulmonary examination shows mildly diminished breath sounds in the right lower lobe with wheezing bilaterally. The patient is unable to follow commands during neurologic examination but moves all his extremities spontaneously. Laboratory results are as follows:

Blood
Sodium 109
Potassium 3.8
Chloride 103
CO_2 33
BUN 17
Creatinine 1.1
Glucose 95
Urine osmolality 600
Plasma osmolality 229
WBC 8,000
Hemoglobin (Hgb) 15.8
Hematocrit (HCT) 45.3
Platelets 410
Arterial blood gas: pH 7.36/ pCO_2 60/ pO_2 285
A chest x-ray (CXR) reveals a large right hilar mass.

---

60. What is the most likely cause of this patient's altered mental status?

   (A) sepsis syndrome with pneumonia
   (B) ischemic stroke
   (C) central pontine myelinolysis
   (D) cerebral edema
   (E) respiratory acidosis

61. Which of the following provides the best explanation for this patient's hyponatremia?

   (A) inappropriate high level of antidiuretic hormone
   (B) increased water intake (psychogenic polydipsia)
   (C) volume depletion due to decreased oral intake over the last week
   (D) the use of a thiazide for the treatment of hypertension
   (E) decreased expression of renal collecting duct "water channels"

62. Which of the following would be the optimal choice of solution to infuse in order to adequately correct this patient's hyponatremia?

   (A) D5W with 20 meq/L KCl at 200 mL/h
   (B) 0.9% saline at 125 mL/h
   (C) 0.45% saline at 100 mL/h
   (D) 3% saline at 35 mL/h
   (E) 0.45% saline with 30 meq/L KCl at 100 mL/h

63. Which of the following is the correct statement regarding the treatment of hyponatremia?

   (A) Desmopressin acetate (DDAVP), used in conjunction with intravenous saline, will help correct the serum sodium.
   (B) Correction of sodium slowly by 3 meq/day will prevent any subsequent neurologic injury.
   (C) Correction of serum sodium by 15 meq over 24 h could lead to permanent neurologic injury.
   (D) Diuretics should be avoided in the treatment of hyponatremia.
   (E) Potassium should always be added to IV saline solutions when treating both hyponatremia and hypokalemia.

Questions 64 through 68

A 53-year-old Black male, with a history of hypertension, hepatitis C, and newly diagnosed nonsmall cell lung cancer, undergoes his first round of chemotherapy, which includes cisplatin. You are called to see this patient 5 days into his hospitalization for oliguria and laboratory abnormalities. Other than the chemotherapy, he is receiving lansoprazole, acetaminophen, and an infusion of D5—0.9% normal saline at 50 mL/h. On examination, his BP is 98/60 and heart rate is irregular, between 40 and 50 bpm. His physical examination shows a middle-aged male in no acute distress. His cardiac examination is unremarkable, his lungs show bibasilar crackles, and the abdominal examination is positive for a palpable spleen tip without any hepatomegaly or abdominal tenderness. He has trace bilateral ankle edema. His distal pulses are irregular. The neurologic examination was unremarkable. His laboratory results are as follows:

(Serum sample)

	Day 1	Day 5
Sodium	135	145
Potassium	4.4	6.8
Chloride	100	108
CO_2	24	20
BUN	15	35
Creatinine	1.5	3.4
Glucose	118	152
Uric acid	6.5	15.3
Phosphate	4.4	8.3
Calcium	9.0	7.5
Lactate dehydrogenase (LDH)	285	994

64. Which electrolyte/acid-base abnormality is most likely responsible for the findings on physical examination?

   (A) hypernatremia
   (B) hyperkalemia
   (C) metabolic acidosis
   (D) hyperphosphatemia
   (E) hyperuricemia

65. What is the mechanism that best explains this patient's hyperkalemia?

   (A) diabetic ketoacidosis
   (B) acute kidney failure leading to an inability to excrete potassium in the urine
   (C) release of potassium from the destruction of neoplastic cells

   (D) chemotherapy-induced hyperkalemia
   (E) type 4 renal tubular acidosis

66. What is the most likely etiology of this patient's acute renal failure?

   (A) renal tubular deposition of uric acid
   (B) calcium oxalate kidney stones causing partial urinary tract obstruction
   (C) renal tubular injury due to cisplatin
   (D) ischemic acute tubular necrosis from a decreased cardiac output
   (E) type II Cryoglobulinemia due to hepatitis C

67. What would be the most likely finding on this patient's ECG?

   (A) shortened P-R segment
   (B) prominent U wave
   (C) widened QRS complexes
   (D) flattened T waves
   (E) atrial fibrillation

68. Which of the following would be a part of the IMMEDIATE treatment strategy in this patient?

   (A) atropine 1 mg IV
   (B) calcium chloride, given IV
   (C) 50 g of Kayexalate, given orally
   (D) 10 units of regular insulin, given subcutaneously
   (E) one ampule of glucagon, given IV

Questions 69 through 72

A 53-year-old White female, with a history of systemic lupus erythematosus, hypertension, and peripheral vascular disease, is admitted to the hospital for chest pain and dyspnea. Her cardiac enzymes were positive for acute myocardial infarction. She subsequently undergoes a cardiac catheterization and stenting of the right coronary artery. Her postcardiac catheterization course is unremarkable, and she is discharged home 3 days later with adequate blood pressure control. Five days later, she is brought to the emergency room by her husband for abdominal pain and nausea. Her medications consist of aspirin, metoprolol, and prednisone. On physical examination, her blood pressure is 190/95 and her heart rate is 85 bpm. In general, she appears nauseated but is in no acute distress. Her cardiac examination reveals a regular rate and rhythm without murmur or rub. Her lung fields are clear bilaterally. The abdominal examination is positive for diffuse discomfort, without guarding or rebound, and normoactive bowel sounds; her stool is positive for occult blood. Her lower extremities have trace edema bilaterally with 2+ distal pulses; moreover, she has a reddish-blue discoloration on both her lower extremities. You retrieve her records from prior hospitalization. The patient's laboratory results are as follows:

Blood	5 Days prior	Now	Urine
Sodium	140	135	
Potassium	4.4	5.2	Na+: 35
Chloride	106	113	Creatinine: 45
CO2	24	20	Specific gravity: 1.012
BUN	15	52	Protein: trace
Creatinine	1.6	3.5	RBCs: 1–3
Glucose	80	115	WBCs: 10–12
Uric acid	6.0	5.8	+ eosinophils
Amylase	90	205	No cellular casts
WBC	8000	12,000	
Hgb	13.5	12.1	
Platelets (PLT)	400,000	370,000	
% Eosinophils	1%	15%	

69. What is the most likely cause of this patient's acute renal failure?

    (A) contrast nephropathy from cardiac catheterization
    (B) acute interstitial nephritis

    (C) prerenal etiology from occult gastrointestinal bleeding
    (D) atheroembolic disease
    (E) lupus nephritis flare

70. Which of the following tests is helpful in distinguishing volume depletion as a possible cause of acute renal failure?

    (A) kidney ultrasound
    (B) calculation of the fractional excretion of sodium
    (C) estimation of the glomerular filtration rate
    (D) examination of the urine sediment under microscopy
    (E) calculation of the anion gap

71. Which of the following is the optimal therapeutic agent for this patient's pain management?
    (A) intravenous Demerol
    (B) intramuscular ketorolac
    (C) oral indomethacin
    (D) intravenous morphine sulfate
    (E) ibuprofen 400 mg orally three times daily as needed

72. Which of the following laboratory findings would be most suggestive of active lupus nephritis?

    (A) urinary red blood cell casts
    (B) urinary white blood cell casts
    (C) >3.5 g of proteinuria on 24 h urine sample
    (D) normal serum complement levels
    (E) urinary eosinophils by Hansel stain

Questions 73 through 77

A 63-year-old Native American male, with a 6-year history of diabetes mellitus, hypertension, and hyperlipidemia, comes to your office as a new patient for a routine examination. He has been experiencing frequent lower back pain and headaches for which he is taking ibuprofen daily for the past 5 weeks. Moreover, he is complaining of mild fatigue. In addition, he is taking aspirin, atorvastatin, verapamil, and glipizide.

His physical examination shows a blood pressure of 165/80 and heart rate of 90 bpm. In general, he is not in any distress. His funduscopic examination reveals no signs of diabetic retinopathy. Cardiac examination reveals a regular rate and rhythm with an S4 gallop. His lungs are clear and abdominal examination is unremarkable without any bruit auscultated. He also has 2+ lower extremity pitting edema. Rectal examination reveals brown stool, negative for occult blood. His laboratory results are as follows:

	Blood	Urine
Sodium	137	Specific gravity: 1.012
Potassium	5.0	Protein: trace
Chloride	115	RBCs: 1–3
CO_2	20	WBCs: 0–3
BUN	30	No cellular casts
Creatinine	1.6	
Glucose	131	24-h specimen: 5.2 g protein
Total protein	8.5	
Albumin	3.0	
AST	15	
Total bilirubin	0.3	
LDL cholesterol	160	
WBC	8700	
Hgb	8.5	
HCT	24	
PLT	245,000	

A kidney ultrasound shows 12 cm kidneys bilaterally (normal = 12 cm).

73. Which of the following is a typical finding in nephrotic syndrome?

    (A) hyperlipidemia
    (B) hypercalcemia
    (C) macrocytic anemia
    (D) elevated thyroxine levels
    (E) hypocomplementemia

74. With regards to the workup of this man's proteinuria, what diagnostic test would you perform next?

    (A) serum and urine protein electrophoresis
    (B) kidney biopsy
    (C) complement levels
    (D) antiglomerular basement membrane (anti-GBM) antibody titer
    (E) glycosylated hemoglobin level

75. Which additional of the following would best help in the determination of the etiology of this patient's nephrotic syndrome?

    (A) fractional excretion of sodium
    (B) anion gap
    (C) estimation of glomerular filtration rate
    (D) fractional excretion of urea
    (E) split 24 h urine for protein

76. Which of the following antihypertensive medications would be best implemented in patients with diabetic nephropathy?

    (A) lisinopril 10 mg orally once daily
    (B) clonidine 0.2 mg orally twice daily
    (C) metoprolol 25 mg orally twice daily
    (D) amlodipine 5 mg orally once daily
    (E) hydralazine 25 mg orally three times daily

77. Which of the following microscopic findings on kidney biopsy is most usually associated with HIV infection?

    (A) pauci-immune crescentic glomerulonephritis
    (B) focal segmental glomerulosclerosis (collapsing variant)
    (C) membranous nephropathy
    (D) membranoproliferative glomerulonephritis
    (E) antiglomerular basement membrane disease

Questions 78 through 80

A patient you see routinely in clinic has elevated liver function tests. Alanine aminotranferase is 89, aspartate aminotransferase is 75, and the total bilirubin and alkaline phosphatase are normal. The patient has no past history of hepatitis, taking medications, or excessive drinking. You order hepatitis serologies. The results are as follows:

Positive: HBsAg and anti-HBc.
Negative: Anti-HBs, anti-HBc IgM, anti-HAV, and anti-HCV

78. What is your interpretation?

   (A) The patient has acute hepatitis B.

   (B) The patient needs a test for IgM antibody to hepatitis A virus to rule out acute hepatitis A.

   (C) The patient needs a test for hepatitis C antigen to exclude acute hepatitis C.

   (D) The patient has chronic hepatitis B.

   (E) If the patient had a negative test for HBsAg, they could be infected with hepatitis delta.

79. What is the most appropriate next step for this patient?

   (A) Verify the diagnosis with a qualitative hepatitis B viral load.

   (B) Vaccinate the patient with hepatitis A vaccine.

   (C) Vaccinate the patient with hepatitis B vaccine.

   (D) Investigate other causes of hepatitis, such as cytomegalovirus (CMV) and Epstein-Barr virus.

   (E) Recommend the patient's spouse receive hepatitis A vaccine.

80. Which statement best describes this clinical situation?

   (A) If the patient was found to be HBe antigen positive, he would be considered highly infectious to spread hepatitis B.

   (B) This patient is in the "window period" because the antibody to hepatitis BsAg is negative.

   (C) This patient is not at risk for delta hepatitis because the patient has antibody to hepatitis B core.

   (D) The low level of transaminase elevations indicates that this patient is not a candidate for hepatitis B antiviral treatment.

   (E) If this patient has antibody to hepatitis Be, he is a candidate for antiviral therapy.

Questions 81 and 82

A 72-year-old diabetic is transferred to your hospital for fever and altered mental status in the late summer. Symptoms started in this patient 1 week prior to admission. On physical examination, the patient was disoriented. There were no focal neurologic findings. There was a fine rash on the patient's trunk. On oral examination, there were tongue fasciculations. A lumbar puncture was performed which showed a glucose of 71 and a protein of 94; microscopy of the cerebrospinal fluid (CSF) revealed 9 RBC and 14 WBC (21 P, 68 L, 11 M). The creatinine phosphokinase was 506. An electroencephalogram and MRI of the brain were normal.

81. What is the best interpretation of these findings?

   (A) The patient may have cryptococcal meningitis.

   (B) The patient may have disseminated candidiasis.

   (C) The patient may have West Nile virus.

   (D) The patient may have *Coccidioides immitis* infection.

   (E) The patient may have rhinocerebral mucormycosis.

82. What further diagnostic test is the most appropriate?

   (A) Perform a West Nile virus IgM on the CSF.

   (B) Perform a serum cryptococcal antigen.

   (C) Perform *C. immitis* complement fixation tests.

   (D) Perform a sinus series.

   (E) Perform a purified protein derivative (PPD) skin test.

83. Beta-lactam antibiotics, such as penicillin, act by:

   (A) interfering with protein synthesis at the ribosome

   (B) attaching to sterols in cell membranes

   (C) inhibiting bacterial cell wall synthesis

   (D) inhibiting the transport of amino acids into bacteria

   (E) inhibiting dihydrofolate reductase

84. Acyclovir-induced nephrotoxicity is caused by:

   (A) the formation of toxic metabolites

   (B) decreased glomerular filtration rate

(C) the precipitation of acyclovir in renal tubules

(D) direct tubular cytotoxic injury

(E) hypersensitivity interstitial nephritis

Questions 85 through 87

A 34-year-old amateur spelunker develops cough, dyspnea, and fever 2 weeks after a caving expedition to caves in Kentucky. On physical examination, the patient's temperature is 102°F and respiratory rate is 24. On pulmonary examination, there are diffuse crackles bilaterally. A CXR is shown in Fig. 1-3.

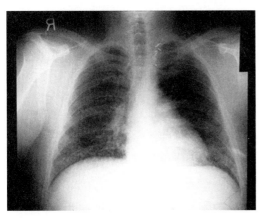

FIG. 1-3 (*Courtesy of Philip C. Johnson, MD.*)

85. Which of the following is the most likely cause of disease in this patient?

(A) The patient likely developed influenza from close contact with the other members of the caving expedition.

(B) The patient likely has disseminated aspergillosis.

(C) The patient likely has miliary tuberculosis.

(D) The patient likely has acute pulmonary histoplasmosis.

(E) The patient likely has *Pneumocystis jiroveci* pneumonia.

86. What diagnostic test would be most appropriate?

(A) serum cryptococcal antigen

(B) fungal serologies

(C) a PPD skin test

(D) an HIV enzyme-linked immunosorbent assay (ELISA) test

(E) arterial blood gas determination

87. Choose the most appropriate statement about infection control of this patient if the patient is hospitalized:

(A) The patient is not likely to need respiratory isolation.

(B) The patient should be placed in respiratory isolation if histoplasmosis is suspected.

(C) The patient should be placed in respiratory isolation if *P. jiroveci* is suspected.

(D) The patient should be placed in respiratory isolation if pulmonary aspergillosis is suspected.

(E) The patient should be placed in respiratory isolation if cryptococcal pneumonia is suspected.

Questions 88 and 89

A 53-year-old insulin dependent diabetic, who underwent a cadaveric renal transplant 1 year prior to admission, presents with fever and cough of 3 weeks duration. He works as a long-haul trucker, carting fruit from McAllen, Texas (on the Texas-Mexico border) to Fresno, California. He does not smoke. His PPD skin test prior to admission was positive. On physical examination, his respiratory rate is 25, his oral temperature is 101°F, his lungs have rhonchi and decreased breath sounds on the left. His CXR is shown in Fig. 1-4.

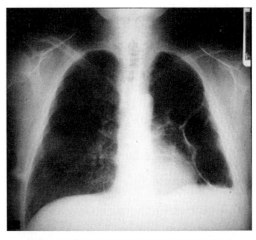

FIG. 1-4 (*Courtesy of Philip C. Johnson, MD.*)

88. What organism besides Mycobacterium tuberculosis leads your differential as a cause of pneumonia in this case?

    (A) *Haemophilus influenza*
    (B) CMV
    (C) *P. jiroveci*
    (D) *C. immitis*
    (E) *Histoplasma capsulatum*

89. What is the best diagnostic approach?

    (A) PPD skin testing
    (B) urine histoplasma antigen testing
    (C) serum cryptococcal antigen testing
    (D) sputum for silver staining for *P. jiroveci*
    (E) fiberoptic bronchoscopy with bronchial alveolar lavage

90. The immunosuppressive properties of tacrolimus include:

    (A) myelosuppression
    (B) inhibition of activation of helper T cells
    (C) inhibition of B-cell formation
    (D) impairment of leukocyte chemotaxis
    (E) macrophage destruction

91. Which of the following antiviral agents has inhibition of reverse transcriptase as its primary mechanism of action?

    (A) ganciclovir
    (B) penciclovir
    (C) amantadine
    (D) zidovudine
    (E) alpha-interferon

92. Aminoglycoside toxicity may be characterized by which of the following untoward effects?

    (A) hepatotoxicity
    (B) nephrotoxicity
    (C) interstitial pulmonary fibrosis
    (D) pulmonary edema
    (E) splenomegaly

93. A 53-year-old fisherman develops pain and swelling of the right hand 8 h after suffering a fish hook injury to the finger. On physical examination the patient's temperature is 102.8oF and the patient appears septic. The patient's hand and a Gram's stain of material aspirated from a bulla are shown in Figs. 1-5 and 1-6.

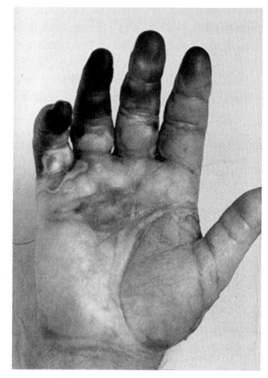

FIG. 1-5 (*Courtesy of Philip C. Johnson, MD.*)

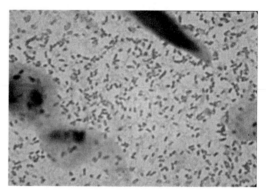

FIG. 1-6 (*Courtesy of Philip C. Johnson, MD.*)

What is the most likely etiology of this bacteremia?

(A) *Staphylococcus aureus* cellulitis
(B) group A, beta-hemolytic *Streptococcus* sepsis

(C) *Pasteurella multocida* cellulitis

(D) *Vibrio vulnificus* sepsis

(E) *Eikenella corrodens* cellulitis

94. In a patient who has *Enterococcus faecalis* bacteremia, which of the following is the best empiric treatment?

(A) treatment with an intravenous first generation cephalosporin

(B) treatment with an intravenous second generation cephalosporin

(C) treatment with an intravenous third generation cephalosporin

(D) treatment with intravenous ampicillin and an aminoglycoside

(E) treatment with intravenous fluoroquinolones

Questions 95 and 96

A 30-year-old female presents to your office for the evaluation of a rash on her back. It has been present and growing for about a week. Along with this rash, she has had a fever, headache, myalgias, and fatigue. Her symptoms started about a week after returning from a camping trip to New England. She denies having any bites from ticks or other insects and exposure to poison ivy and has had no wounds to her skin. On examination, her temperature is 99.5°F and her vital signs are otherwise normal. Her rash is as shown in Fig. 1-7. Her examination is otherwise unremarkable.

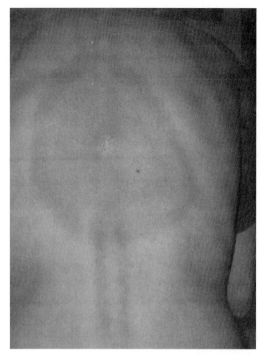

FIG. 1-7 Also see color plate.

95. What is the most likely cause of her rash?

(A) contact dermatitis secondary to plant exposure

(B) infection transmitted by tick bite

(C) infection transmitted by mosquito bite

(D) group-A *Streptococcus* suprainfection of small puncture wound

(E) allergic reaction to ingested (i.e., food) allergen

96. You order IgM and IgG ELISA testing for *Borrelia burgdorferi* and the results return as negative. Which of the following management options would be most appropriate?

(A) Treat the patient with a topical steroid for presumed contact dermatitis.

(B) Treat the patient with oral steroids for a presumed systemic allergic reaction.

(C) Treat the patient with oral cephalexin for streptococcal cellulitis.

(D) Treat the patient with doxycycline for Lyme disease.

(E) No medication at present, but have the patient return in 6–8 weeks for repeat serologic testing and treat for Lyme disease if positive at that time.

Questions 97 and 98

A 39-year-old HIV+ male presents for routine follow-up. He is on highly active antiretroviral therapy. A CD4 count is 150/μL. His vital signs are within normal limits and his examination is normal.

97. Which of the following management options is most appropriate at this time?

   (A) Continue with current regimen without change.
   (B) Add azithromycin for *Mycobacterium avium* complex prophylaxis.
   (C) Add trimethoprim/sulfamethoxazole (Bactrim DS) for *Pneumocystis carinii* prophylaxis.
   (D) Give the varicella vaccine, regardless of history of chicken pox, as his immunity to varicella is likely to be reduced.
   (E) Start ganciclovir for CMV prophylaxis.

98. He has a PPD placed and follows up in 48 h. At the site of the injection you find 6 mm of induration. A CXR is normal. He has never been treated for tuberculosis or a positive PPD before. Which management option is most appropriate?

   (A) collect sputum samples for 3 days to send for AFB staining
   (B) empirically start 4-drug therapy for active tuberculosis
   (C) empirically start isoniazid daily for 9 months
   (D) have the patient return in 1 week for a second PPD to assess for the presence of a "booster" phenomenon; treat with isoniazid if ≥10 mm induration
   (E) no intervention at this time but repeat the test in 6 months

99. While visiting a neighbor, a 14-year-old girl is bitten on the left hand by the neighbor's pet cat. The cat is an indoor pet and has had all of the required routine vaccinations. You see the girl in the office approximately 1 h after the injury. On the dorsum of the left hand you see two shallow puncture wounds that are not actively bleeding. She has full range of motion of her hand, normal capillary refill, and sensation.

You see in the chart that the patient had a diphtheria/tetanus (dT) booster vaccine last year. What is the most appropriate management at this time?

   (A) Recommend local care at home with hydrogen peroxide and topical antibiotics.
   (B) Give a booster dT and start oral cephalexin.
   (C) Give an intramuscular (IM) dose of penicillin and emergently refer to a hand surgeon for debridement.
   (D) Irrigate the wounds and prescribe oral amoxicillin/clavulanic acid (Augmentin).
   (E) Start oral ciprofloxacin and refer to the health department for rabies prophylaxis.

Questions 100 through 103

A 29-year-old woman complains of fatigue and decreased exercise tolerance. She takes no medications and denies changes in the color of the stool. Physical examination is significant for pale skin and conjunctivae. Stool was negative for blood. Laboratory evaluation revealed hemoglobin of 7.8 gr/dL, reticulocytopenia, microcytosis, and hypochromia.

100. Which of the following would most likely be found on further laboratory testing?

	MCV	Ferritin	Erythrocyte protoporphyrin	Folate	B_{12}
(A)	N or D	N or I	I	N or D	N
(B)	D	D	I	N	N or D
(C)	I	N	N	D	N or I
(D)	I	N	N	N or I	D
(E)	D	N	N	N	N

N = normal, I = increased, D = decreased

101. In iron deficiency anemia, which of the following statements is correct?

   (A) The largest amount of iron is found in plasma bound to proteins like lactoferrin and transferrin.
   (B) The average dietary iron intake is about 40–50 mg a day but only 1–5% is absorbed.

(C) Under normal conditions the body requires 0.5 mg of iron a day.

(D) When iron stores are low, aconitase, an enzyme in the Krebs cycle, undergoes a conformational change functioning as an iron response protein-1 (IRP-1) modulating iron absorption.

(E) When iron stores are low, there is an increased synthesis of apoferritin and decreased synthesis of transferrin receptors.

102. In vitamin B12 or folate deficiency, which of the following statements is correct?

(A) High serum levels of homocysteine and decreased levels of methylmalonic acid are reliable indicators of cobalamin deficiency.

(B) The recommended amount of dietary folate is 800 μg/day

(C) The peripheral smear in patients with cobalamin deficiency is identical to that found in folate deficiency.

(D) The most common cause of cobalamin deficiency is hypersecretion of gastric acid (i.e., Zollinger-Ellison syndrome)

(E) Because body folate stores are high, individuals with low consumption of folate will take several years to become anemic.

103. Which of the following is the most appropriate next step in the management of the anemia in this woman?

(A) Start iron therapy as soon as possible.

(B) Transfuse red blood cells and start iron therapy.

(C) Start B_{12} and folate replacement.

(D) Identify the cause of the anemia with a thorough history and physical examination.

(E) Start iron therapy and B_{12} replacement.

104. An 18-month-old boy is taken to his family doctor for evaluation of easy bruising and decreased range of motion of the right knee. On examination he has multiple large ecchymoses, mostly in the lower extremities, and a right knee hemarthrosis. He has not had surgery and there is no family history of a bleeding disorder. The doctor orders screening tests that reveal a prolonged activated partial thromboplastin time (aPTT) with a normal prothrombin time (PT) and platelet count.
What further tests should be ordered to make a diagnosis in this boy?

(A) factor VII

(B) factors II, VII, IX, and X

(C) bleeding time

(D) factors XI, IX, VIII

(E) factor I and II

105. Which of the following antipsychotic agents has agranulocytosis as a prominent adverse reaction?

(A) haloperidol

(B) chlorpromazine

(C) risperidone

(D) thioridazine

(E) clozapine

106. Which drug can be used as a treatment for warfarin toxicity?

(A) heparin

(B) allopurinol

(C) coumarin

(D) vitamin E

(E) vitamin K

107. Rapid reversal of the anticoagulant effect of heparin is produced by administration of:

(A) cimetidine

(B) heparinase

(C) clofibrate

(D) protamine sulfate

(E) vitamin K

108. Which of the following would be least likely to interfere with platelet aggregation?

(A) aspirin

(B) celecoxib

(C) naproxen

(D) indomethacin

(E) ketorolac

109. A 58-year-old woman is concerned about her risk for osteoporosis and is seen by her general internist. Her mother was diagnosed with osteoporosis and had a hip fracture at age 84. She has no personal or family history of kidney stones or ulcer disease, and she has never had a fracture. She had a hysterectomy at age 48 and took estradiol for 2 years, but discontinued because of a fear of adverse effects. She does not have any vasomotor symptoms. She takes 1500 mg of calcium carbonate and 400 IU vitamin D daily. She is not on any other medications. On examination, she appears well developed and there is no evidence of kyphosis. A bone mineral density test is performed that demonstrates a T score in the spine of –3.5 and in the hip of –2.8. CXR and mammogram are normal. Further evaluation demonstrates the following:

Serum calcium	11.4 mg/dL	(9.5–10.5)
Phosphate	2.1 mg/dL	(2.5–4.5)
24-h urine calcium	405 mg	(100–250)
Serum magnesium	1.8 meq/L	(1.3–2.1)
Serum creatinine	0.7 mg/dL	(0.5–1.4)
Hemoglobin	14 g/L	(12–16)

Which of the following is the most likely diagnosis?

(A) milk-alkali syndrome
(B) primary hyperparathyroidism
(C) sarcoidosis
(D) secondary hyperparathyroidism
(E) osteomalacia

110. Vitamin D supplementation can be helpful in treating which disease?

(A) hyperparathyroidism
(B) hypoparathyroidism
(C) alcoholic neuritis
(D) pernicious anemia
(E) scurvy

111. A 34-year-old woman was found to have a 2-cm right thyroid nodule at the time of a well woman examination. The remainder of the thyroid was palpably normal and there were no lymph nodes palpable. There was no history of thyroid disease or radiation therapy to her head or neck. She was clinically euthyroid. Thyroid stimulating hormone (TSH) was normal. Which of the following tests would be the most useful in establishing a specific diagnosis?

(A) ultrasound of the thyroid
(B) nuclear scan of the thyroid
(C) thyroid antibody studies
(D) fine needle aspiration of the nodule
(E) CT of the neck

112. Propylthiouracil is effective in treating hyperthyroidism because:

(A) It interferes with the incorporation of iodine into thyroglobulin.
(B) It interferes with the concentration of iodide by the thyroid gland.
(C) It inhibits the inositol phosphate signaling pathways within the thyrocyte.
(D) It destroys thyroid tissue.
(E) It antagonizes thyroid hormones at receptor sites.

113. A 40-year-old woman presents with nausea, vomiting, and weakness. She has been amenorrheic since the birth of her last child 1 year ago and has not felt well since that time. On examination, she appears chronically ill, her thyroid is not palpable, and there is no galactorrhea. Laboratory studies on admission include:

Sodium	120 meq/L	
Glucose	55 mg/dL	
Total T4	2.0 µg/mL	(normal 4.5–12)
TSH	1.0 µU/mL	(normal 0.4–5.0)

The most appropriate next step is to start treatment with which of the following?

(A) hydrocortisone
(B) fluid restriction
(C) desmopressin
(D) glucagon
(E) fludrocortisone

114. A 32-year-old woman complains of episodic confusion in the morning for the past 6 months. During one of these episodes, she was brought to the emergency room and her serum glucose was found to be 40 mg/dL. She was given intravenous dextrose and her symptoms resolved within 15 min. She has gained approximately 25 lb during the past year. Which of the following would be the most appropriate next step?

(A) measure serum insulin and proinsulin 2 h after a mixed meal
(B) MRI of the pancreas
(C) measure insulin, c-peptide, and sulfonylurea level on the initial blood sample in emergency room
(D) octreotide scan
(E) advise a high protein diet with frequent feedings

115. Diuretic agents that reduce potassium loss by an aldosterone-independent mechanism include:

(A) chlorothiazide
(B) spironolactone
(C) acetazolamide
(D) ethacrynic acid
(E) triamterene

116. Which of the following insulin preparations is longest acting?

(A) insulin lispro
(B) lente
(C) regular Humulin
(D) Ultralente Humulin U
(E) neutral protamine Hagedorn (NPH)

117. A 54-year-old man presents with a 3-cm right thyroid nodule that was found incidentally by the patient while shaving. He denies any pain or discomfort. He denies any history of thyroid disease, any family history of thyroid disease, and any history of head/neck irradiation. He notes a 10-lb weight loss over the past 6 months. His examination is only remarkable for the firm right thyroid nodule. The remainder of the thyroid is not palpable. There is no adenopathy. Heart rate is 90/min and regular.

The skin is warm and moist, and a fine tremor is present when he holds his hands out. TSH level is <.02 µU/mL. Which of the following is the most appropriate next step?

(A) thyroid ultrasound
(B) anti-thyroid peroxidase antibodies
(C) thyroid stimulating immunoglobulins
(D) fine needle aspiration of the nodule
(E) thyroid nuclear scan

118. A 19-year-old woman who is 2 months postpartum complains of palpitations, heat intolerance, tremulousness, weight loss, and fatigue. Her thyroid is prominent and firm but nontender. Serum TSH level was undetectable. A nuclear medicine radioactive iodine uptake is performed and shows no uptake of iodine in the neck. Which of the following is the most appropriate next step?

(A) administer radioactive iodine
(B) initiate glucocorticoid therapy
(C) initiate levothyroxine therapy
(D) initiate propranolol therapy
(E) initiate methimazole therapy

119. A 60-year-old man with a history of severe chronic obstructive pulmonary disease (COPD), which is steroid dependent, is admitted to the intensive care unit with pulmonary infiltrates and a sepsis syndrome. His hospital course is complicated by acute renal insufficiency and respiratory failure. Therapy includes glucocorticoids and dopamine. He has no history of thyroid disease. Several weeks into his hospital course, the following laboratory studies are performed:

Total T4	2.2	(5–12 µg/dL)
T3-resin uptake	55%	(25–35%)
Free thyroid index	1.2	(1.2–4.2)
TSH	0.20	(0.45 µU/mL)
Total T3	<30	(80–220 ng/dL)
Reverse T3	500	(80–250 ng/L)

Based on these laboratory studies, which of the following is the most appropriate next step?

(A) initiate levothyroxine therapy

(B) discontinue glucocorticoid therapy

(C) initiate methimazole therapy

(D) order MRI of the pituitary

(E) supportive treatment only

Questions 120 and 121

A 28-year-old woman presents for evaluation of primary infertility. She has had fewer than four periods per year since menarche at age 14, facial hirsutism, acne, and weight gain. On examination, she has a BP 150/100. Her BMI is 40. *Acanthosis nigricans* is noted along the posterior surface of her neck.

120. Which of the following laboratory studies is most likely to be abnormal in this patient?

(A) TSH

(B) prolactin

(C) glucose tolerance test

(D) growth hormone

(E) cosyntropin (Cortrosyn) stimulation test

121. Which of the following would be her most likely fasting lipid profile?

(A) high triglycerides, high HDL

(B) low triglycerides, low HDL

(C) high triglycerides, low HDL

(D) high LDL cholesterol

(E) normal lipid profile

122. A 21-year-old male presents with a 3-day history of widespread blisters that rupture to leave painful cutaneous erosions. On examination, the patient is febrile and tachycardic. There is desquamation of his skin with oral mucosal erosions. He has widespread tense bullae and large superficial erosions see Fig. 1-8(A) and (B). A skin biopsy done for rapid frozen section reveals a subepidermal split. The most likely diagnosis is:

(A) staphylococcal scalded skin syndrome (SSSS)

(B) scarlet fever

(C) pemphigus vulgaris

(D) toxic epidermal necrolysis (TEN) due to clindamycin

(E) TEN due to Bactrim

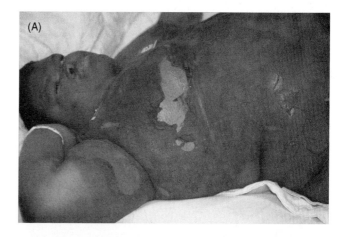

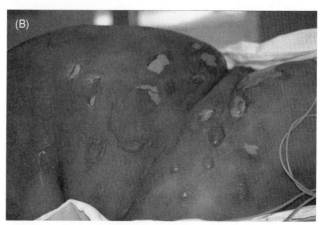

FIG. 1-8 Also see color plate. *(A) and (B) (Courtesy of Steven Mays, MD.)*

123. A 40-year-old diabetic female is admitted for treatment of a lower extremity cellulitis. On the third day of admission, the patient develops a tender vesicular eruption on the buttocks (see Fig. 1-9). The patient reports having had this eruption on two previous occasions. The most likely diagnosis is:

(A) bullous impetigo

(B) shingles

(C) herpes simplex

(D) fixed drug reaction

(E) scabies

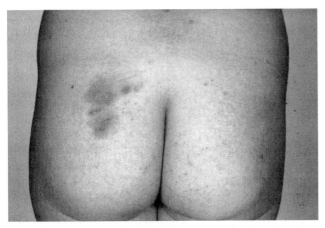

FIG. 1-9 (*Courtesy of Steven Mays, MD.*)

124. The most common malignancy in the United States is:

(A) prostate cancer

(B) lung cancer

(C) breast cancer

(D) basal cell carcinoma

(E) cervical cancer

125. An 18-year-old male presents for evaluation of facial acne. On examination, he has 30 comedones on the forehead, nose, cheeks, and chin. He has no pustules. The most appropriate therapy is:

(A) tretinoin 0.025% cream

(B) clindamycin lotion

(C) oral minocycline

(D) oral Accutane

(E) erythromycin gel

126. A 30-year-old female presents with a 1-day history of a painful nodule on her forehead and central facial erythema (see Fig. 1-10). She is febrile. An appropriate next step would be:

(A) outpatient therapy with oral clindamycin

(B) outpatient therapy with oral valacyclovir

(C) outpatient therapy with oral prednisone

(D) CT scan of the orbit

(E) lumbar puncture

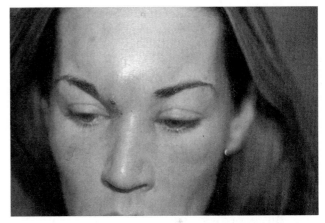

FIG. 1-10 Also see color plate. (*Courtesy of Steven Mays, MD.*)

127. A 53-year-old male presents for evaluation of psoriasis. His past medical history is significant for hypertension and four prior treated basal cell carcinomas of the face and chest. On physical examination, he has widespread plaque psoriasis involving 50% of his body surface area, including the palms and soles. He has no evidence of psoriatic arthritis. Which of the following single therapies is appropriate?

(A) topical therapy with a medium-potency corticosteroid cream

(B) topical therapy with a medium-potency corticosteroid cream and calcipotriene (Dovonex) cream

(C) phototherapy

(D) oral methotrexate

(E) oral prednisone

128. A 45-year-old male has received intravenous contrast dye prior to computer tomography of the abdomen. Twenty minutes later the patient reports severe pruritus. He denies respiratory distress, syncope, or palpitations. His blood pressure is 98/54, pulse is 90, and respiratory rate is 22. On physical examination, he has widespread urticaria. His lungs are clear to auscultation. The next appropriate step would be:

(A) administration of 0.5 mL of 1:1000 epinephrine subcutaneously

(B) administration of 0.5 mL of 1:100,000 epinephrine subcutaneously

(C) administration of 25 mg of diphenhydramine subcutaneously

(D) administration of intravenous glucocorticoids

(E) careful observation but no medications

Questions 129 and 130

129. A 20-year-old male has had a recent wide local excision of a 0.7-mm melanoma from the right ankle. There is no evidence of metastatic disease. The most important prognostic factor for this patient is:

(A) the Breslow depth of the tumor

(B) the Clark level of the tumor

(C) the location of the tumor

(D) the age of the patient

(E) the number of prior severe blistering sunburns

130. One year later, the patient develops a palpable right inguinal lymph node. Inguinal lymph node dissection reveals one node positive for metastatic melanoma; the remaining nodes are negative. A complete restaging workup shows no evidence of any additional metastatic disease. The correct stage for this patient is:

(A) stage I

(B) stage IIa

(C) stage IIb

(D) stage III

(E) stage IV

131. A 43-year-old patient presents with his fourth episode of culture-proven shingles in a T7 distribution. The most likely associated underlying condition is:

(A) leukemia

(B) lymphoma

(C) acquired immunodeficiency syndrome (AIDS)

(D) chronic prednisone therapy

(E) diabetes mellitus

132. Epinephrine is often administered along with local anesthetics because it:

(A) prolongs and increases the depth of local anesthesia

(B) neutralizes the irritant action of the local anesthetic agent

(C) increases the rate of systemic absorption and therefore hastens the onset of action of the anesthetic agent

(D) increases the pH of the anesthetic so that less anesthetic is required to produce nerve block

(E) blocks neurotransmitter release (thus decreasing pain perception) via stimulation of presynaptic alpha-adrenergic receptors

133. C1 deficiency has three subcomponents, of which the most common is deficiency of C1q. Most of those patients will have clinical and serological findings typical of:

(A) polymyositis

(B) rheumatoid arthritis

(C) systemic lupus erythematosus

(D) recurrent *Streptococcus pneumoniae* infections

(E) recurrent *Haemophilus influenza* type B infections.

Questions 134 and 135

A 21-year-old Asian female, with past medical history of exertional asthma, comes to your office complaining of mild low back pain. It started after her working out in the gym 3 days ago. The pain is 2–4 out of 10 in intensity, has no radiation, increases with bending or lying down for a long time, and improves with warm showers. You examine the patient, diagnose her with paravertebral muscle spasm, and give her prescriptions for cyclobenzaprine and naproxen to use as needed for pain and stiffness.

You receive a call from your patient 2 h later. She is having generalized itching, dizziness, and swelling of the tongue and lips. She is having difficulty breathing. She tells you that she took the first dose of the medication you prescribed about 30 min ago.

134. At this time you should:

    (A) Advise patient to use her albuterol inhaler as she is having an asthma attack.
    (B) Advise her to take another dose of naproxen and stop cyclobenzaprine for now.
    (C) Assure her that this is a common side effect to cyclobenzaprine; she will get used to it as she takes the next dose.
    (D) Ask her to return to your clinic for evaluation.
    (E) Ask her to call 911 immediately.

135. The most beneficial immediate intervention for this patient would be:

    (A) oxygen
    (B) albuterol nebulizer treatment
    (C) IV fluids
    (D) epinephrine
    (E) diphenhydramine

136. Which of the following antibiotics would be contraindicated in a patient who has had a previous anaphylactic reaction to penicillin?

    (A) tetracycline
    (B) cefotaxime
    (C) sulfamethoxazole
    (D) erythromycin
    (E) trimethoprim

137. In persons suffering from severe anaphylactic shock, the drug of choice for restoring circulation and relaxing bronchial smooth muscle is:

    (A) epinephrine
    (B) norepinephrine

    (C) isoproterenol
    (D) phenylephrine
    (E) dopamine

Questions 138 through 140

A 19-year-old male who moved to your city 3 months ago comes to your office complaining of dry cough for the past 2–3 months. Along with the cough, he has had some shortness of breath with exertion. He denies fever, chills, nausea, vomiting, wheezing, and sneezing. The cough occurs mostly in the morning and improves as the day goes on. He denies similar complaints in the past and has no history of allergies. He says that his father had eczema and an allergy to eggs.

138. You order a CXR. Which of the following are you most likely to find?

    (A) normal
    (B) diffuse pulmonary congestion
    (C) increased bronchial wall markings
    (D) cardiomegaly
    (E) flattening of the diaphragm

139. The pulmonary function test that is most likely to be diagnostic in this patient is:

    (A) increased total lung capacity
    (B) increased functional residual capacity
    (C) increased residual volume
    (D) decreased forced expiratory volume in 1 s
    (E) decreased forced inspiratory volume

140. What is the single best treatment for preventing symptoms in this patient?

    (A) long-acting β_2 agonists
    (B) an inhaled steroid
    (C) an inhaled anticholinergic
    (D) leukotriene modifiers
    (E) long-acting oral bronchodilators

Questions 141 through 143

A 63-year-old male presents to your office with palpitations for the past 3 weeks. He has had no chest pains or dyspnea. He has no significant medical history and takes no medications. He does not smoke cigarettes and a recent lipid panel was normal. On examination, he is in no apparent distress. His pulse is 115 bpm and irregular. His BP is 125/77. His lungs are clear and his cardiac examination reveals an irregularly irregular rhythm with no murmurs, rubs, or gallops.

141. Which of the following is most likely to be found on an ECG?

(A) saw-tooth p waves

(B) wide QRS complexes

(C) absent p waves

(D) Q waves in leads II, III, and aVF

(E) peaked T waves

142. An abnormal result of which of the following laboratory tests would be most likely to explain the cause of this condition?

(A) thyroid stimulating hormone

(B) troponin T

(C) BUN and creatinine

(D) serum glucose

(E) arterial blood gas

143. Which of the following studies would be most appropriate to order at this time?

(A) radionuclide ventriculography

(B) exercise stress test

(C) echocardiogram

(D) cardiac catheterization

(E) electrophysiologic studies

144. Which of the following can produce a potentially lethal drug interaction when administered with thiazide diuretics?

(A) uricosuric agents

(B) quinidine

(C) insulin

(D) vitamin D

(E) sulfonylureas

145. Which of the following would reduce the effectiveness of warfarin by facilitating its metabolism?

(A) chloramphenicol

(B) hydrochlorothiazide

(C) phenobarbital

(D) penicillin G

(E) digoxin

146. During therapy for angina, reflex tachycardia and exacerbation of symptoms are concerns most closely associated with the use of:

(A) propranolol

(B) nitroglycerin

(C) verapamil

(D) dobutamine

(E) isoproterenol

147. Which of the following has been found to increase the survival rate following myocardial infarction?

(A) flecainide

(B) timolol

(C) quinidine

(D) digoxin

(E) nitroglycerin

Questions 148 through 150

A 55-year-old male is brought to the emergency department, by ambulance, because of crushing chest pain radiating to his left shoulder and arm that started 1 h ago. He has a history of hypertension, high cholesterol, and has smoked a pack of cigarettes a day for 30 years. He has never had symptoms like this before.

148. Which of the following would be most likely to be seen on an ECG?

(A) Q waves

(B) P-R interval depression diffusely

(C) S-T segment elevation in anterior and inferior leads

(D) S-T segment elevation in anterior leads with reciprocal S-T segment depression in inferior leads

(E) normal ECG

149. While monitored in the ER, the patient's rhythm suddenly converts to ventricular tachycardia, and he becomes pulseless and unresponsive. Which of the following would be the most appropriate initial management of this situation?

   (A) defibrillation
   (B) synchronized cardioversion
   (C) IV amiodarone
   (D) IV lidocaine
   (E) IV epinephrine

150. The patient's rhythm converts to asystole. What is the most appropriate first action to take?

   (A) IV epinephrine
   (B) IV atropine
   (C) discontinuation of resuscitation
   (D) direct current (DC) cardioversion
   (E) check a second monitor lead

151. A principal advantage of low molecular weight heparin compared to standard heparin is:

   (A) a more predictable pharmacokinetic profile
   (B) inhibition of clotting factor synthesis
   (C) direct inhibition of thrombin
   (D) intravenous administration
   (E) does not cross placental membrane

152. Overdose with tricyclic antidepressants can result in lethal toxicity associated with:

   (A) coma
   (B) respiratory depression
   (C) paralysis
   (D) hyperthermia
   (E) cardiac arrhythmias

153. Which of the following is effective in treating heart failure by increasing the force of ventricular contraction?

   (A) digoxin
   (B) verapamil
   (C) propranolol

   (D) captopril
   (E) furosemide

154. Which of the following pharmacologic agents is most useful in treating acute pulmonary edema associated with CHF?

   (A) propranolol
   (B) diltiazem
   (C) furosemide
   (D) mannitol
   (E) spironolactone

155. A 60-year-old male undergoes a cardiac catheterization for unstable angina. He is found to have a 70% narrowing of the left main coronary artery and an ejection fraction of 50%. Which of the following would be the most appropriate management of this condition?

   (A) angioplasty and stenting of the left main coronary artery
   (B) medical management with a beta-blocker, statin, and aspirin
   (C) medical management with an angiotensin-converting enzyme (ACE) inhibitor, statin, and aspirin
   (D) referral for coronary artery bypass grafting (CABG)
   (E) placement of a cardiac defibrillator

Questions 156 through 158

A 70-year-old male is seen in the office for chest pain. He reports that he is getting substernal chest pain, without radiation, when he mows his lawn. The pain resolves with 10–15 min of rest. He has never had pain at rest. He has no other cardiac complaints and his review of systems is otherwise negative. He has an unremarkable medical history and takes only a baby aspirin a day. On examination, his blood pressure is 160/70, pulse 85, and respiratory rate 16. His cardiac examination is notable for a harsh, 3/6 systolic ejection murmur along the sternal border that radiates to the carotid arteries. His carotid pulsation is noted to rise slowly and is small and sustained. His lungs are clear. The remainder of his examination is normal.

156. Which of the following would be most likely to be seen on an ECG?

 (A) S-T segment elevations in the precordial leads
 (B) Q waves in the precordial leads
 (C) low-voltage QRS complexes
 (D) left ventricular hypertrophy pattern
 (E) normal ECG

157. Which of the following would be the most appropriate test to order next?

 (A) echocardiogram
 (B) exercise stress test
 (C) cardiac catheterization
 (D) 24-h Holter monitor
 (E) electrophysiologic studies

158. Subsequent workup confirms the diagnosis of critical aortic stenosis. Which of the following treatments would be most appropriate at this time?

 (A) a beta-blocker
 (B) an ACE inhibitor
 (C) a long-acting nitrate with as needed sublingual nitroglycerin
 (D) balloon valvuloplasty
 (E) aortic valve replacement

159. Cholestyramine adversely affects the absorption of:

 (A) lipid-soluble vitamins
 (B) carbohydrates
 (C) amino acids
 (D) hydrophilic molecules
 (E) ethanol

160. Which of the following would most likely induce the cardiac arrhythmia pictured in Fig. 1-11?

 (A) adenosine
 (B) lidocaine
 (C) phenytoin
 (D) flecainide
 (E) quinidine

161. Which of the following antihypertensive drugs is most commonly associated with reflex tachycardia?

 (A) clonidine
 (B) sodium nitroprusside
 (C) metoprolol
 (D) labetalol
 (E) hydrochlorothiazide

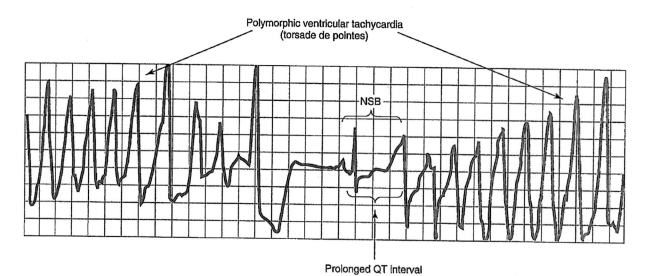

FIG. 1-11 (*From Katzung BG, (ed). Basic & Clinical Pharmacology, 9th ed. New York. NY: Mc-Graw-Hill, 2004.*)

162. Which of the following drugs is most effective for treating supraventricular arrhythmias?

   (A) quinidine
   (B) lidocaine
   (C) adenosine
   (D) bretylium
   (E) procainamide

163. Which of the following concerning digoxin is true?

   (A) It has a high margin of safety.
   (B) It has a number of effects on cardiac electrophysiology.
   (C) It increases atrioventricular (AV) nodal conduction.
   (D) It blocks calcium channels.
   (E) It is eliminated primarily through hepatic metabolism.

164. Which of the following is associated with ACE inhibitors?

   (A) cough
   (B) inhibition of angiotensin I synthesis
   (C) adjunctive treatment for rheumatoid arthritis
   (D) causes agranulocytosis
   (E) blockade of beta-2 receptors

Questions 165 through 167

A 17-year-old male presents for evaluation of shortness of breath. He has episodes where he will audibly wheeze and have chest tightness. His symptoms worsen if he tries to exercise, especially when it is cold. He has used an over the counter inhaler with good relief of his symptoms, but he finds that his symptoms are worsening. He now has episodes of wheezing three or four times a week and will have wheezing and coughing, on average, three or four times a month. You suspect a diagnosis of asthma.

165. Which of the following would confirm your suspicion of the diagnosis of asthma?

   (A) presence of expiratory wheezing on examination
   (B) presence of neutrophils on a sputum sample
   (C) a CXR showing hyperinflation
   (D) increase in forced expiratory volume in 1 second (FEV_1) of 15% after giving inhaled albuterol
   (E) history of allergic rhinitis

166. Your diagnostic workup confirms the diagnosis of asthma. What clinical classification of asthma does this patient have?

   (A) exercise-induced asthma
   (B) mild asthma
   (C) mild persistent asthma
   (D) moderate persistent asthma
   (E) severe persistent asthma

167. Which of the following is your most appropriate management?

   (A) Continue the as needed use of over-the-counter Primatene.
   (B) Prescribe an albuterol inhaler for use every 6 h
   (C) Prescribe an ipratropium inhaler for use every 8 h
   (D) Prescribe an inhaled steroid and albuterol inhaler
   (E) Prescribe an inhaled steroid, a long-acting bronchodilator and albuterol inhaler

168. Which of the following would be most effective in relieving the bronchoconstriction of an acute asthma attack without cardiac stimulation?

   (A) theophylline
   (B) cromolyn
   (C) albuterol
   (D) fluticasone
   (E) epinephrine

Questions 169 through 171

A 48-year-old woman presents for evaluation of progressively worsening dyspnea. She relates the onset of symptoms to a "walking pneumonia" that she had a year ago. Her breathing has worsened progressively since that time. She has a "smoker's cough" productive of some clear or white phlegm, for which she frequently sucks on cough drops. She started smoking regularly at the age of 18. She currently smokes about a pack of cigarettes a day, down from as much as two packs per day. She is not on any medications regularly. She has no history of heart disease and has always had normal blood pressure.

169. Which of the following physical examination findings are you most likely to find in this patient?

   (A) prolonged expiratory phase of respiration
   (B) supraclavicular adenopathy
   (C) rales one-quarter of the way up in both lungs
   (D) clubbing of fingers
   (E) prominent first heart sound

170. Which of the following is most likely to be found on a CXR?

   (A) cardiomegaly
   (B) residual infiltrate from inadequately treated pneumonia
   (C) a pulmonary mass with hilar adenopathy
   (D) hyperinflation of the lungs
   (E) Kerley B lines

171. You recommend smoking cessation to your patient. She asks why, at this point, she should quit. Which of the following statements is true?

   (A) Her pulmonary function will improve 50% or more if she quits.
   (B) Quitting will not affect her pulmonary status but may reduce her risk of having a heart attack.
   (C) At this point, quitting will not improve her survival.

   (D) She is going to require supplemental oxygen and smoking will represent a significant fire hazard.
   (E) If she is able to stay off of cigarettes, her rate of decline of lung function in the future can revert to that of a nonsmoker.

172. Antineoplastic drugs that are alkylating agents have as their primary mechanism of action:

   (A) inhibition of purine and pyrimidine synthesis
   (B) binding of tubulin
   (C) cross-linking of deoxyribonucleic acid (DNA)
   (D) intercalation into DNA
   (E) inhibition of dihydrofolate reductase

173. In postmenopausal women with an intact uterus, estrogen replacement therapy without progestin is most frequently associated with an increased risk in:

   (A) breast cancer
   (B) endometrial cancer
   (C) ovarian cancer
   (D) hepatic cancer
   (E) lung cancer

174. In treating patients on cancer chemotherapy with a medication to prevent hyperuricemia from tumor lysis, which of the following is effective in reducing the synthesis of uric acid?

   (A) indomethacin
   (B) colchicine
   (C) allopurinol
   (D) probenecid
   (E) sulfinpyrazone

175. Which of the following is a consideration in selecting particular drugs when designing drug regimens to treat cancer?

   (A) The drugs should have the same side-effect profile.
   (B) Only one or two of the drugs need to have activity against the particular tumor.

(C) The drugs should have different mechanisms of action.

(D) Drugs should be selected that maximize the time between dosing.

(E) The drugs selected, when administered in combination, should destroy 100% of the tumor cells with a single course.

Questions 176 and 177

176. A 37-year-old White executive secretary comes to you after she found a lump in her right breast while she was showering. She describes a lesion beneath her right nipple. You question her about her personal and family history. She began menarche at age 12, and she is still having regular menstrual periods. She has had two children; the first was born when she was 25 years old. She has no family history of breast, ovarian, or colon cancer on either her maternal or paternal side. You perform a physical examination including a careful examination of her breasts. You note that her breasts contain many small cysts bilaterally. However, you also palpate a localized, firm, nontender mass below the right areola. You also describe a peau d'orange appearance of the areola. What should you advise her?

(A) She appears to have fibrocystic disease and that she should return for a repeat physical examination in 6 months.

(B) Ask her to make another appointment to see you in 2 months.

(C) Order a mammogram.

(D) Obtain serum markers Ca 27/29 and CEA.

(E) Order a breast ultrasound.

177. A mammogram is performed; however, the mammogram demonstrates no abnormality involving either breast. What next should be done?

(A) Tell your patient to feel reassured and return if the mass enlarges.

(B) Tell her to stop drinking caffeine, not to eat chocolate, and to reduce the stress in her life.

(C) Return for another physical examination and mammogram in 6 months.

(D) Order an ultrasound of the right breast and lymph node basin.

(E) Order a CT scan of the breast, chest, and axilla.

Questions 178 and 179

A 56-year-old Black male construction worker comes for evaluation of a worsening, nonproductive cough that he first noticed 2 months before. During the last week the cough has worsened and has become productive of yellow, blood-tinged sputum. He reports his appetite is poor, and he has lost approximately 15 lb over the past 2 months. You take a social history and find out he has smoked two packs of cigarettes a day since he was 16 years old. He states that he drinks approximately 10 beers per week. You perform a physical examination. He appears chronically ill; however, his vital signs are normal. The head and neck examination is within normal limits. There are decreased breath sounds in the left upper chest. Breath sounds are distant in the other lung fields. The diaphragms are low. There is no palpable hepatosplenomegaly. You order a posterior-to-anterior (PA) and lateral CXR. The chest radiogram shows opacity of the left upper lobe. There are no pleural effusions. The cardiac silhouette is not enlarged. The mediastinum does not appear enlarged.

178. What next should be ordered?

(A) Culture sputum, blood, and urine; administer a broad-spectrum antibiotic; order apical lordotic x-ray views.

(B) Culture sputum, blood, and urine; order a spiral CT scan of the chest.

(C) Culture sputum, blood, and urine; order an MRI of the chest.

(D) Treat with broad spectrum antibiotics for pneumonia, and tell him to come back in 3 months to repeat the chest radiography.

(E) Culture sputum, blood, and urine; order a positron emission tomographic (PET) scan.

179. The patient has the follow-up test that you recommend. It shows a 5-cm mass compressing the left upper lobe bronchus with consolidation of the left upper lobe. Two 1 cm peribronchial lymph nodes near the left main stem bronchus and several 1.5–2.0 cm mediastinal lymph nodes are seen. The hilar nodes do not appear enlarged. There are no enlarged lymph nodes visualized in the right chest. There are no lesions seen in the right lung. There are emphysematous changes involving both lungs. A biopsy of the lung mass shows a small cell carcinoma. What should be done next?

(A) MRI of the brain with and without gadolinium contrast

(B) complete pulmonary function studies followed by a left pneumonectomy

(C) left upper lobectomy

(D) radiation of the left upper lobe mass and the mediastinal lymph nodes

(E) chemotherapy

Answers and Explanations

1. **(E)**

2. **(D)**

3. **(A)**

Explanations 1 through 3

Although this is the first time that your patient has been noted to have an elevated blood pressure reading, given his family history and obesity, it is important to consider the coexistence of other cardiovascular risk factors. His evaluation should include, among other things, screening for diabetes mellitus and dyslipidemia along with an ECG. It is reasonable to ask the patient to submit himself to a strict diet (low in fat and salt) and to increase his exercise and activity, since these lifestyle modifications will likely result in weight loss, decreased blood pressure and improve his risk profile for cardiovascular disease. Nonetheless, it is rarely enough to normalize blood pressure in all but the earliest stages of hypertension. Provided that no other comorbidities exist, the patient should return to clinic in no more than 2 months for a repeat blood pressure check. There is no need to consider secondary causes of hypertension, given his age and presentation. You should not start antihypertensive medications until further evaluation is completed, and a second elevated reading confirms your diagnosis of hypertension.

In the initial evaluation of hypertension (as per JNC VII, 2003) it is important to evaluate the patient for end organ damage. This should include the heart, kidneys, eyes, and nervous system. It is recommended to obtain a urinalysis to assess for proteinuria, glucosuria, or hematuria; to obtain an ECG to evaluate the heart for potential hypertrophy or early signs of cardiovascular disease; to obtain a fasting lipid profile, particularly after the age of 35, to assess the cardiovascular risk profile; and to check the patient's renal function to assess for damage or dysfunction. Thyroid function tests are only indicated in the workup of secondary causes of hypertension.

Although the recently published ALLHAT trial showed that diuretics are equally effective as other more expensive antihypertensive medications in most populations, your patient suffers from concomitant DM. In this population it is currently recommended that an ACE inhibitor be chosen as the first-line therapy, provided that there are no contraindications. You are given no evidence of such contraindications; therefore, given the effectiveness of this class of drug and its renoprotective properties in diabetes, it is the most appropriate choice. Except for central acting alpha-blockers, which are considered second-line choice, the other classes are reasonable first choices in the general population according to JNC VII. *(The 7th report of the joint national committee on the prevention, detection, evaluation, and treatment of high blood pressure. NIH publication No. 03-5233, May 2003)*

4. **(C)**

5. **(B)**

Explanations 4 and 5

Although the most common cause of chronic cough in adults is the postnasal drip syndrome (not a choice in this question), the patient's cough is present only in the recumbent position and at night. This sign, as well as the fact that he has recently gained considerable amount of weight, point toward the correct diagnosis of GERD. All of the other answers are also potential causes of chronic cough among adults. The history and examination give some clues that point toward GERD (constant clearing of the throat, worse during recumbence, normal nasal mucosa, and worse after meals) and give some others that would make the alternative diagnoses less likely. While 4 months period is too long for a common cold, other infectious agents (including TB) are not likely given the lack of risk factors. It would be unusual for a patient to develop asthma at this age without other symptoms, and chronic bronchitis is even less likely given the remote history of smoking only a few cigarettes per day. Although nervous cough is also possible, this occurs more often as an escape from socially awkward situations or as a stress relieving method.

Because the symptoms are due to GERD, they should be treated with a PPI as initial therapy. Although weight loss and exercise may be beneficial in relieving GERD symptoms, they should be considered additional therapies and not curative. Antibiotics are not necessary since the patient does not show signs or symptoms of bacterial or fungal infection. The use of cough suppressants and expectorants would temporarily improve the cough but would do nothing to address the underlying disorder. Inhaled bronchodilators such as beta-2 agonist play no role in the treatment of GERD, unless the patient was to develop pneumonitis and dyspnea. (*Harrison's Principles of Internal Medicine*, pp. 203–205)

6. **(B)** We are dealing here with a rare disease and certainly one that you most likely will not encounter in clinical medicine. However, to answer the question correctly you must only recognize that we are dealing with an autosomal recessive disease (a positive family history in either side of the family and the mandatory unaffected parents are normally hints). In order to be unaffected by the disease and to have a child who is affected, both parents must be carriers of one copy of the autosomal recessive gene. If we call the recessive gene for this disorder "p" and the normal, dominant gene "P," then we can create a 2 × 2 table demonstrating the likelihood of having a child with the two recessive genes necessary to develop the disease.

		Maternal	
		P	p
Paternal	P	PP	Pp
	p	pP	pp

We can see that there is a one-in-four chance of a child acquiring the two recessive genes necessary to develop the disease. All other answers are incorrect since they represent either an autosomal dominant disease (a 50:50 chance) or are inaccurate for recessive diseases (there is no chance that the child will be affected).

7. **(A)**

8. **(B)**

Explanations 7 and 8

Despite recent findings from the Women's Health Initiative (WHI) study, which show that HRT may not be cardioprotective and may increase the risk for cardiovascular events (MI and stroke) in postmenopausal women with a known history of cardiovascular disease, HRT remains an effective way to treat and alleviate vasomotor instability and reduce the risk of osteoporosis and bone fractures (particularly hip fractures). In addition, there is evidence to support that this effect, along with improvement in affect and mood stability, is long lived and persists during the course of therapy. The incidence of endometrial cancer appears to be reduced in those taking HRT. The use of HRT in those with risk factors for cardiovascular disease must be made on an individual case base, with careful consideration of the risks versus the potential benefits of the intervention.

The WHI study has demonstrated an added risk for developing cardiovascular events, such as MI and stroke, among those with known coronary disease or populations at high risk for CAD. A significant family history of CAD (father died at early age of an MI) would place this patient in the category of higher risk. Although patients taking HRT are at an increased risk for developing venous thromboembolism, this would not preclude its use unless the patient had a known history of the disease. The incidence of breast cancer in women on HRT remains controversial and, in our patient's case, we are told that there is a negative family history, hence making it less of a concern. Bloating and breast tenderness may develop in patients taking HRT, but its occurrence would not be a reason not to start therapy on our patient. *(Women's Health Initiative Investigators. Risks and benefits of estrogen plus progestin in healthy postmenopausal women. JAMA 2002; 288: 321–333)*

9. **(C)** The symptoms of polydipsia, polyuria, and weight loss are suggestive of new onset diabetes in this young man. A diagnosis of DM can be made in any of the following ways: (1) A plasma glucose level of >126 mg/dL after fasting, (2) a nonfasting plasma glucose level >200 mg/dL, or (3) a glucose tolerance test that yields a plasma glucose level >200 mg/dL after 2 h. The American Diabetes Association (ADA) does not recommend the routine use of glycosylated hemoglobin (A1C) in the diagnosis of diabetes. In any case, the level would have to be >6% in order to suggest a diagnosis of diabetes, not 5%. *(American Diabetes Association. Diagnosis and classification of diabetes mellitus. Diabetes Care 27:S5–S10, 2004)*

10. **(B)**

11. **(E)**

Explanations 10 and 11

The history of acute coronary syndrome and diabetes places this patient at high risk for cardiovascular complications (MI or stroke). His diabetes, as well as all other risk factors, must be better controlled in order to decrease this risk. Statins (HMG-CoA reductase inhibitors) have been shown to lower cardiovascular morbidity and mortality in the primary and secondary prevention of cardiovascular complications. While niacin would indeed likely raise his HDL, data are still insufficient to recommend this as the main goal in reduction of cardiovascular events in patients with known CAD. The main goal at this point should be to lower LDL levels and total cholesterol to at least the recommended levels for patients at the highest risk

for cardiovascular complication, with an emphasis on lowering the LDL to <100 mg/dL and total cholesterol to <200 mg/dL.

Although both hypothyroidism and diabetes are well known causes of secondary hyperlipidemia, the case makes no mention of depressed thyroid function in this patient. Hence it would be unreasonable to start hormone supplementation without evidence of hypothyroid state. Although beneficial in cardiovascular disease and stroke, controlling blood pressure has no known direct effect on lipid profile. Controlling diabetes would therefore be the only choice that would directly contribute to positively affecting his lipid profile, by lowering LDL and TG levels and, therefore, decreasing total cholesterol. Sleeping, although healthy and beneficial to general well being, has no direct effect on lipid metabolism. *(The third report of the national cholesterol education program expert panel on the detection, evaluation, and treatment of high blood cholesterol in adults. NIH Publication No. 01-3670, May 2001)*

12. **(B)**

13. **(C)**

14. **(B)**

Explanations 12 through 14

The patient has clinical and biochemical evidence of gallstone pancreatitis including epigastric pain, a history suggestive of prior biliary colic, elevated transaminases and bilirubin (suggestive of an obstructing common bile duct stone), and an elevated amylase and lipase. Gastroenteritis would not be expected to alter liver chemistries. Drug-induced pancreatitis is possible as furosemide has been shown to cause pancreatitis, but would not result in the abnormal liver chemistries. Acute cholecystitis and cholangitis would likely be associated with an elevated leukocyte count, right upper quadrant abdominal pain, and fever.

An abdominal ultrasound could assess the gallbladder for the presence of stones and signs of cholecystitis, such as gallbladder wall thickening or pericholecystic fluid. It could also look for a dilated biliary tree or an obstructing stone in the common bile duct. An abdominal x-ray could reveal a localized ileus ("sentinel loop") or calcifications suggestive of chronic pancreatitis, but would be of significantly lesser yield. A CT or MRI of the abdomen would provide images of the pancreas and liver, but are often clinically unhelpful early in the course of acute pancreatitis. An ERCP is not indicated at this point, as only one set of liver chemistries is available. Should the bilirubin rise or fail to fall, an ERCP might be warranted to decompress the biliary tree.

The patient has a common bile duct stone causing biliary obstruction. This stone likely caused the patient's acute pancreatitis as well. Papillotomy (also known as sphincterotomy) will allow endoscopic removal of the stone. The stone cannot be removed through the native papilla, as the sphincter of Oddi musculature would not allow such a large stone to pass. Thus, sphincterotomy must be performed to disrupt the sphincter musculature. Papillary balloon dilation is possible but is associated with an increased risk of pancreatitis. A biliary stent is a viable option to provide drainage, but is inferior to sphincterotomy and stone extraction. No manipulation of the pancreatic duct is warranted. The stone should not be left in place as it could lead to recurrent pancreatitis or cholangitis. (*Harrison's Principles of Internal Medicine,* pp. 1639, 1792–1797)

15. **(C)** The biological half-life of a drug is the time required for 50% of the dose to be eliminated. This value is useful in determining the duration of a drug's effect and therefore proper drug dose regimes. (*Hardman et al., p. 18*)

16. **(C)** The liver has a well-known sensitivity to the interaction of alcohol and acetaminophen. One of the metabolites of acetaminophen is a highly reactive intermediate. In therapeutic doses, the intermediate is inactivated via conjugation. However, in high doses, the intermediate will react with hepatic cellular proteins resulting in necrosis. Alcohol potentiates this adverse effect. (*Hardman et al., p. 704*)

17. **(C)**

18. **(C)**

19. **(B)**

Explanations 17 through 19

The patient has chronic diarrhea superimposed on a long history of loose stools, steatorrhea, and significant weight loss. While these features could be seen in several diseases, the presence of the pruritic vesiculopapular lesions on his extensor surfaces makes the diagnosis highly likely to be celiac sprue, with its frequently accompanying skin manifestation *dermatitis herpetiformis*. Crohn's disease is not usually associated with steatorrhea, and ulcerative colitis is often associated with bloody stools. Chronic pancreatitis and Whipple's disease could cause a similar clinical picture but would not have the associated skin findings.

A small bowel biopsy would confirm histopathologic features consistent with celiac sprue, such as villous atrophy and crypt hyperplasia. A small bowel biopsy could also diagnose or rule out Whipple's disease by looking for the pathognomonic PAS positive organism *Tropheryma whippelii*. Colonic biopsies would be unhelpful in celiac sprue. A fecal fat quantification would likely confirm and assess the degree of steatorrhea, but would offer little other diagnostic information. A small bowel x-ray is too nonspecific to confirm the diagnosis and an abdominal CT scan would likely be normal unless the patient had developed a complication of advanced sprue, such as intestinal lymphoma.

Patients with celiac sprue are at increased risk for malignancies of the small bowel with adenocarcinoma and lymphoma being the two most commonly encountered. Patients with celiac sprue are not at greatly increased risk of the other malignancies listed. Limited data suggest that strict adherence to a gluten-free diet may decrease the incidence of malignancy in these patients. (*Harrison's Principles of Internal Medicine, pp. 1673–1675*)

20. (B)

21. (E)

22. (E)

Explanations 20 through 22

Oral corticosteroids are a mainstay of first-line treatment for moderate to severe ulcerative colitis. Starting doses of 40 mg po qd of prednisone, with a slow taper, are often effective in reducing colonic inflammation, although some patients are unable to wean steroids or maintain remission once achieved. The patient does not have dysplasia in any biopsy specimens, nor does he have signs of systemic toxicity, so a colectomy would be premature. Oral metronidazole is ineffective in ulcerative colitis. Cortisone enemas would be helpful if the patient had isolated left sided disease, but it is doubtful that enema therapy would reach his hepatic flexure. Intravenous cyclosporine would be used in severe colitis as a last measure before colectomy but this patient is not yet sick enough to warrant such therapy.

PSC occurs in approximately 3% of patients with ulcerative colitis and is its major liver complication. It is a chronic inflammatory condition of the biliary tree. It can typically manifest with elevated alkaline phosphatase and bilirubin levels, and results in diffuse stricturing and pruning of the biliary tree. Wilson's disease, hereditary hemochromatosis and alpha-1 antitrypsin deficiency are not associated with ulcerative colitis and are not cholestatic liver diseases. Primary biliary cirrhosis could account for these laboratory findings, but is rare in both males and patients with ulcerative colitis.

Patients with PSC are at increased risk of developing cholangiocarcinoma but not the other liver tumors mentioned. Patients with celiac sprue are at increased risk for small bowel cancers (adenocarcinoma, lymphoma). Patients with familial adenomatous polyposis are at increased risk to develop desmoid tumors. *(Harrison's Principles of Internal Medicine, pp. 1682–1688)*

23. (E)

24. (B)

Explanations 23 and 24

The patient should undergo screening colonoscopy, especially with his strongly positive family history of first degree relatives developing colon cancer before age 50. Colonoscopy is the only test that can directly evaluate the entire colon and rectum. Most polyps can be removed completely at colonoscopy, and large lesions or masses can be directly biopsied. Virtual colonoscopy and barium enema combined with flexible sigmoidoscopy are good tests, but any positive findings on either of these tests would warrant further examination with colonoscopy. Barium enema alone is insufficient for screening. Fecal occult blood testing is helpful as a screening tool, but would be inadequate alone in this patient given his family history.

The patient satisfies criteria for HNPCC, a syndrome seen in patients with germline mutations in DNA mismatch repair (MMR) genes. He has three first degree relatives with cancer of the colorectum, endometrium, small bowel, ureter, or renal pelvis (all of whom are first degree relatives of each other). The colorectal cancers involve at least two generations and at least one case was diagnosed before age 50. FAP involves a mutation of the APC gene and results in dense colonic polyposis, mandibular osteomas, and universal colon cancer at a young age unless colectomy is performed. Peutz-Jeghers syndrome results in hamartomatous polyps of the gut as well as mucocutaneous pigmentation changes. Cronkhite-Canada syndrome manifests as gastrointestinal polyposis, alopecia, cutaneous hyperpigmentation, malnutrition, and dystrophic fingernails. Turcot's syndrome is a variant of FAP in which patients can also develop medulloblastoma, glioblastoma multiforme, and hypertrophy of retinal pigmented epithelium. *(Harrison's Principles of Internal Medicine, pp. 582–583)*

25. (C)

26. (E)

27. (B)

Explanations 25 through 27

The patient has a peptic stricture, seen in the setting of longstanding untreated gastroesophageal reflux with esophagitis. The history of progressive solid food dysphagia without weight loss is typical. Tobacco, alcohol, thiazide diuretics, and spicy foods do not predispose to benign esophageal strictures.

The patient has developed a peptic stricture, a serious complication of gastroesophageal reflux disease. The patient needs esophageal dilation (either with mechanical or pneumatic dilators) and maximal acid suppression. PPI therapy is superior to histamine receptor antagonist therapy in terms of healing erosive esophagitis.

Patients with longstanding GERD are at increased risk of developing Barrett's esophagus, a risk factor for esophageal adenocarcinoma. GERD is not a risk factor for esophageal squamous cell cancer, gastric cancer, or duodenal cancer. Patients with chronic *Helicobacter pylori* infection (which this patient did not have) are at increased risk for a form of gastric lymphoma known as a MALT-oma. *(Harrison's Principles of Internal Medicine, pp. 1645–1647)*

28. (C)

29. (D)

30. (B)

31. (A)

32. (E)

Explanations 28 through 32

The patient's history and examination are worrisome for pancreatic disease, and he has strong signs of pancreatic insufficiency. His long history of alcohol use suggests the possibility of chronic pancreatitis or pancreatic cancer. Fecal fat studies would only confirm or quantify his steatorrhea. A CT scan would image the pancreas for changes consistent with chronic pancreatitis (duct dilation, calcifications, pseudocysts) and could look for a neoplasm of the pancreas as well. ERCP is not indicated as a first-line test in patients with abdominal pain given its risk of causing acute pancreatitis. Upper endoscopy would be helpful to rule out peptic ulcer disease and other gastric complaints, but would not provide more global information about the abdomen.

The patient has greasy stools and weight loss, findings seen in patients with steatorrhea due to chronic pancreatitis. Patients with steatorrhea malabsorb fat soluble vitamins (vitamins A, D, E, and K). "Night blindness" (poor night vision) due to vitamin A deficiency is common among patients with advanced chronic pancreatitis and likely led to this patient's motor vehicle accident.

The patient has diabetes mellitus as a consequence of pancreatic endocrine insufficiency, another feature of chronic pancreatitis. Diabetes develops when greater than 80–90% of the gland has been destroyed. Patients with chronic pancreatitis have a coexisting loss of glucagon from islet cells and, thus, often become brittle diabetics, with hypoglycemia seen after insulin administration. Vitamin K and B_{12} deficiency, which the patient may have, do not cause hypoglycemia. The patient was previously noted to eat well, so inadequate oral intake is unlikely. Diabetic education should decrease the rate of chronic insulin overdosage.

The patient has pancreatic exocrine insufficiency and thus cannot produce enough pancreatic enzymes to digest his food. Pancreatic enzyme replacement therapy in tablet form is a mainstay of therapy for chronic pancreatitis. It can rapidly reverse this problem by providing exogenously produced pancreatic enzymes to break down fats, carbohydrates, and proteins for absorption in the small bowel. The patient would not benefit from additional oral feedings without enzyme supplementation and would only worsen his steatorrhea by doing so. He can take food orally, so feeding via gastrostomy, TPN, or PPN are not indicated.

The patient's worsening pain and weight loss despite therapy is worrisome for the development of pancreatic cancer. Cancer antigen 19-9 is frequently (but not universally) elevated in pancreatic cancers, although it can be elevated in cholangiocarcinoma as well. PSA is associated with prostate cancer. CEA is associated with colon cancer. CA-125 is associated with ovarian cancer. AFP is associated with hepatocellular carcinoma. *(Harrison's Principles of Internal Medicine, pp. 1799–1803)*

33. (D)

34. (C)

Explanations 33 and 34

DEXA is the newest, least expensive, and quickest method of assessing bone mineral density. The precision of DEXA is approximately 1–2%. Standard radiography is inadequate for accurate bone mass assessment. Single-photon absorptiometry is used to scan bone which is in a superficial location with little adjacent soft tissue (e.g., radius). It may not be an accurate reflector of the density in the spine or hip, which are the sites of greatest potential risk for fracture. The quantitative CT scan and dual photon absorptiometry take more time, expose the patient to more radiation, and, in the case of quantitative CT scanning, significantly increase costs, when compared to DEXA.

The major risk factors for osteoporosis are family history, slender body build, fair skin, early menopause, sedentary lifestyle, cigarette smoking, medications (corticosteroids or L-thyroxine), more than two drinks a day of alcohol or caffeine, and low calcium intake. The current recommendation for oral calcium in men and premenopausal women is 1000 mg a day. Postmenopausal women and patients with osteoporosis should have 1500-mg calcium a day and 400–800 IU of vitamin D, which promotes intestinal calcium absorption. This patient's intake of calcium and vitamin D is not a risk factor for osteoporosis. *(Ruddy, pp. 1635–1637)*

35. (C)

36. (B)

37. (A)

Explanations 35 through 37

Reactive arthritis (previously called Reiter's syndrome) consists of a triad of nonspecific urethritis, conjunctivitis, and asymmetric arthritis, usually involving the large joints of the lower extremities. Genitourinary causes of reactive arthritis include *Chlamydia* or *Ureaplasma*. Gastrointestinal infections due to *Salmonella, Shigella, Yersinia, Klebsiella,* and *Campylobacter* can also cause reactive arthritis. Gout attacks are typically monoarticular and begin abruptly (often during the night or early morning) with the affected joint being exquisitely painful, warm, red, and swollen. These attacks often spontaneously resolve in 3–10 days. While the symptoms from pseudogout may mimic those of gout, they tend to be less painful and take longer to reach peak intensity. Gonococcal arthritis is seen more often in females, is associated with migratory arthralgia, tends to favor the upper limbs and knees and may be associated with cutaneous lesions (pustules). The absence of attacks and joint distribution makes gout and pseudogout less likely. The history of conjunctivitis and association with diarrhea makes the diagnosis of reactive arthritis more likely than resistant gonococcal arthritis. His clinical symptoms do not suggest ankylosing spondylitis, although if he was HLA-B27 positive he would be at increased risk of developing spondylitis.

This patient has the classic symptoms and exposure risk (gastrointestinal infection) to suggest reactive arthritis. For the articular symptoms, reduction of inflammation and restoration of function can be achieved with nonsteroidal anti-inflammatories alone. A sufficient number of patients with reactive arthritis will not be HLA-B27 positive, thus rendering this test useless as a screening test. However, it may be useful when the clinical picture is incomplete (such as absence of antecedent infection or lack of extraarticular features). Once an antecedent infection has triggered reactive arthritis, it is unlikely that antibiotics will affect the course of the illness (except in the case of chlamydia-associated urogenital disease where a trial of prolonged antibiotic therapy may be reasonable). Systemic corticosteroids are usually ineffective in reactive arthritis, but may be tried for resistant disease or conditions such as AIDS in which cytotoxic therapy is contraindicated. Given the absence of skin lesions, penile discharge, or urogenital symptoms, one would be hard-pressed to challenge the patient's statement that he has not engaged in unprotected sex at the risk of jeopardizing the physician-patient relationship.

Reactive arthritis may be the first manifestation of HIV infection. Therefore, HIV antibody status should be determined when the appropriate risk factors and/or clinical features are present. As mentioned previously, systemic steroids are usually ineffective for reactive arthritis and, with the possibility of joint infection, would necessitate ruling out infection by arthrocentesis of the affected joints. Joint infection can not be ruled out based on his presentation, and joint sepsis must be excluded prior to corticosteroid injection. The clinical presentation is classic for reactive arthritis, and the absence of systemic symptoms makes the likelihood of disseminated bacterial infection low. Indomethacin, at a dose of 150–200 mg a day, is the prototypic nonsteroidal anti-inflammatory medication (NSAID) for treatment of reactive arthritis. Doses higher than this are associated with significant gastrointestinal complications and do not improve efficacy in a patient resistant to the standard dose. In the event that the patient does not respond to 200 mg of indomethacin or alternative NSAIDs, disease-modifying antirheumatic drugs (DMARD) such as methotrexate, azathioprine, or sulfasalazine may be used, provided that HIV test results are negative, as these immunosuppressants have been reported to precipitate the onset of AIDS in HIV positive patients. *(Ruddy, pp. 1055–1062)*

38. **(D)** Probenecid is used in the management of hyperuricemia. Its mechanism of action is related to its ability to enhance the excretion of uric acid by inhibiting urate reabsorption from the renal tubule fluid. Small doses of the drug, however, may actually raise blood urate levels. *(Katzung, pp. 597–598)*

39. **(C)** Indomethacin inhibits the prostaglandin synthesis that facilitates the inflammation of acute gout and inhibits the phagocytosis of urate crystals by leukocytes. This inhibits the cell lysis and release of cytotoxic factors that initiate the inflammatory cascade. Allopurinol (an inhibitor of urate synthesis) and probenecid and sulfinpyrazone (promoters of urate excretion) are useful for preventing gout but are not effective during an acute attack. Aspirin is inappropriate in the treatment of gout since it can inhibit urate elimination and therefore increase hyperuricemia, the underlying metabolic abnormality in gout. *(Katzung, pp. 596–599)*

40. **(D)** Teriparatide is a recently approved recombinant form of parathyroid hormone that stimulates bone formation, rather than inhibiting resorption, and which is associated with a marked reduction in the incidence of bone fractures. Estrogen and the estrogen receptor modulator raloxifene, alendronate, and calcitonin all inhibit bone resorption and increase bone mineral density, but the percent increase in bone density is less than occurs with teriparatide.

41. **(C)** Leukocoria, a white pupillary reflex, can be caused by several conditions. The most serious, and potentially life threatening, is retinoblastoma. Retinoblastoma is a malignant neoplasm of the retina that may appear as a white mass extending into the vitreous, a mass lesion underlying a retinal detachment or as a diffusely spreading lesion. Retinoblastomas may be unilateral, bilateral, or multifocal. The diagnosis is usually made between 1 and 2 years of age. Other causes of leukocoria may include retinopathy of prematurity, congenital cataracts, toxocarisis (a nematode infection), or Coats' disease (a retinal vascular abnormality). The treatment of retinoblastoma may involve

surgery, chemotherapy, or other modalities such as cryotherapy and photocoagulation. (*Wills eye manual, Sec. 8.1*)

42. (E)

43. (D)

44. (A)

Explanations 42 through 44

Papilledema is optic disc swelling and implies raised intracranial pressure. Headache is a common associated symptom. The initial evaluation of papilledema should involve imaging, either by MRI or CT scan with and without contrast, to exclude mass lesions. If these studies are negative, then the subarachnoid opening pressure should be measured by lumbar puncture. An erythrocyte sedimentation rate is unlikely to be diagnostic in this case. It would be more important in the evaluation of vision loss or headache in a person over the age of 50. Neither a pregnancy test nor a glucose tolerance test would provide information on the cause of increased intracranial pressure.

Pseudotumor cerebri is a condition of idiopathic intracranial hypertension. It is a diagnosis of exclusion that would be made in the presence of papilledema, normal imaging studies and elevated opening pressure on lumbar puncture with normal CSF studies. The majority of patients with pseudotumor cerbri are young, female, and obese. This condition is treated with a carbonic anhydrase inhibitor, such as acetazolamide, which lowers intracranial pressure by reducing the production of CSF. Weight reduction, while important, is often unsuccessful in improving the condition by itself. Steroids, tetracycline, pregnancy, and oral contraceptives are not associated with the development of pseudotumor cerbri. (*Harrison's Principles of Internal Medicine, pp. 171–172*)

45. (B)

46. (B)

Explanations 45 and 46

Persons with diabetes mellitus are 25 times more likely to become legally blind than persons without diabetes. Blindness is primarily the result of progressive diabetic retinopathy and clinically significant macular edema. The presence of retinal vascular microaneurysms, blot hemorrhages, and cotton wool spots mark the presence of nonproliferative diabetic retinopathy. Increased retinal vascular permeability, alterations in blood flow, and abnormal microvasculature lead to retinal ischemia. In response to the ischemia, new blood vessels may form at the optic nerve and/or macula (neovascularization). This marks the presence of proliferative diabetic retinopathy. These new vessels rupture easily and may lead to vitreous hemorrhage, fibrosis, and retinal detachment. (*Harrison's Principles of Internal Medicine, p. 2121*)

47. (E)

48. (A)

49. (C)

Explanations 47 through 49

The presence of headache, eye pain, nausea, and vomiting should prompt the consideration of the diagnosis of acute angle closure glaucoma. This is a rare but serious condition in which the aqueous outflow is obstructed, and the intraocular pressure abruptly rises. Susceptible eyes have a narrow anterior chamber and when the pupil becomes dilated, the peripheral iris blocks the outflow via the anterior chamber angle. Edema of the cornea occurs, resulting in cloudiness on examination. Diagnosis is made by measuring the intraocular pressure during an acute attack. Treatment includes medications to induce miosis in an effort to relieve the blockage or, if that fails, surgical intervention.

In some patients, the headache or gastrointestinal symptoms can overshadow the ocular symptoms, resulting in a delay in diagnosis and unnecessary workup for other conditions. In this case, the lack of findings on abdominal examination makes appendicitis or perforated bowel unlikely. Diabetic ketoacidosis can present with primarily GI symptoms, but would not explain the ocular symptoms. Similarly, cerebellar or other brain tumors may cause headache, nausea, and vomiting, but would not be causes of a painful, red eye. (*Harrison's Principles of Internal Medicine, p. 170*)

50. **(C)** Primidone is an anticonvulsant used to treat epilepsy. It is metabolized to both phenobarbital and phenylethylmalonamide. Both of these compounds contribute to the overall anticonvulsant activity of primidone. (*Katzung, pp. 386–387*)

51. **(C)** Nitrous oxide is primarily used during surgery as an adjuvant to more potent anesthetic gases. This is because, when administered in combination with halogenated anesthetics such as enflurane, lower concentrations of the more potent agents may be administered to achieve surgical anesthesia. Therefore, the incidence of respiratory and circulatory depression is reduced and recovery is more rapid. As a single agent, nitrous oxide is an effective analgesic; however, it cannot reliably induce surgical anesthesia without being administered under hyperbaric pressures. Cyclopropane is no longer utilized because of its flammability. D-Tubocurarine is not an anesthetic, but a neuromuscular blocker that has no anesthetic properties. (*Hardman et al., pp. 394–395*)

52. **(D)** All benzodiazepines have hypnotic effects at appropriate doses. Although these agents may decrease the time required for a person to fall asleep, they have been shown to alter REM sleep patterns. The onset and duration of action of these agents depend on their absorption, metabolism to inactive or active products, and extent of accumulation in the body. Some agents (e.g., temazepam) are absorbed slowly from the gastrointestinal tract; peak plasma levels may not be obtained for 2 h or more after a dose. Therefore, these agents should be administered well before bedtime. Flurazepam is extensively metabolized to active metabolites; one of these metabolites is excreted very slowly from the body. The accumulation of this metabolite appears to enhance the sedative–hypnotic effects of flurazepam by approximately the second or third night of administration. The prolonged use of benzodiazepines will result in dependence and withdrawal symptoms. (*Hardman et al., pp. 400–409*)

53. **(B)** Fluoxetine is an atypical antidepressant with little anticholinergic activity. Because of its high specificity as a serotonin uptake inhibitor, fluoxetine does not have many of the symptoms linked to muscarinic blockade, such as dry mouth, tachycardia, and drowsiness, which are typical of tricyclic antidepressants. (*Hardman et al., p. 466*)

54. **(B)** The mechanism of action for lithium effects in bipolar disorder is not well understood. It may inhibit the phosphatase responsible for the intracellular release of inositol; however, the connection to manic behavior remains uncertain. Lithium is useful in treating acute manic episodes, but is also utilized prophylactically to decrease the occurrences of mania and to decrease the intensity of the depression phase. Neuroleptic drugs such as haloperidol can be effective in treating an acute manic episode. The other drugs are effective in treating depression but not bipolar disorder (*Katzung, pp. 476–478*)

55. **(A)** Cimetidine inhibits the metabolism of other drugs by affecting hepatic microsomal enzyme activity. Therefore, serum levels should be monitored when cimetidine is used concomitantly with drugs with a low therapeutic index, such as warfarin, phenytoin, and theophylline. Phenobarbital, ethyl alcohol, and methylcholanthrene induce liver enzymes. (*Katzung, pp. 1035–1038*)

56. **(D)** Memantine, the only drug approved for the treatment of moderate to severe Alzheimer's disease, is an *N*-methyl-D-aspartate (NMDA) receptor antagonist and the first Alzheimer drug of this type approved in the United States. It blocks the activity of glutamate, a neurotransmitter involved in information processing, storage, and retrieval. NMDA receptors facilitate calcium influx into

neurons. Too much calcium, though, can result in cell death. All of the other drugs are acetylcholinesterase inhibitors that increase the concentration of acetylcholine in the brain. *(Katzung, pp. 1010–1011)*

57. **(E)** Buspirone is a nonsedating anxiolytic agent that is a partial agonist at 5-HT_{1A} receptors. Unlike benzodiazepines, such as diazepam and oxazepam (Serax), it has no hypnotic, anticonvulsant, or muscle relaxant properties. Amitriptyline and doxepin have also been used to treat anxiety, especially when associated with depression; however, these drugs are also sedating. *(Katzung, p. 360)*

58. **(A)** Sildenafil is a phosphodiesterase inhibitor effective in the treatment of erectile dysfunction whose mechanism of action is related to an increase in intracellular cyclic guanosine monophosphate (GMP). The antianginal agent nitroglycerin increases cyclic GMP via the activation of guanylyl cyclase. When the two drugs interact, there can be a dramatic fall in blood pressure related to extreme vasodilation. The other selections can reduce blood pressure; however, since their mechanisms of action are not associated with the intracellular concentration of cyclic GMP, there is no synergistic interaction with sildenafil *(Hardin et al., pp. 850–851)*

59. **(A)** Local anesthetics exist in solution in both uncharged base and charged cationic forms. The base diffuses across the nerve sheath and membrane and then reequilibrates within the axoplasm. It is intracellular penetration of the cation into, and attachment to a receptor at a site within the sodium channel, that leads to inhibition of sodium conductance and ultimate conduction blockade. Bupivacaine is typical of amide-linked local anesthetics with high anesthetic potency and long duration of action (class III). Procaine is typical of class I agents that are ester linked and have low anesthetic potency and short duration of action. Important features of group III compounds include: (1) high degree of lipid solubility or high partition coefficient that aid in penetration of the drug, (2) high degree of protein binding that aids in

attachment of the drug once it has penetrated the cell, and (3) pK_a closer to pH = 7.4 so that more of the drug is in the un-ionized form and is free to penetrate the membrane. Ester-linked anesthetics, such as procaine, are rapidly metabolized by pseudocholinesterases, whereas bupivacaine is slowly degraded by hepatic enzymes. *(Hardman et al., pp. 331–339)*

60. **(D)**

61. **(A)**

62. **(D)**

63. **(C)**

Explanations 60 through 63

The patient has hypotonic hyponatremia, which can lead to increased water shifting into the brain, resulting in cerebral edema. This patient has nothing in history or physical examination to suggest a stroke or the presence of sepsis as the etiology of his altered mental status. Central pontine myelinolysis is a potentially devastating neurologic complication that can result from the treatment of hyponatremia, not hyponatremia itself. While respiratory acidosis could potentially contribute to this patient's change in mental status, cerebral edema due to hypotonicity is the most likely etiology.

The patient's laboratory studies indicate a low plasma osmolality with an inappropriately increased urine osmolality. With this degree of hypotonicity, the urine should be maximally dilute (osmolality of <100 mOsmol/kg H_2O). The high urine osmolality suggests the presence of antidiuretic hormone. In psychogenic polydipsia, the urine would be maximally dilute. Answer C is unlikely since his physical examination does not suggest volume depletion; furthermore, the patient is taking a calcium channel blocker, not a diuretic, for the treatment of his hypertension. Decreased expression of renal collecting duct water channels would lead to water wasting and, thus, the development of diabetes insipidus and hypernatremia.

The patient has symptomatic hypotonic hyponatremia with signs of cerebral edema. This requires immediate attention. Choices A, C, and E are essentially hypotonic solutions which should be withheld in patients with hyponatremia. The serum sodium in this case should be increased by at least 5% for the treatment of cerebral edema. The use of 0.9% saline would require nearly 5 L of infusate to address this cerebral edema. This could lead to pulmonary edema and volume overload. The use of hypertonic saline (3% saline) is the ideal solution to use in this scenario, as the infusion of 3% saline will correct the symptoms while avoiding volume overload. As in all cases of hyponatremia management, frequent serum sodium assays are necessary in order to avoid too rapid of a correction, which could result in neurologic injury—pontine myelinolysis.

The optimal rate of correction to avoid pontine myelinolysis is controversial; however, correction should not exceed 8–12 meq/L in the first 24 h or 25 meq/L in the first 48 h. DDAVP is of no clinical use in the management of hyponatremia. Loop diuretics can be of use in the treatment of hyponatremia, especially in hypervolemic hyponatremia, as they result in a hypotonic diuresis and aid in the removal of excess water. Answer B is not accurate, as too slow of a correction in symptomatic hyponatremia can result in neurologic injury through the persistence of cerebral edema. Answer E is incorrect, as hypokalemia can usually be corrected by oral intake of potassium, making IV supplementation not always necessary. *(Brenner & Rector, pp. 896–903)*

64. **(B)**

65. **(C)**

66. **(A)**

67. **(C)**

68. **(B)**

Explanations 64 through 68

The patient has tumor lysis syndrome. The destruction of malignant cells by chemotherapeutic agents will lead to the release of intracellular contents, including potassium, phosphorus, and uric acid (from nucleic acids). This can result in hyperkalemia, hyperuricemia, and hyperphosphatemia.

Hyperkalemia will produce significant ECG abnormalities, including peaked T waves and widened QRS complexes. The presence of bradycardia and irregular heart rate on physical examination are suggestive of the cardiac effects of hyperkalemia, which can lead to life-threatening arrhythmias if not addressed.

Patients with tumor lysis syndrome can develop a severe hyperuricemia. The kidneys are responsible for the excretion of uric acid. In acidic urine, the uric acid can crystallize in collecting tubules, resulting in intratubular obstruction and acute kidney failure. Calcium oxalate stones are not a part of this entity. Cisplatin can cause renal potassium and magnesium losses, which is not the case in this patient. The laboratory data suggest the release of intracellular contents (high LDH, uric acid, potassium, and phosphate) and the diagnoses of urate nephropathy as the cause of his acute kidney failure.

As mentioned before, hyperkalemia will produce significant ECG abnormalities, including peaked T waves and widened QRS complexes. Prominent U waves are found in hypokalemia, not hyperkalemia. Atrial fibrillation is not a typically seen in hyperkalemia.

This patient is having hemodynamic instability because of life-threatening hyperkalemia. Calcium chloride, in this case, is necessary to help stabilize the myocardium from the effects of hyperkalemia, although it will not have an effect on the serum potassium itself. Intravenous insulin, given in conjunction with dextrose (in order to prevent hypoglycemia), is the first-line treatment for hyperkalemia, as it will promote the movement of potassium intracellularly. Albuterol is also effective in the treatment of hyperkalemia, as a β agonist will promote the cellular uptake of potassium. Kayexalate binds potassium in the large intestine and helps remove total body potassium; however, this is not immediately helpful in treating life-threatening hyperkalemia because of the increased time to onset of action. *(Brenner & Rector, pp. 1006–1007, 1022, 1635–1636)*

69. (D)

70. (B)

71. (D)

72. (A)

Explanations 69 through 72

This patient has atheroembolic disease, most likely from the dislodging of arterial plaque during or after the cardiac catheterization, with subsequent kidney embolization. The findings in her history and physical examination that would suggest this are the presence of significant hypertension, abdominal pain, the red-blue rash on her extremities (livedo reticularis), and eosinophilia with urinary eosinophils. Furthermore, the time course of the development of acute renal failure is suggestive of atheroembolic disease. The typical time course for contrast nephropathy is of an immediate onset, usually with subsequent recovery. However, in patients with atheroembolic disease, the kidney failure can occur much later after the procedure. Contrast nephropathy is not associated with the laboratory abnormalities and physical examination findings seen in this case. Interstitial nephritis is unlikely, as is a lupus nephritis flare, given her classic presentation for emboli.

Calculation of the fractional excretion of sodium (FeNa) is helpful in differentiating between "prerenal" causes (FeNa <1%) of acute renal failure versus intrinsic causes (FeNa >1%). A kidney ultrasound is helpful in determining the presence of urinary tract obstruction. Neither the anion gap nor calculation of glomerular filtration rate is helpful in determining if volume depletion is a possible etiology of acute renal failure. Examination of urine sediment would be helpful in determining the presence of a glomerular etiology of acute renal failure, not a prerenal etiology.

Demerol and metabolites can accumulate in patients with depressed kidney function, leading to increased levels and, potentially, convulsions. NSAIDs should be avoided in patients with acute kidney failure, as these drugs are potential nephrotoxins and could prevent a recovery of kidney function. Ketorolac, indomethacin, and ibuprofen are all NSAIDs. Therefore, morphine is the best option of those given.

White blood cell casts are suggestive of pyelonephritis. High levels of proteinuria are significant for the diagnosis of nephrotic syndrome, but not lupus nephritis specifically. Urine eosinophils are usually seen in patients with acute interstitial nephritis or atheroembolic disease. Lupus nephritis is usually associated with depressed serum complement levels. Of these tests, red blood cell casts are the most suggestive of glomerulonephritis. *(Brenner & Rector, pp. 1079–1084, 1382–1388)*

73. (A)

74. (A)

75. (B)

76. (A)

77. (B)

Explanations 73 through 77

Nephrotic syndrome is usually associated with edema, hypoalbuminemia, urine protein losses >3.5 g/day and hyperlipidemia. While some forms of nephrotic syndrome can be associated with hypocomplementemia, this is not a typical finding. Other abnormalities often seen in nephrotic syndrome include microcytic, hypochromic anemia (due to transferrin loss), hypocalcemia (due to vitamin D deficiency), and low thyroxine levels (due to loss of thyroxine-binding globulin [TBG]). *(Harrison's Principles of Internal Medicine, pp. 1584–1585)*

This patient has history, physical and laboratory findings that suggest possible multiple myeloma. For example, his history is pertinent for lower back pain and headaches. Moreover, Bence-Jones protein is not usually detected by urine dipstick but will be detected during a 24-h urine collection. This would explain why there is relatively little urine protein detected on dipstick but over 5 g on the 24-h urine. Lastly, multiple myeloma should be considered in an older patient with unexplained anemia. Given these findings, a serum and urine protein electrophoresis would be the best test to order next. A kidney biopsy would usually be diagnostic, but is unnecessary if the electrophoresis is positive. Complement levels and anti-GBM titer would not be of any use at the present time. Checking glycosylated hemoglobin will inform you of the adequacy of glucose control, but will be of little use with regards to the workup of the nephrotic syndrome.

This patient has a low anion gap due to the presence of unmeasured cations in the blood. In this case, they arise from circulating immunoglobulins. The fractional excretion of sodium and urea can be helpful in differentiating prerenal causes from other etiologies of acute renal failure. A split 24-h urine for protein is helpful in determining the presence of orthostatic proteinuria.

Initiation of ACE inhibitors or angiotensin receptor blockers is the best option in patients with diabetic nephropathy, as these medications have been shown to slow the progression of kidney disease. The other medications listed may be used adjunctively, with an ACE inhibitor or angiotensin receptor blocker, if adequate blood pressure control could not be achieved with monotherapy.

HIV-associated nephropathy is typically associated with a collapsing glomerulopathy, a variant of focal segmental glomerulosclerosis. Membranous nephropathy is associated with a number of other infections, including syphilis, hepatitis B, and hepatitis C virus. Membranoproliferative glomerulonephritis has also been associated with hepatitis C virus. (*Brenner & Rector, p. 1441*)

78. (D)

79. (B)

80. (A)

Explanations 78 through 80

This patient has chronic hepatitis B. The different serologic studies for hepatitis B are shown in Figs. 1-12 and 1-13. The patient does not have acute hepatitis B because the IgM antibody to hepatitis B core is negative, and the total antibody to hepatitis B core is positive. Antibody to hepatitis B core occurs prior to the development of antibody to hepatitis B surface. IgM is found in acute infections; primarily IgG is seen in chronic infections.

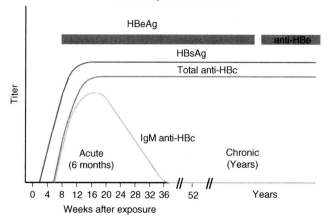

Acute Hepatitis B with Recovery

FIG. 1-12

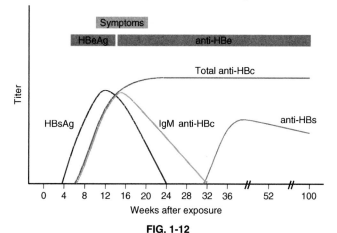

Chronic Hepatitis B Infection

FIG. 1-13

The presence of antibody to hepatitis B core with a positive hepatitis B surface antigen is indicative of chronic infection. Delta hepatitis infection requires the hepatitis B surface antigen. Delta hepatitis can occur concurrently with acute hepatitis B infection or later in the setting of chronic hepatitis B infection (Figs. 1-14 and 1-15). There is no test for hepatitis C antigen. This is not a presentation of acute hepatitis A, which usually has very high transaminases. The antibody to hepatitis A virus occurs after 1 month and is associated with high transaminases (Fig. 1-16).

Hepatitis A Virus Infection

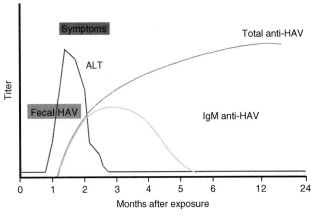

FIG. 1-16

HBV - HDV Coinfection

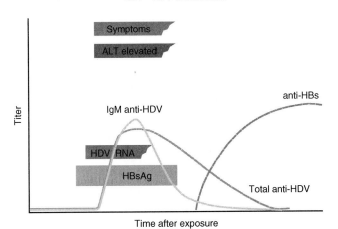

FIG. 1-14

HBV - HDV Superinfection
Typical Serologic Course

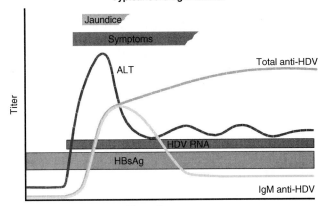

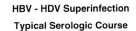

FIG. 1-15

Hepatitis A vaccine is indicated for patients with chronic liver disease. If this patient had had hepatitis C, then hepatitis B vaccine would also be indicated. Hepatitis B vaccine is essentially hepatitis B surface antigen that causes the production of hepatitis B surface antibody. Since this patient has hepatitis B surface antigen already, answer C would be incorrect. Verifying the diagnosis with a qualitative hepatitis B viral load is not necessary. A quantitative hepatitis B viral load might be useful to evaluate for potential antiviral therapy. The only reason hepatitis A would be recommended for the patient's spouse would be if the patient had acute hepatitis A. Investigating for other causes of hepatitis is not necessary as the diagnosis of chronic hepatitis B is already established.

If the patient was found to be HBeAg positive, he would be considered highly infectious for the spread of hepatitis B. Hepatitis Be antigen is the DNA polymerase that shows active replication of the hepatitis B virion. These patients are 100 times more infectious than those lacking the hepatitis Be antigen. The window period is a situation where a patient is just recovering from hepatitis B. Hepatitis Bs antigen is negative and the antibody to hepatitis Bs has not developed. The diagnosis is made by antibody to hepatitis B core. This is seen in Fig. 1-17. Any patient who is hepatitis B surface antigen positive is at risk for delta hepatitis. This patient would be at risk for delta hepatitis by virtue of having a positive hepatitis B surface antigen. There is no level of transaminases, even normal transaminases, which would preclude antiviral therapy. The level of viral production indicated by the hepatitis B quantitative viral load, along with an assessment of the underlying liver pathology, is the best indication of need for treatment. As mentioned above, antibody to hepatitis Be would show the patient is less infectious and likely have a lower viral load. *(Mandell, pp. 300–305, 1671, 1934–1936)*

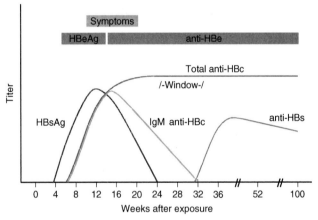

Acute Hepatitis B with Recovery

FIG. 1-17

81. (C)

82. (A)

Explanations 81 and 82

This is a clinical presentation of West Nile virus infection. The tongue fasciculations go along with an inflammation at the base of the brain. The patient is at the right age for West Nile virus infection and he is immunocompromised due to diabetes. The diagnosis can be made by performing a West Nile virus IgM titer on the CSF. Diabetics can have cryptococcal meningitis. Lumbar puncture in this setting is usually normal with increased opening pressure, and rhabdomyolysis is not a feature of this disease. Diabetics are more at risk for candidiasis.

However, the patient has no history of instrumentation, IV catheters, or other situations that would lead to disseminated candidiasis. Diabetics are at increased risk for *C. immitis* infection, but we have no history of the patient living in an area endemic for this organism. Diabetics are at increased risk for rhinocerebral mucormycosis. An MRI of the head might have shown involvement of the sinus. However, this patient's presentation is not consistent with rhinocerebral mucormycosis. *(Huhn GD, et al. West Nile virus in the United States: Update on an emerging infectious disease. Am Fam Physician 2003; 68: 653–660, 671–672)*

83. (C) Cephalosporin and penicillin antibiotics act by interfering with the late stages of bacterial cell wall synthesis, although the precise biochemical reactions are not entirely understood. Peptidoglycan provides mechanical stability to the cell wall because of its high degree of cross-linking with alternating amino pyranoside sugar residues (*N*-acetylglucosamine and *N*-acetylmuramic acid). The completion of the cross-linking occurs by the action of the enzyme transpeptidase. This transpeptidase reaction, in which the terminal glycine residue of the pentaglycine bridge is joined to the fourth residue of the pentapeptide (D-alanine) thereby releasing the fifth residue (D-alanine), is inhibited by beta-lactams. *(Hardman et al., pp. 1190–1191)*

84. (C) Acyclovir is a useful antiviral drug. When used intravenously, acyclovir can precipitate in renal tubules, resulting in nephrotoxicity. This adverse effect especially occurs in dehydrated individuals. *(Hardman et al., p. 1318)*

85. (D)

86. (E)

87. (A)

Explanations 85 through 87

The patient has diffuse interstitial infiltrates on CXR that correspond in time and presentation to acute inhalation histoplasmosis. This would be seen in a patient, such as an amateur spelunker, who has been in a cave with bats. It is the act of crawling through the cave that disturbs the spores of histoplasmosis that grow in the bat guano. The incubation period for influenza is 1–2 days. It is passed primarily by secretions from the nose spread by hands. The other members of the expedition were not sick, as they might be with influenza. Disseminated aspergillosis occurs in immunocompromised patients who have defects in both cell mediated and humoral immunity. This patient does not have this. While the CXR could mimic miliary tuberculosis, the association with caving 14 days before would make tuberculosis less likely and histoplasmosis more likely. There is no history that the patient is immunocompromised with HIV and would be at risk for *P. jiroveci* pneumonia.

Fungal serologies would establish the diagnosis, but acute and convalescent serologies would take 3 weeks for results. These are only useful in outbreak investigations. The other choices do not fit due to the reasons above. Treatment of acute respiratory histoplasmosis is based on severe hypoxia and would require arterial blood gases to establish the need for therapy.

None of the fungal infections mentioned are transmissible person to person, therefore respiratory isolation would not be necessary. Histoplasmosis is a dimorphic fungus that grows as a yeast at body temperature and a mold at room temperature. The mold produces the spores that are infectious. A similar situation occurs for *Cryptococcus neoformans*. *Coccidioides immitis* and aspergillosis are not transmitted from person to person. *(Mandell, pp. 2720–2723)*

88. **(D)**

89. **(E)**

Explanations 88 and 89

The clinical picture is most consistent with disease caused by *C. immitis*. This is due both to the nature of the cavitary lesion on CXR and the endemic area. Figure 1-4 shows a peripheral,

thin-walled cavitary lesion on CXR as well as a right lower lobe infiltrate. As a renal transplant recipient 1 year out, this patient is likely to have infections with tuberculosis and disseminated fungal infections. It is interesting that the route that he travels is through the lower Sonoran life zone where coccidiomycosis is endemic. CMV produces a diffuse interstitial infiltrate pattern on CXR, as does *Pneumocystis* and *Histoplasma capsulatum*.

Fiberoptic bronchoscopy with bronchial alveolar lavage should be performed in any patient with this clinical presentation who is immunocompromised because of the lack of ability to produce a good sputum specimen. We know that the patient is PPD positive, so skin testing is not useful. The patient is not mentioned to be in the endemic area for histoplasmosis. Serum cryptococcal antigen testing is a remote possibility. While *Cryptococcus* can produce a pulmonary disease with cavitary lesions, in immunocompromised hosts such as this, the patient more likely would present with meningitis. *(Mandell, pp. 2749–2752)*

90. **(B)** Tacrolimus (FK506) inhibits T-cell activation by binding to a specific protein FKBP. The result is inhibition of calcineurin-dependent activation of lymphokine gene expression, apoptosis, and degranulation. Cyclosporin has a similar mechanism, but binds to a different cytoplasmic protein (cyclophilin). *(Hardman et al., p. 1469)*

91. **(D)** Zidovudine (AZT) is the prototype antiviral agent utilized against retroviruses such as HIV. AZT is sequentially phosphorylated to the triphosphate, which then can competitively inhibit reverse transcriptase by substituting for thymidine triphosphate. Ultimately, AZT is incorporated into DNA and causes inhibition of viral DNA polymerase. Amantadine inhibits viral uncoating and also viral assembly. Alpha-interferon contributes to viral resistance by stimulating the synthesis of a number of proteins which ultimately have antiviral action. *(Hardman et al., pp. 1353–1354)*

92. **(B)** Aminoglycosides accumulate in the proximal tubular cells of the kidney, resulting in a

defect in renal concentrating ability and reduced glomerular filtration after several days. Impairment of renal function is almost always reversible. Streptomycin, in particular, may damage the optic nerve. Aminoglycosides may also cause ototoxicity that can be unilateral or bilateral and is often irreversible. *(Hardman et al., p. 1229)*

93. **(D)** *V. vulnificus* is associated with sepsis in patients with liver disease who eat raw oysters or those with salt water contamination of wounds, like those caused by fish hooks. *Pasteurella multocida* is a cause of cellulitis caused by exposure to cat saliva as a result of a bite or a clawing injury. *Eikenella corrodens* is associated with cellulitis caused by a human bite. *Staphylococcus* and *Streptococcus* are the most common causes of cellulitis. The Gram's stain shows gram-negative, comma-shaped organisms typical for vibrios. *(Mandell, p. 2274)*

94. **(D)** No cephalosporin is appropriate for the treatment of *Enterococcus faecalis*. This organism is occasionally sensitive to fluoroquinolones, but this choice is unreliable. The combination of ampicillin and an aminoglycoside is synergistic for susceptible *E. faecalis*. *(Mandell, p. 2151)*

95. **(B)**

96. **(D)**

Explanations 95 and 96

Lyme disease is the most common vector-borne disease in the United States. It is caused by infection with *B. burgdorferi*, a spirochete that is transmitted to humans through the bite of ticks of the *Ixodes* family. These ticks are very small, so frequently the victim is unaware of having been bitten. After an incubation of 3–30 days, a red macule or papule develops at the site of the bite, which expands to form a large annular lesion with partial central clearing or several red rings within an outside ring. The lesion, erythema migrans, is often said to resemble a "bull's-eye" target. Within a few days or weeks of this, the patient often complains of flu-like symptoms—fever, chills, myalgias, headache, fatigue—caused by the hematogenous spread of the

spirochete. Lyme disease has been found in most of the United States, but is most common in the New England states, where over 20% of *Ixodes* ticks are infected with the spirochete. Left untreated, patients may progress to develop multiple complications, including neurologic, musculoskeletal, or cardiac involvement.

Lyme disease is usually diagnosed by recognition of the symptoms and signs, along with serologic testing. However, serologic tests may be negative for several weeks after infection. IgG and IgM should be tested in acute and convalescent samples. Only 20–30% of exposures will have positive acute antibody responses, whereas 70–80% will have positive convalescent titers. Samples that are positive by ELISA assay should be confirmed by western blot testing. Empirical antibiotic therapy, preferably with doxycycline, is recommended for patients with a high probability of Lyme disease—such as those with erythema migrans. Doxycycline is the preferred antibiotic for treatment of early stage Lyme disease in adults because of its effectiveness against Lyme disease and other infections, such as human granulocytic ehrlichiosis, which is also transmitted by *Ixodes* ticks. Waiting to treat until convalescent titers become positive would not be recommended in this patient, who has a high likelihood of having Lyme disease, as it may result in more complications developing and necessitate the need for longer and more intensive treatment. For more advanced stages of disease, such as the presence of nervous system involvement or third degree heart block, parenteral antibiotic treatment is necessary. Ceftriaxone is the treatment of choice in this setting. *(Harrison's Principles of Internal Medicine, pp. 1061–1064)*

97. **(C)**

98. **(C)**

Explanations 97 and 98

Guidelines for the prevention of opportunistic infections in persons with HIV recommend institution of trimethoprim/sulfamethoxazole DS 1 tablet daily for *Pneumocystis carinii* pneumonia prophylaxis when the CD4 count falls below 200/μL. Azithromycin or clarithromycin are recommended for *M. avium* complex when the CD4 count falls below 50/μL. The varicella vaccine is a live-virus vaccine and, as such, is contraindicated in the presence of HIV disease with a reduced CD4 count. If the patient did not have a history of chicken pox or varicella immunization and had a significant exposure to chicken pox, the use of varicella immune globulin would be recommended. Ganciclovir would be recommended for CMV prophylaxis if there were a history of prior end-organ disease. *(Harrison's Principles of Internal Medicine, p. 1881)*

In a patient with HIV, a PPD is considered positive if there is 5 mm of induration. In a patient with a normal CXR, no symptoms of active disease and no history of treatment for a prior positive PPD, the recommended treatment would be isoniazid for 9 months. In the absence of a suspicious appearing CXR or symptoms, AFB testing would be unnecessary. A booster test would also be unnecessary, as the initial test is already positive. Multidrug therapy would be indicated only for confirmed or suspected active tuberculosis. *(www.cdc.gov)*

99. **(D)** Animal bites, most commonly from pet dogs and cats, result in over 1 million wounds in the United States each year. Bites and scratches from cats are prone to infection with organisms that are normally found in the animal's oropharynx. These infections tend to be polymicrobic and include alpha-hemolytic streptococci, staphylococci, and *Pasteurella* species, among others. *Pasteurella* infections tend to spread rapidly, often within hours. Cat bites may also result in the transmission of rabies and tetanus. In the setting of a well cared for indoor house pet, rabies would be unlikely and rabies vaccine unnecessary, although reporting the injury to the health department may be required (depending on local statute). A dT booster would not be necessary, as she had one within a year. Surgical debridement would not be necessary for a shallow wound with normal hand function. If there were signs of tendon, nerve, or vascular injury, then sur-

gical evaluation would be mandatory. Local care alone would not be appropriate because of the propensity for cat bite wounds to become infected. Antibiotic prophylaxis is recommended for most cat bite wounds, particularly those involving the hands. The recommended first line agent is a combination of beta-lactam and beta-lactamase inhibitor, such as amoxicillin/clavulanic acid. An alternative regimen includes clindamycin with either TMP-SMZ (Bactrim DS) or a fluoroquinolone. *(Harrison's Principles of Internal Medicine, pp. 817—819)*

100. **(B)**

101. **(D)**

102. **(C)**

103. **(D)**

Explanations 100 through 103

Iron deficiency anemia is characterized by a low mean corpuscular volume (MCV), low ferritin, and a high erythrocyte protoporphyrin in serum. Microcytosis and hypochromia are the hallmark in the peripheral smear. Elevated erythrocyte protoporphyrin in serum can also be seen in anemia of chronic disease and chronic lead poisoning.

Most iron in the body is stored in red cells. The smallest amount of iron is found bound to proteins like transferrins and lactoferrins. Men have an average iron storage of about 1 g and women about 600 mg. An average dietary intake of iron is 10–20 mg, of which only 5–10% is actually absorbed. In normal conditions the body requirement of iron is 1 mg/day to compensate for normal losses.

The most common cause of cobalamin deficiency is pernicious anemia. Rarely, hypersecretion of gastric acid (i.e., Zollinger-Ellison syndrome) results in cobalamin deficiency. The peripheral smears in folate and cobalamin deficiency are indistinguishable, showing macrocytosis and hypersegmented neutrophils. Both methylmalonic acid and homocysteine levels become elevated with cobalamin deficiency. Folate deficiency is caused by decreased intake, increased utilization, or impaired absorption. Because body stores of folate are low, persons who have an inadequate consumption will become anemic in several months. The recommended amount of dietary folate is 400 µg a day.

Anemia is not a diagnosis in itself; it is an objective sign of the presence of a disease. It is always secondary to an underlying condition. In most cases a thorough history and physical examination can help elicit the pathogenesis of the anemia and direct appropriate treatment. (Hoffman, pp. 397–406, 446–470)

104. **(D)** The aPTT measures components of the intrinsic (contact factors, FXII, FXI, FIX, FVIII) and common pathways (FX, FII, FV, and fibrinogen). The PT is a measure of extrinsic (FVII) and common pathway factors. In this case, having an isolated aPTT prolongation, the most likely diagnosis is a deficiency of FXI, FIX, or FVIII. Patients with FXII deficiency have no bleeding diathesis. (Hoffman, p. 1843)

105. **(E)** Suppression of the bone marrow, including agranulocytosis, is associated with the use of clozapine. The incidence approaches 1% within several months of treatment, independent of dose. Patients should be monitored closely. Mild leukocytosis and other blood dyscrasias occur much less frequently with other antipsychotic drugs. (Hardman et al., p. 503)

106. **(E)** Warfarin acts as a vitamin K antagonist by blocking the regeneration of the reduced form of the vitamin. The result is a decrease in clotting factors II, VII, IX, and X leading to an increase in bleeding time. Warfarin toxicity can be alleviated by increasing the availability of vitamin K. (Hardman et al., pp. 1526–1530)

107. **(D)** Protamine sulfate is a strongly basic molecule that is thought to inhibit acidic heparin electrostatically. It may not, however, affect heparin-induced platelet aggregation. Cimetidine is an H_2-antagonist that increases the anticoagulant response by an as yet unknown mechanism. Clofibrate is an agent used to reduce plasma lipid levels. Vitamin K is used to reverse the effect of warfarin. Heparinase is not used clinically. (Katzung, p. 548)

108. **(B)** Celecoxib is selective for the inhibition of mediators of inflammation synthesized via the enzyme cyclooxygenase (COX) II isoform. COX I is expressed constitutively in most tissues including platelets, while COX II is not. In platelets, COX I mediates the synthesis of the eicosanoid thromboxane, which promotes platelet aggregation. Unlike older NSAIDs, which are nonselective for COX isoforms and increase bleeding time by inhibiting the synthesis of thromboxane via inhibition of COX I, celecoxib does not have this effect. (Katzung, pp. 582–583)

109. **(B)** Primary hyperparathyroidism is common in postmenopausal women and more than 80% present without any symptoms. The most common findings are bone loss, usually in association with estrogen deficiency. The elevated calcium, decreased phosphate, and increased urinary calcium are typical of this disorder. Milk-alkali syndrome is primarily a historical disease occurring in patients receiving large quantities of calcium and alkali, and presenting with renal insufficiency, elevated phosphate, and alkalosis. Her normal renal function and relatively low dose of calcium exclude this entity. Familial hypocalciuric hypercalcemia is autosomal dominant and is diagnosed by a low urinary calcium clearance. The lack of renal insufficiency excludes secondary hyperparathyroidism. The normal CXR and hemoglobin make sarcoidosis and multiple myeloma unlikely. Postmenopausal osteoporosis and osteomalacia are excluded by the elevated calcium level. (Larsen, pp. 1323–1332)

110. **(B)** Vitamin D is actually a hormone that, along with parathyroid hormone and calcitonin, regulates plasma calcium concentration. One action of vitamin D is to increase plasma Ca^{2+}, which can be reduced in hypoparathyroidism. Scurvy is associated with vitamin C deficiency. Alcoholic neuritis is associated with thiamine deficiency (Hardman et al., pp. 1731–1732)

111. **(D)** In evaluating a sporadic thyroid nodule in a patient who is euthyroid, it is critical to

determine whether the nodule is malignant or benign. The most diagnostic test is the fine needle aspiration. Ultrasound will only distinguish between cystic and solid structures, and most nodules have some solid component. The nuclear scan will demonstrate a photopenic area in over 85% of patients. Neither these tests nor CT scan will reliably separate benign from malignant nodules. Thyroid antibody studies do not play a role in the evaluation of a thyroid nodule in a euthyroid patient. They are sometimes used in the evaluation of thyroiditis. (*Harrison's Principles of Internal Medicine, p. 2083*)

112. **(A)** Drugs used to treat hyperthyroidism can be divided into four categories: (1) antithyroid drugs, which interfere directly with thyroid hormone synthesis, such as propylthiouracil; (2) ionic inhibitors such as thiocyanate, which block iodide transport mechanisms; (3) high dose iodide administration, which decreases the release of thyroid hormones; and (4) radioactive iodide, which destroys thyroid tissue via gamma radiation. In particular, propylthiouracil inhibits the incorporation of iodine into tyrosyl residues of thyroglobulin and also inhibits the coupling of iodotyrosyl residues to form iodothyronines. These effects are the result of inactivation of the enzyme peroxidase, which occurs when the heme moiety is in the oxidized state. (*Hardman et al., pp. 1580–1582*)

113. **(A)** The patient has Sheehan's syndrome, necrosis of the pituitary associated with childbirth. She has panhypopituitarism, but the most urgent hormone to replace is hydrocortisone. Thyroid hormone should not be replaced until after glucocorticoids are administered. The hyponatremia will correct with glucocorticoids and saline. The patient is not deficient in mineralocorticoids, as she does not have primary adrenal insufficiency; therefore, fludrocortisone is not indicated. (*Larsen, p. 258*)

114. **(C)** The patient appears to have significant hypoglycemia and neuroglycopenia. The differential diagnosis includes medications such as sulfonylureas; alcohol; endocrine deficiency syndromes such as adrenal insufficiency, hypopituitarism, and hypothyroidism; surreptitious

insulin administration; and insulinoma. The best way to establish the diagnosis is to measure the levels of each of these levels on the critical sample demonstrating hypoglycemia. (*Larsen, pp. 1599–1604*)

115. **(E)** Triamterene interferes with the transport of sodium in the collecting ducts of the nephron, which results in a modest increase in Na^+ excretion. Since Na^+ is normally exchanged for K^+ in this segment of the nephron, decreased sodium transport results in decreased potassium excretion. The actions of this diuretic are similar to those of spironolactone, but do not involve aldosterone receptor blockade. (*Hardman et al., pp. 777–779*)

116. **(D)** Preparations of insulin are divided into four categories according to their onset and duration of action after subcutaneous administration: rapidly acting, short acting, intermediate acting, and long acting. The rapidly acting preparations include insulin lispro and insulin aspart. The two long-acting insulins, insulin glargine (Lantus) and Ultralente have durations of action that extend up to 24 h. Intermediate-acting insulins (NPH and Lente) have an onset and duration of action intermediate between those of regular and protamine zinc insulins. (*Katzung, pp. 696–701*)

117. **(E)** The very low TSH suggests that the patient is hyperthyroid, most likely because of an autonomously functioning thyroid adenoma or hot nodule. In general, these nodules are more than 3 cm in diameter in order to be associated with hyperthyroidism. They are associated with a very low rate of malignancy and do not require fine needle aspiration. The diagnosis would be confirmed by the finding of uptake in the area of the nodule on scan with suppression of uptake in the rest of the thyroid. (*Harrison's Principles of Internal Medicine, p. 2083*)

118. **(D)** The patient has the clinical features of hyperthyroidism due to postpartum thyroiditis. This is caused by an autoimmune process with leakage of stored thyroid hormone from the gland. The hyperthyroidism is self-limited and is not associated with new synthesis of

thyroid hormone. Therefore, methimazole is not indicated. The thyroid is not painful, as it is in subacute (de Quervain's) thyroiditis, so glucocorticoids are not indicated. The radioactive iodine uptake is low, so radioactive iodine treatment is not indicated. Symptom control with propranolol is the only therapy needed during this phase of the illness. (*Harrison's Principles of Internal Medicine, p. 2075*)

119. **(E)** The patient exhibits the typical features of the nonthyroidal illness syndrome. The total thyroxine level is low, but TBG is also low (based on the elevated T3 resin uptake), so that the free thyroid index is still in the normal range. The low TBG is related to the patient's nutritional deficiency. The low T3 and TSH levels are related to his illness and the use of both glucocorticoids and dopamine, which decrease TSH. The reverse T3 level is high because of the blockade of T4 to T3 conversion caused by the illness. This finding excludes hypopituitarism as an underlying cause. There is no specific therapy for this problem other than treating the underlying illness. (*Harrison's Principles of Internal Medicine, p. 2075*)

120. **(C)**

121. **(C)**

Explanations 120 and 121

The patient has the typical features of polycystic ovarian syndrome (PCOS) associated with insulin resistance and the metabolic syndrome. The presence of hyperandrogenism and oligomenorrhea, without other known causes (such as congenital adrenal hyperplasia), makes the diagnosis of PCOS. The hirsutism and acne are the result of the hyperandrogenism associated with PCOS. Thyroid disorders and hyperprolactinemia can contribute to menstrual disturbances but would not be expected to cause the signs of androgen excess or *acanthosis nigricans*. A cosyntropin stimulation test would be used for the diagnosis of adrenal insufficiency. Growth hormone levels may be elevated in acromegaly or in some pituitary tumors. Women with PCOS have a high risk of

glucose intolerance, diabetes, dyslipidemia, and hypertension. Individuals with insulin resistance syndromes typically exhibit hypertriglyceridemia with low HDL levels. (*Larsen, pp. 627–633*)

122. **(E)** TEN is a severe mucocutaneous drug reaction caused by sulfonamides, Lamictal, Dilantin, allopurinol, penicillin, and other drugs. Patients present with fever and erosions of one or more mucosal surfaces. There are widespread dusky red cutaneous macules, as well as bullae that rupture to leave large erosions. In TEN, the erosions involve greater than 30% of the body surface area. In the milder form, Stevens-Johnson syndrome, the involved area is <10%. Skin biopsy shows a subepidermal split. Clindamycin is not a common cause of TEN.

The main differential diagnosis for TEN is SSSS mediated by *Staphylococcus aureus* exfoliative toxins A and B. Affected patients have widespread tender erythema and superficial cutaneous erosions. The oral mucosa is spared. Skin biopsy shows an intraepidermal split.

Pemphigus vulgaris is an autoimmune blistering disease caused by IgG autoantibodies against keratinocyte adhesion molecules. Affected patients have flaccid blisters of the oral mucosa and skin. Skin biopsy shows an intraepidermal split. (*Harrison's Principles of Internal Medicine, pp. 321, 109, 311*)

123. **(C)** The classic presentation of herpes simplex is clustered vesicles or pustules on an erythematous base. The most common sites of infection are the lips and the genitalia; however, the sacral area is not an unusual site of infection. The classic presentation of shingles is clustered vesicles or pustules on an erythematous base, usually in a unilateral dermatomal pattern. Recurrent episodes of shingles may occur in AIDS patients but are extremely rare in all other patient populations. (*Harrison's Principles of Internal Medicine, pp. 1037–1038, 1115; Fitzpatrick p. 2077*)

124. **(D)** Nonmelanoma skin cancer is the most common type of cancer in the United States: approximately 80% are basal cell carcinomas,

while 20% are squamous cell carcinomas. Excluding nonmelanoma skin cancer, the three most common malignancies in the US women are breast, lung, and colorectal; in men, they are prostate, lung, and colorectal. *(Harrison's Principles of Internal Medicine, p. 497; American Cancer Society website 2003)*

125. **(A)** The most effective topical therapy for comedonal acne is topical retinoids such as tretinoin (Retin A). Topical and oral antibiotics have more efficacy against pustular acne. Oral Accutane is indicated for severe nodulocystic acne that is unresponsive to other therapies.

126. **(D)** This patient has a bacterial abscess of her central forehead. She has an associated erythema and edema of her eyelids that is suggestive for orbital cellulitis. Proper management includes obtaining blood cultures, initiating broad-spectrum intravenous antibiotics and imaging of the orbit. Orbital cellulitis may also arise from an associated bacterial sinusitis. *(Harrison's Principles of Internal Medicine, p. 173)*

127. **(D)** This patient has severe psoriasis in that the disease affects a high percentage of his body surface area and his hand and feet. Topical agents are not effective against palmoplantar psoriasis or against very widespread psoriasis (i.e., >10% body surface area). Phototherapy is relatively contraindicated in this patient given his history of multiple prior cutaneous malignancies. Oral methotrexate is often very effective in the treatment of severe psoriasis and has FDA approval for that indication.

Psoriasis is usually a lifelong disease. Oral prednisone is not a therapeutic option due to the multiple severe side effects associated with chronic prednisone therapy. Life-threatening pustular psoriasis may occur in this patient population when prednisone is withdrawn. *(Harrison's Principles of Internal Medicine, p. 292)*

128. **(A)** Anaphylaxis is an acute multisystem allergic reaction to a particular antigen in a sensitized patient. The reaction may be mild or severe. Clinical manifestations may include urticaria and angioedema; laryngeal edema with dyspnea; bronchospasm; tachycardia and hypotension; and vomiting and diarrhea. The correct initial step in the treatment of mild anaphylaxis is the administration of 0.3–0.5 mL of 1:1000 epinephrine subcutaneously. *(Harrison's Principles of Internal Medicine, pp. 1949–1950)*

129. **(A)**

130. **(D)**

Explanations 129 and 130

In patients who have melanoma that is confined to the skin (i.e., no evidence of metastatic disease), the most important prognostic factor is the Breslow histologic depth of the tumor. The age of the patient and location of the tumor also play a role in prognosis, but to a lesser degree. The forearm and leg tend to have a better prognosis; scalp, hands, feet, and mucous membranes have a worse prognosis. Older persons tend to have poorer prognoses, as well.

Melanoma patients who have metastases confined to the regional lymph node basin are stage III. Patients who have metastases beyond the regional lymph node basin are stage IV. *(Harrison's Principles of Internal Medicine, 15th ed., p. 555)*

131. **(C)** The incidence and severity of shingles is increased in most immunosuppressed patients. This population includes patients with lymphoma, leukemia, or HIV; patients who have received bone marrow transplantation; and patients on chronic immunosuppressive therapy. However, HIV patients are notable for their tendency to suffer multiple recurrences of shingles. *(Fitzpatrick, p. 2077)*

132. **(A)** The duration of action of a local anesthetic is proportional to its contact time with the nerves. Therefore, if the drug can be localized at the nerve, the period of analgesia should be prolonged. Using a vasoconstrictor such as epinephrine decreases the systemic absorption of the local anesthetic. Once the absorption is decreased, the anesthetic remains longer at the desired site and is systemically absorbed at a

slower rate, which allows destruction by enzymes and less systemic toxicity. *(Hardman et al., pp. 372–373)*

133. **(C)** Deficiency of C1q, along with other C1, C2, and C4 deficiencies, results in immune complex syndromes that are clinically similar to lupus. Deficiencies of C5, C6, C7, and C8 often result in recurrent, invasive *Neisseria (meningitidis* or *gonorrhoea)* infections. *(Harrison's Principles of Internal Medicine, p. 1826)*

134. **(E)**

135. **(D)**

Explanations 134 and 135

This patient is exhibiting signs and symptoms of an anaphylactic reaction, likely to one of the medications that she recently took. Angioedema is occurring (swelling of the lips and tongue). Her dyspnea may be a manifestation of laryngeal edema or of bronchospasm. She is at high risk for respiratory compromise and, therefore, of the options listed, having her activate the emergency medical system is the most appropriate. Calling 911 from your office would be another option.

Of the interventions listed, epinephrine would provide the most benefit in correcting the underlying problem. The alpha- and beta-adrenergic effects result in vasoconstriction, bronchial smooth-muscle relaxation, and reduction on vascular permeability. Oxygen may be required if the patient is hypoxic, IV fluids may be necessary for persistent hypotension and albuterol may benefit the treatment of bronchospasm, but epinephrine would most immediately address the multiple systemic effects of anaphylaxis. *(Harrison's Principles of Internal Medicine, pp. 1915–1916)*

136. **(B)** Cross-sensitivity between penicillin and cephalosporins ranges from 5 to 20%. Cephalosporins all have a beta-lactam ring, which is the major determinant of penicillin allergy. All cephalosporins should be avoided by persons with severe previous hypersensitivity reactions to penicillin. Since none of the other agents are structurally related to penicillin, cross-reactivity would not be a concern with their use. *(Hardman et al., pp. 1203–1205)*

137. **(A)** Epinephrine is the drug of choice for treating severe anaphylactic shock because it is active at both alpha- and beta-adrenergic receptors. The alpha-adrenergic effects constrict the smaller arterioles and precapillary sphincters, thereby markedly reducing cutaneous blood flow. Veins and large arteries also respond to epinephrine. The beta-adrenergic effects of epinephrine cause relaxation of the bronchial smooth muscle and induce a powerful bronchodilation, which is most evident when the bronchial muscle is contracted, as in anaphylactic shock. Neither norepinephrine nor dopamine would be the drug of choice since neither has action on the $beta_2$ receptors and therefore would not cause the bronchodilation needed for treating anaphylactic shock. Isoproterenol has a powerful action on all beta receptors but almost no action on the alpha receptors, so vasodilation instead of vasoconstriction would be produced. Phenylephrine would be a poor drug for anaphylactic shock because it has little effect on the beta receptors and causes no bronchodilation. *(Hardman et al., pp. 223–225)*

138. **(A)**

139. **(D)**

140. **(B)**

Explanations 138 through 140

This patient is manifesting symptoms consistent with asthma. With the history of recently moving to a new area, along with a family history of allergies and eczema, his asthma may be further classified as allergic asthma. Episodic symptoms of cough, dyspnea, and wheezing are likely to occur. The diagnosis of asthma is made by demonstrating reversible airway obstruction. Airway obstruction is likely to be manifested by a reduction in the forced expiratory volume in 1 second (FEV_1). An increase in the FEV_1 of 15% after the use of a bronchodilator is the definition of reversibility. A CXR is most likely to be normal. Numerous cardiac conditions, such as CHF, cardiomyopathies, or pericardial effusions, may result in cardiomegaly on a CXR. Diffuse infiltrates may be seen with infections, interstitial lung disease, or other conditions. Flattened diaphragms would be consistent with prolonged obstructive lung disease, such as emphysema.

The treatment of choice for the prevention of symptoms in all stages of asthma other than mild intermittent is inhaled steroid. All patients with asthma should also have a short-acting bronchodilator for acute symptomatic relief. A leukotriene modifier would be an alternative recommendation and might be a good addition to an inhaled steroid, as they also have FDA indications for patients with allergic rhinitis. (*Harrison's Principles of Internal Medicine, pp. 1456–1463*)

141. (C)

142. (A)

143. (C)

Explanations 141 through 143

Atrial fibrillation is the most common sustained clinical arrhythmia. It occurs in approximately 4% of the population over the age of 60. It is diagnosed by the presence of irregularly irregular QRS complexes on an ECG with an absence of p waves. The QRS complex is most commonly narrow, as this is a supraventricular arrhythmia. Wide QRS complexes can occur if there is an underlying conduction abnormality, such as Wolff-Parkinson-White syndrome or a bundle branch block. Saw-tooth p waves occur in atrial flutter, another atrial arrhythmia that may present similarly to atrial fibrillation but which is less common. The saw-tooth p waves, or flutter waves, are representative of an atrial rate typically in the range of 300–350/min. Not infrequently, atrial flutter will lead to atrial fibrillation. Q waves in II, III, and aVF would be seen if there had been a previous inferior myocardial infarction. Peaked T waves are seen in certain conditions, such as hyperkalemia,

but are not routinely associated with atrial fibrillation.

Atrial fibrillation may be precipitated by both cardiac and noncardiac conditions. Among the noncardiac conditions are metabolic abnormalities, which include hyperthyroidism. Of the tests listed, a suppressed thyroid stimulating hormone level, consistent with hyperthyroidism, would be most likely to be causative of atrial fibrillation. Troponin may be elevated in acute myocardial ischemia. Atrial fibrillation can occur following a myocardial infarction, particularly when complicated by CHF. This is not consistent with the clinical scenario presented. Renal disease and diabetes may contribute to some of the conditions that can predispose to the development of atrial fibrillation, such as metabolic derangements or coronary artery disease (CAD). Acute and chronic pulmonary disease may also precipitate atrial fibrillation. In the setting of a man who is otherwise healthy and without significant medical history, new onset atrial fibrillation would be less likely to be the initial presentation of diabetes, renal failure, or pulmonary disease than hyperthyroidism. For this reason, option (A) is the single best answer of those provided.

The initial evaluation of atrial fibrillation should generally include a detailed history and physical examination, ECG, CXR, thyroid function tests, and an echocardiogram. The echo would provide information on the overall ventricular function and evidence of valvular disease. It would also allow for the measurement of atrial size, which provides prognostic information on the ability to achieve and maintain a sinus rhythm. The presence of atrial thrombus could also be determined. An exercise stress test may be useful if the arrhythmia was precipitated by exercise. Electrophysiologic studies are usually reserved for the setting of disease that is refractory to medical management. Cardiac catheterization would be appropriate in the setting of confirmed or suspected ischemic heart disease as a cause of the condition. Radionuclide ventriculography would provide significantly less overall information than an echocardiogram in this setting and would not be as useful as an initial test. *(Goldman and Braunwald, 333–339)*

144. (B) Quinidine can prolong the Q-T interval resulting in the development of polymorphic ventricular tachycardia (torsade de pointes). Hypokalemia, a side effect of thiazide diuretics, increases the risk of torsade de pointes, which can then degenerate into fatal ventricular fibrillation. Thiazide diuretics may decrease the effectiveness of uricosuric agents, insulin, and sulfonylureas and may increase the effects of vitamin D. However, these effects tend not to be life-threatening. *(Hardman et al., pp. 877, 965–966)*

145. (C) The cytochrome P-450 enzyme is an important component of the mixed-function oxidase primarily located in the smooth endoplasmic reticulum of the liver. This enzyme, and others, is important in catalyzing drug inactivation by oxidation, reduction, and conjugation. Phenobarbital is a potent stimulator of cytochrome P-450 and causes enhanced metabolism of this agent as well as other drugs (e.g., warfarin). Chloramphenicol is capable of inhibiting this enzyme; penicillin, hydrochlorothiazide, and digoxin have no known effects on cytochrome P-450. *(Hardman et al., p. 13)*

146. (B) The goal of treatment of angina is to relieve symptoms and prolong exercise capacity by improving the relationship of oxygen demand and supply. Nitroglycerin is a smooth muscle relaxant that produces both venodilation (reduced preload) and arteriolar dilation (reduced afterload). Although the combined effect is to reduce myocardial oxygen demands, the potential exists for reflex tachycardia and increased contractility. These reflexes tend to increase oxygen demands as well as potentially reduce coronary blood flow and should be avoided. Avoidance can be accomplished by carefully titrating the dose of nitroglycerin or the concurrent use of a beta-blocker such as propranolol. Verapamil is a calcium channel blocker that is particularly useful in primary angina. It has minimal ability to reduce afterload and thus is usually not associated with

reflex tachycardia. This is in contrast to nifedipine, which has disadvantages similar to those of nitroglycerin. Isoproterenol would be contraindicated in angina because, by itself, it may increase myocardial oxygen demands. Similarly, dobutamine, an analogue of dopamine, is a beta$_1$ adrenoreceptor agonist and would not be used to treat angina. *(Katzung, pp. 186–197)*

147. (B) Beta-blockers have been found to decrease the mortality rate in patients who survive myocardial infarction. The mechanism is thought to be suppression of arrhythmias, but this has not been established. Other antiarrhythmic drugs such as flecainide and quinidine, although effective in suppressing arrhythmias, may actually increase mortality. Digoxin and nitroglycerin, although effective at increasing cardiac output and decreasing workload on the heart, do not necessarily prolong survival. *(Katzung, pp. 154–156)*

148. (D)

149. (A)

150. (E)

Explanations 148 through 150

The clinical scenario described is classic for an acute myocardial infarction. The patient has multiple risk factors, including smoking, hypertension, and elevated cholesterol. His symptoms of crushing chest pain radiating to the left arm is commonly seen in this setting. Often the first electrocardiographic sign of acute ischemia is the development of hyperacute T waves. The ECG will usually show S-T segment elevations in the area of the involved occluded vessel, with reciprocal S-T segment depressions in uninvolved areas. This can be followed by the eventual resolution of S-T segment abnormalities and the development of T wave inversions and Q waves. Diffuse P-R depressions are often the initial manifestation of pericarditis, a less common cause of acute chest pain. This often progresses to diffuse S-T segment elevations, the presence of which helps to distinguish pericarditis from the focal S-T elevations more classically associated with a thrombosed coronary artery. Q waves would be unlikely to occur within 1 h of the onset of symptoms. In this clinical setting, a normal ECG, while possible, would be less likely to occur. *(Goldman and Braunwald, 262–263)*

Ventricular arrhythmias, both tachycardia and fibrillation, are recognized complications of acute myocardial infarction. The presence of ventricular fibrillation or pulseless ventricular tachycardia should lead to the primary "ABCD" survey, as outlined in the American Heart Association's ACLS protocols. The mnemonic stands for airway, breathing, circulation, defibrillation. Epinephrine, lidocaine, or amiodarone are reserved for the setting where defibrillation is ineffective. Synchronized cardioversion would be used in efforts to convert a patient's rhythm in the setting of a stable tachycardia. *(American Heart Association, ACLS provider manual, 2001. pp. 75–90)*

According to ACLS protocols, the primary survey for asystole is "ABCCD"—airway, breathing, circulation, confirmation of true asystole and defibrillation (or recognition that asystole is not a shockable rhythm). In a patient monitored in an emergency or telemetry setting, confirmation of true asystole would include checking a second lead, confirming that the leads are attached to the patient, and that cables are correctly attached. The use of epinephrine and atropine, or the consideration of discontinuation of resuscitation, would be appropriate after the confirmation of true asystole. *(ACLS provider manual, 109–122)*

151. **(A)** The principal advantage of low molecular weight heparin is a more predictable pharmacokinetic profile that facilitates subcutaneous dosing without laboratory monitoring. Therefore, the drug can be administered in an outpatient setting. Warfarin, not heparin, inhibits clotting factor synthesis. Low molecular weight heparin works mainly by facilitating the inhibition of factor X_a rather than thrombin. Heparins, including low-molecular-weight heparins, do not cross the placental barrier. *(Hardman et al., pp. 1522–1523)*

152. **(E)** Some of the more serious symptoms of toxicity associated with tricyclic antidepressant overdose include anticholinergic symptoms, coma, seizure, and cardiac arrhythmias. Cardiac toxicity characterized by supraventricular tachycardia and/or QRS widening can be especially difficult to manage. Children may be especially vulnerable to overdose resulting in death. *(Hardman et al., p. 466)*

153. **(A)** Digoxin increases ventricular muscle contraction by inhibiting the sodium/potassium ATPase pump. The ultimate result is in an increase in intracellular calcium that facilitates myocardial contraction. Verapamil, propranolol, captopril, and furosemide can all be effective in treating heart failure by decreasing the workload on the heart. Verapamil is a calcium channel blocker, propranolol is a beta-adrenergic antagonist, captopril is an ACE inhibitor, and furosemide is a loop diuretic. *(Hardman et al., pp. 916–920)*

154. **(C)** Furosemide is effective in treating the acute pulmonary edema associated with CHF by virtue of its potent diuretic action, which rapidly eliminates excess body fluid volume. Both propranolol and verapamil may decrease cardiac output and thus exacerbate congestion. Mannitol tends to increase vascular fluid volume, which can result in increased congestion. Spironolactone is not potent enough as a diuretic to be effective in treating this condition. *(Hardman et al., pp. 904, 924)*

155. **(D)** Significant stenosis (>50%) of the left main coronary artery, in the setting of both stable and unstable angina, is an indication for CABG surgery. Other strong indications for CABG include "left main equivalent" disease of stenosis of the proximal left anterior descending and circumflex arteries or three vessel disease, especially with reduced ejection fraction. The outcomes from bypass surgery in these settings are superior to any form of medical therapy. Angioplasty of the left main coronary artery is considered by the American Heart Association to have evidence ineffectiveness or, potentially, harm. Left main CAD is not, in and of itself, an indication for defibrillator implantation. *(Braunwald, pp. 1353–1361)*

156. (D)

157. (A)

158. (E)

Explanations 156 through 158

Aortic stenosis is one of the most common valvular abnormalities found in adults. It can be congenital—such as a unicuspid or bicuspid valve—or acquired. In young adults, acquired aortic stenosis is often seen as a consequence of rheumatic fever. This is becoming less common in developed nations. In adults over the age of 65, the most common cause of aortic stenosis is age related degenerative, calcific aortic stenosis. The valvular cusps are immobilized and the stenosis caused by calcium deposits along the flexion lines of the valves. Acquired aortic stenosis typically has a prolonged asymptomatic period. During this time the stenosis may be found incidentally by auscultation of the characteristic harsh, holosystolic murmur in the aortic valve area that radiates to the carotid arteries. There may also be a slow, small, and sustained arterial pulsation (pulsus parvus and tardus) due to the relative outflow obstruction. The cardinal symptoms of aortic stenosis that signal advancing disease, and increased risk of mortality, are angina, heart failure, and syncope. An ECG will show left ventricular hypertrophy in approximately 85% of symptomatic cases of aortic stenosis. A normal ECG is possible but would be more likely in early, asymptomatic stages. S-T segment elevation would be more consistent with acute cardiac ischemia and Q waves would be more consistent with a completed myocardial infarction. Low voltage QRS complexes can be seen in several conditions, including pericardial effusion, chronic obstructive pulmonary disease (COPD), or obesity.

When considering the diagnosis of aortic stenosis, the initial diagnostic test of choice would be echocardiography. It would provide information on both the structure (bicuspid, tricuspid, and the like) and the function (valve area, pressures) of the valve. The size and function of the left ventricle can also be determined. If aortic stenosis is found on echocardiogram and the patient is symptomatic, the next test would be cardiac catheterization. This would allow for direct measurement of the pressure gradient across the valve. It would also allow for evaluation of the status of the coronary arteries in order to determine whether coronary artery bypass grafting would need to be performed along with valve replacement. Exercise stress testing is relatively contraindicated in the setting of symptomatic aortic stenosis. Holter monitoring would only be useful if there were a concomitant arrhythmia. Electrophysiologic studies would not play a role in the typical evaluation of aortic stenosis.

The management of symptomatic critical aortic stenosis is surgical. If the patient is a surgical candidate, the treatment of choice is aortic valve replacement. Balloon valvuloplasty would be an option either as a temporizing measure when surgery could not be immediately performed or when the patient is not a surgical candidate. A high percentage of patients develop recurrent stenosis within 6 months of this procedure. Antihypertensive and vasodilating medications must be used with extreme caution, and usually should be avoided, as they can impair the ability of the ventricle to create the pressure needed to pump blood across the narrowed aortic valve. *(Braunwald, pp. 1671–1680)*

159. (A) Cholestyramine, a bile acid sequestrant, reduces plasma cholesterol levels by decreasing concentrations of low-density lipoproteins. Orally administered drugs (especially those that are lipid soluble) may be bound by cholestyramine as well. This problem may be avoided to a large extent by administering other drugs at least 1 h before or 4 h after cholestyramine. Steatorrhea may be another side effect, impairing absorption of fat soluble vitamins. If this condition develops, vitamin supplementation is recommended. *(Hardman et al., pp. 989–990)*

160. (E) Quinidine is a class IA cardiac antiarrhythmic drug which prolongs the duration of the action potential, as reflected in a lengthening of the Q-T interval. This effect is associated with torsade de pointes in approximately 2–8% of patients administered quinidine and can even be induced at plasma levels of the drug that are subtherapeutic. Lidocaine and phenytoin shorten the duration of the action potential. Adenosine and flecainide do not alter Q-T interval. *(Katzung, pp. 225–228)*

161. (B) Sodium nitroprusside is a potent vasodilator of both arteries and veins. However with a fall in blood pressure, the sympathetic nervous system will become activated and increase heart rate. Agents that block the activity of the sympathetic nervous system, such as clonidine (an alpha-2 antagonist), labetalol (an alpha- and beta-receptor antagonist), metoprolol (a selective beta-1 antagonist), or hydrochlorothiazide (a diuretic), do not induce reflex tachycardia. *(Katzung, pp. 164–175)*

162. (C) Adenosine produces marked hyperpolarization and suppression of calcium-dependent action potentials. It directly inhibits AV nodal conduction and increases AV nodal refractory period. It is currently the drug of choice to treat paroxysmal supraventricular tachycardia. The other drugs have relatively modest or no usefulness in treating supraventricular arrhythmias. *(Katzung, pp. 228, 236)*

163. (B) Digoxin has a number of effects on cardiac electrophysiology related to its mechanism of action, inhibition of the sodium/potassium ATPase pump. The result is enhanced intracellular concentrations of calcium, which leads to increased force of contraction (positive inotropic effect), as well as much of its toxicity. Digoxin also has vagotonic effects that result in decreased AV nodal conduction. Unlike digitoxin, which is both longer acting and primarily eliminated through hepatic metabolism, over 80% of digoxin is eliminated unchanged in the urine. *(Hardman et al., pp. 916–922)*

164. (A) ACE inhibitors inhibit the metabolism of angiotensin I to angiotensin II. Angiotensin II is one of the most potent endogenous vasoconstrictors. Therefore, ACE inhibitors lower blood pressure and are effective in treating CHF via a decrease in peripheral resistance and by lowering afterload. Moreover, ACE inhibitors lessen salt and water retention by decreasing the release of aldosterone. One of the most common side effects associated with ACE inhibitors is cough, which is thought to result from an increase in autacoids such as bradykinin. *(Katzung, pp. 177–178)*

165. (D)

166. (C)

167. (D)

Explanations 165 through 167

Asthma is a chronic lung disease characterized by inflammation of the airways, causing recurrent symptoms. The characteristic symptoms are wheezing, chest tightness, shortness of breath, or cough. Symptoms often worsen in the face of certain triggers, which include allergens, cold air, exercise, or other irritants. Physical examination may reveal hyperexpansion of the thorax, expiratory wheezing with a prolonged expiratory phase of respiration, and signs of allergies or atopic dermatitis. Asthma can be diagnosed by a history of episodic symptoms of airway obstruction (wheeze, dyspnea, cough, chest tightness), establishing the presence of airflow obstruction that is at least partially reversible and ruling out other causes of these symptoms/signs. Airflow obstruction can be shown by spirometry revealing an FEV_1 of <80% predicted or an FEV_1/forced vital capacity of <65% of the lower limit of normal. Reversibility can be shown by an FEV_1 increase of ≥15% and at least 200 mL with the use of a short-acting beta agonist. Wheezing on examination, the presence of allergic rhinitis and hyperinflation on a CXR are often seen in asthma, but are not specific for asthma. Eosinophils on a sputum sample are suggestive of asthma, while the presence of neutrophils is more consistent with a bacterial infection.

Asthma is classified as mild, mild persistent, moderate persistent, or severe based on the frequency of symptoms and the degree of airflow obstruction (see Table 1-1). Based on this patient's frequency of symptoms, he falls into the mild persistent class. Treatment recommendations are based on the severity of the disease. Mild persistent asthma should be treated with an anti-inflammatory. The preferred treatment is a low dose inhaled steroid with a short-acting beta agonist for as needed symptom relief. Alternative treatments include nedocromil, cromolyn, leukotriene modifiers, or sustained release theophylline. A stepwise approach to asthma therapy is advocated by many expert panels (see Table 1-1).

168. **(C)** Albuterol is a selective beta-2 adrenergic agonist that, in therapeutic doses, will dilate bronchi without significant cardiac stimulation. Because Epinephrine stimulates both beta-1 and beta-2 receptors, bronchodilation is accompanied by cardiac stimulation. Theophylline and other methylxanthines are known to alter intracellular calcium availability and also inhibit cyclic nucleotide phosphodiesterases; however, at therapeutic levels, the main effect of these drugs seems to be inhibition of adenosine receptors. They are potent cardiac stimulants. Cromolyn and fluticasone can decrease the frequency of asthma attacks, but are less effective in treating bronchoconstriction once it has occurred. *(Katzung pp. 323–331)*

169. **(A)**

170. **(D)**

171. **(E)**

Explanations 169 through 171

COPD is a group of chronic and progressive pulmonary disorders that cause reduced expiratory

TABLE 1-1   CLASSIFICATION OF ASTHMA SEVERITY

Classification	Days with symptoms	Nights with symptoms	PEF or FEV$_1$ (PEF is % of personal best; FEV$_1$ is % of predicted)	PEF variability	Treatment
Severe persistent	Continual	Frequent	≤60%	>30%	Preferred: high dose inhaled steroid and long-acting beta agonist AND, if needed, corticosteroid tablets or syrup
Moderate persistent	Daily	≥5/month	>60–<80%	>30%	Preferred: low-to-medium dose inhaled steroid and long-acting beta agonist Alternative: increase inhaled steroid within medium dose range OR low-to-medium dose inhaled steroid and leukotriene modifier or theophylline if needed (particularly in patients with recurring severe exacerbations): Preferred: increase inhaled steroid within medium dose range and long-acting beta agonist Alternative: increase inhaled steroid within medium dose range and add leukotrienemodifier or theophylline
Mild persistent	3–6/ week	3–4/month	≥80%	20–30%	Preferred: low dose inhaled steroid Alternative: cromolyn, nedocromil, leukotriene modifier, or theophylline
Mild intermittent	≤2/week	≤2/month	≥80%	<20%	No daily medication needed severe exacerbations may occur, separated by long periods of normal function and no symptoms. A course of systemic corticosteroids is recommended

All patients: Short-acting bronchodilator as needed for symptoms
Source: (Reproduced from) Practical Guide for the Diagnosis and Management of Asthma, NIH: National Heart, Lung and Blood Institute, 1997; NAEPP Expert Panel Report; Guidelines for the Diagnosis and Management of Asthma–Update on Selected Topics, 2002; NIH: National Heart, Lung and Blood Institute, 2002.

flow. Most of the obstruction is fixed, although some reversibility can be found. COPD affects approximately 16 million Americans and smoking is, by far, the greatest risk factor. Onset is typically in the fifth decade and the typical presenting symptoms are dyspnea and cough. Patients often relate these to an acute illness (walking pneumonia in this case) but the decline in pulmonary function has been present for some time prior to the onset of symptoms. The physical examination has poor sensitivity and may, in early disease, only show wheezing on forced expiration and a prolonged expiratory phase of respiration. Clubbing is not typically a manifestation of COPD and its presence should lead to a search for another cause, such as lung cancer. In the setting of pulmonary hypertension, sometimes one can hear a pronounced pulmonic component to the second heart sound, although hyperinflation may obscure this finding. Bilateral pulmonary crackles would be more consistent with pulmonary edema. Supraclavicular adenopathy should lead to a workup to exclude cancer, especially of breast, lung, ovarian, or GI origin.

Hyperinflation of the lungs is the most likely CXR finding in this case. This would manifest as flattened diaphragms with elongated lungs and a long, narrow cardiac shadow. Kerley B lines would be more characteristic of pulmonary edema from left-sided heart failure, rather than COPD. A pulmonary mass with adenopathy would be more consistent with lung cancer—certainly a possibility in a long-time smoker, but much less common than COPD. A residual infiltrate from pneumonia a year ago would be highly unlikely.

Smoking cessation should always be recommended when COPD is diagnosed. It has been shown that the rate of decline of the FEV_1 can revert back to that of a nonsmoker. While pulmonary function may improve some, it likely will not improve dramatically. Quitting smoking can prolong survival and delay the onset of disability along with reducing the risk of malignancy and cardiovascular disease development. *(Harrison's Principles of Internal Medicine, 15th ed., 1491–1499)*

172. **(C)** The antineoplastic alkylating agents work by covalently binding to DNA strands, linking them together. The result is strand breakage leading to inhibition of cell replication. The drugs of this class tend to be nonspecific and relatively toxic, but there is little cross resistance with other anticancer medications. Thus, alkylating agents are frequently administered in combination therapies with other classes of antineoplastic drugs. *(Hardman et al., pp. 1389–1399)*

173. **(B)** The administration of estrogens alone is associated with an increase in endometrial cancer of 1.7- to 15-fold. The risk varies with both the dose administered and the duration of treatment. The coadministration of progestins with estrogen reduces the risk of endometrial cancer even below that of nonusers. Most studies report no increase in the risk of breast cancer for women who take estrogen alone or in combination with progestin, although continued use for longer than 10 years may be associated with a slight increase in risk. Oral contraceptive use appears to slightly lessen the risk of ovarian cancer. Hepatocellular carcinoma is a rare complication of oral contraceptives. *(Katzung, p. 668)*

174. **(C)** All of the drug choices in the question are useful in the management of gout, a condition resulting from hyperuricemia. However, allopurinol reduces the synthesis of uric acid by blocking the metabolism of xanthine and hypoxanthine to uric acid via xanthine oxidase inhibition, making it useful in reducing the risk of hyperuricemia from tumor lysis. Urinary alkalinization and aggressive hydration are also components of treatment. Probenecid and sulfinpyrazone enhance urate excretion by blocking the reabsorption of urate from the proximal tubule. Colchicine is effective in treating acute gout attacks by inhibiting leukocyte migration and phagocytosis. Indomethacin, and other NSAIDs, can be effective in treating acute gout attacks by inhibiting urate crystal phagocytosis. However, low dose aspirin may actually increase the risk of acute gout. *(Katzung, pp. 596–599)*

175. **(C)** Drug regimens to treat cancer should utilize agents that have different mechanisms of action to facilitate a synergistic killing effect against the tumor cells. Agents should also have different toxicity profiles to minimize adverse reactions. The regimen should be designed so that the drugs can be administered as frequently as possible to discourage tumor regrowth. Because each cycle of chemotherapy may allow more than 1% of the tumor cells to survive, it is always necessary to repeat treatments in multiple cycles. *(Harding et al., p. 1386)*

176. **(C)**

177. **(D)**

Explanations 176 and 177

Any new palpable breast lesion in females (or males) of any age necessitates a mammographic evaluation and biopsy. Delay is inadvisable. Serum tumor markers, such as CA 27/29 (or even less specifically CEA), are useful to follow tumor response to therapy; however tumor markers are not reliable as diagnostic tools in breast cancer because of a relatively low sensitivity. Lobular carcinomas are frequently not visualized on mammogram, particularly standard mammograms; ultrasound however detects these tumors and should be ordered when a palpable lesion is not detected on a mammogram. *(UK trial of early detection of breast cancer group. 16-year mortality from breast cancer in the UK trial of early detection of breast cancer. Lancet 1999; 343: 1909–1914; J Clin Oncol. 2001 Mar 15; 19(6):1865–78. Erratum in: J Clin Oncol 2001 Nov 1; 19(21): 4185–4188. J Clin Oncol 2002 Apr 15; 20(8): 2213; Berg WA, et al. Diagnostic Accuracy of Mammography, Clinical Examination, US, and MR Imaging in Preoperative Assessment of Breast Cancer. Radiology. 2004 Oct 14)*

178. **(B)**

179. **(A)**

Explanations 178 and 179

Because there is a smoking history, it is appropriate to order a spiral CT scan to better delineate whether the mass is a tumor, an infectious process, or both. Tumor blocking a bronchus can frequently be associated with a pneumonia involving lung behind the compressed bronchus; therefore, the evaluation should include collecting the appropriate cultures along with the further imaging. *(Petty T, Ann Intern Med. 2004; 141: 649–650)*

The full staging of small cell lung cancer is very important both for prognosis to relate to the patient and his family and to define the most appropriate therapy. Therefore, it is appropriate to order the MRI studies of the head along with CT scans with contrast of the abdomen and pelvis, a bone scan and a bone marrow aspirate and biopsy to determine if the disease is limited to the thorax or has metastasized to other organs. Small cell lung cancer limited to the thorax is potentially a disease that can achieve complete, long-term remissions with appropriate therapy. Small cell lung cancer metastatic beyond the chest can be well palliated but, at this time, our current treatments are unable to induce a long-term disease-free remission. Surgery alone is not an appropriate treatment for small cell lung cancer. Even with a successful complete tumor resection, without systemic therapy (chemotherapy), the small cell lung cancer recurs in 100% of cases within months to several years. *(Devita VT, et al., Cancer Principles and Practice of Oncology, 2001: 6th ed., 983–1018)*

BIBLIOGRAPHY

Braunwald E, et al. *Harrison's Principles of Internal Medicine*, 15th ed. New York, NY: McGraw-Hill, 2001.

Brenner BM. *Brenner & Rectors's The Kidney*, 7th ed. Philadelphia, PA: W.B. Saunders, 2004.

Freedberg IM, Eisen AZ, Wolff K, et al., (eds). *Fitzpatrick's Dermatology in General Medicine*. New York, NY: McGraw-Hill, 2003.

Goldman L, Braunwald E. *Primary Cardiology*. Philadelphia, PA: W.B. Saunders, 1998.

Hardman JG, Limbird LE, Molinoff PB, et al., (eds). *Goodman & Gilman's The Pharmacological Basis of Therapeutics*, 10th ed. New York, NY: McGraw-Hill, 2001.

Hoffman R, et al. *Hematology: Basic principles and practice*, 3d ed. New York, NY: Churchill Livingstone, 2000.

Kaspar DL, Braunwald E, Fauci AS, et al., (eds). *Harrison's Principles of Internal Medicine*. New York, NY: McGraw-Hill, 2005.

Katzung BG, (ed). *Basic & Clinical Pharmacology*, 9th ed. New York, NY: McGraw-Hill, 2004.

Kunimoto DY, et al. *The Wills Eye Manual: Office and Emergency Room Diagnosis and Treatment of Eye Disease*, 4th ed. Philadelphia, PA: Lippincott Williams & Wilkins, 2004.

Larsen PR, et al. *Williams Textbook of Endocrinology*, 10th ed. Philadelphia, PA: W.B. Saunders, 2003.

Mandell GL, Bennett JE, Mandell DR. *Mandell, Douglas and Bennett's Principles and Practice of Infectious Diseases*, 5th ed. Philadelphia, PA: Churchill Livingstone, 2000.

Ruddy S, et al. *Kelley's Textbook of Rheumatology*, 6th ed. Philadelphia, PA: W.B. Saunders, 2001.

CHAPTER 2

Surgery
Questions

1. A 22-year-old male presents to the emergency department (ED) with complaints of right-sided chest pain and dyspnea. He has no other significant medical history. There is no history of trauma. On examination he has a pulse of 95, BP of 110/70, and SpO$_2$ of 95% on 2 L. A chest x-ray reveals a large right pneumothorax. Which of the following statements is true?

   (A) Since the patient is hemodynamically stable, he can be observed with oxygen supplementation, pain control, and serial chest x-rays.

   (B) The patient is likely to have a tall, thin habitus.

   (C) This condition is probably due to small lacerations in the apex of the right lung.

   (D) His risk of recurrence is 10%.

   (E) Recurrences are usually on the contralateral side since adhesions prevent recurrence on the ipsilateral side.

2. A 10-month-old male child presents with 12-h history of episodes of crying, holding his stomach, and bending over in pain. The parents report one reddish stool. He has no past medical history or episodes of similar events. He did have 24 h of viral symptoms that resolved a few days ago. The following study was obtained (see Fig. 2-1). Which of the following statements is true?

   (A) The initial treatment for this child involves emergent laparotomy.

   (B) Air contrast enema can be diagnostic AND therapeutic.

   (C) Colonic mass is the usual source of this problem in a child.

   (D) "Dance's" sign is the appearance on x-ray of "telescoped" intestine.

   (E) Recurrence is likely after treatment.

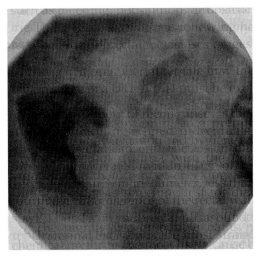

FIG. 2-1 (*Courtesy of H.J. Kim, MD.*)

3. A 4-week-old previously healthy male child presents with projectile emesis after feeds. Mother states that he has had 2 weeks of post-prandial emesis which became projectile in the past 2 days. She states that it looks like formula and has never been bilious. Which of the following statements is true?

   (A) Physical examination is almost always normal in patients with this condition.

   (B) Upper GI contrast study is the best diagnostic option.

   (C) This patient should be taken emergently to the operating room once the diagnosis is made.

   (D) If uncorrected, these infants will progress to complete obstruction.

   (E) Surgical therapy involves bypassing the site of obstruction.

4. A 1-month-old female child presents after an episode of bilious emesis. She became irritable 12 h ago, had the emesis 6 h ago, and is now lethargic. She had one small stool that was somewhat bloody 2 h ago. Which of the following statements is true?

   (A) An upper GI contrast study should be obtained immediately.

   (B) The most likely explanation is pyloric stenosis.

   (C) The patient should be admitted with IV fluids and observation. If she does not improve over the next 24 h, a surgical consult should be obtained.

   (D) An air contrast enema is the most appropriate next step.

   (E) A nasogastric tube should be inserted and IV antibiotics started to treat probable necrotizing enterocolitis.

5. Which of the following statements is true concerning Meckel's diverticulum?

   (A) It is found within 2 in of the ileocecal valve.

   (B) It represents a remnant of the embryonic vitelline duct.

   (C) Ectopic colonic epithelium is found in it.

   (D) Diagnosis is best made by computed tomographic (CT) scan.

   (E) The diverticulum is usually found on the mesenteric border of the bowel.

Questions 6 and 7

6. A 55-year-old man with hepatic cirrhosis from alcohol abuse presents with a massive hematemesis. This is his third admission for GI bleed in the past 2 months. He is currently receiving appropriate therapy for liver failure (including beta-blocker and diuretics). He is lethargic and confused. His pulse is 100 and blood pressure is 85/40. His initial hematocrit is 20. Which of the following steps is the most appropriate management strategy?

   (A) The transplant team should be called immediately.

   (B) The bleeding is probably secondary to an uncontrolled duodenal ulcer related to his alcohol use.

   (C) Red blood cells should be administered immediately, but fresh frozen plasma should be withheld if possible.

   (D) Endoscopic control options, including sclerotherapy and banding.

   (E) Transjugular intrahepatic portal systemic shunt (TIPS) is not an option in the immediate period.

7. Your attempts to control the bleeding are initially successful, but the patient has a recurrent bleed 2 days later. The medicine team obtains a surgical consult for a surgical shunt. Which of the following statements is true?

   (A) The best shunts are nonselective, meaning that they divert all blood from the portal system.

   (B) Synthetic graft materials should never be used because of the risk of infection.

   (C) A mesocaval shunt involves connecting the superior mesenteric vein (SMV) to the inferior vena cava (IVC).

(D) Encephalopathy rarely worsens after the placement of the shunt. In fact, it often improves in these patients.

(E) Postoperative mortality for emergency shunts is related more to the type of shunt placed rather than the degree of hepatic failure in the patient.

8. A 55-year-old female presents to your office with a right breast mass found by self-examination. She has no history of breast disease in herself or her family. Her last mammogram was at age 45 and was normal. On examination, there is a firm, 1.5-cm mass in the upper outer quadrant of her right breast which is nontender. There is no palpable lymphadenopathy. Which of the following statements is true?

(A) Mammogram alone is sufficient for diagnosis.

(B) Ductal carcinoma in situ (DCIS) will probably not be seen on mammogram.

(C) If this mass is a cancer, in the tumor, node, metastasis (TNM) staging protocol, this 1.5-cm mass would be a T2 lesion.

(D) The upper outer quadrant is an unusual location for a breast cancer.

(E) A biopsy of this lesion is warranted.

9. Which of the following is a contraindication to sentinel lymph node biopsy in breast cancer?

(A) clinically negative axillary examination

(B) multicentric disease

(C) lesion under the nipple

(D) history of previous breast biopsy

(E) patient preference for breast conservation measures

10. A 45-year-old male was involved in a motor vehicle collision. He was a restrained passenger in a high speed, head on collision with a death at the scene. He is brought to the ED unresponsive with a pulse of 140, a BP of 70/30, and a SpO$_2$ of 80%. He has multiple facial lacerations, a dilated right pupil, a contusion on his chest, and a distended abdomen. The medic team has placed two large-bore IVs and given him 2 L of lactated ringers. The initial step in the care of this patient is:

(A) Given the mechanism, low oxygen saturation, and the presence of a contusion on his chest, the patient likely has a pneumothorax. A chest tube should be placed immediately.

(B) The patient should be taken to the operating room immediately for laparotomy since he is hemodynamically unstable with abdominal distension indicating an abdominal source.

(C) The patient should be intubated using in-line traction to protect his cervical spine before continuing the assessment.

(D) Because of the facial lacerations, there is a possibility of facial fractures making endotracheal intubation risky. An emergent cricothyroidotomy should be performed.

(E) A central line should be placed immediately to continue the resuscitation.

11. An 18-year-old male is brought to the ED after sustaining a stab wound to the left chest that is medial and superior to the nipple. He was unresponsive at the scene and was intubated by the emergency medical technician (EMT) team. His pulse is 140 and BP is 60/30 after receiving 1 L of lactated ringers and two units of blood during his transport. He has no breath sounds on the left. His trachea is midline. He has no evidence of neck vein distension. Which of the following statements is true?

(A) Cardiac tamponade is unlikely since there is no evidence of neck vein distension.

(B) A left chest tube should be placed immediately.

(C) Given the probability of a cardiac injury, an emergent thoracotomy should be performed in the ED.

(D) An aortic angiogram should be ordered immediately to assess for aortic injury.

(E) No intervention should be performed until a chest x-ray is completed to provide more information.

12. A 12-year-old female sustains a closed fracture of the tibia and fibula after falling from a tree house. The leg is distended and feels tight. The ED physician is concerned about an anterior compartment syndrome. Which of the following is the first sign of a compartment syndrome?

    (A) severe pain in the calf muscles
    (B) unable to dorsiflex foot
    (C) absence of pulses in the foot
    (D) numbness between the first and second toe
    (E) firm calf on examination

13. A 23-year-old male is brought by ambulance to the emergency room after being found in a house fire. He was in a closed room with a large amount of smoke and has sustained burns to his face, torso, arms, and legs. His pulse is 120, BP 110/55, and SpO$_2$ 92% on 2 L of oxygen by nasal cannula. Which of the following statements is true?

    (A) The burns should be covered in cool, moist dressings.
    (B) An inhalation injury is unlikely since he is able to oxygenate on minimal supplementation.
    (C) Fluids should be limited to prevent pulmonary edema after his smoke inhalation.
    (D) This patient meets criteria for transfer to a dedicated burn center.
    (E) Depth of the burn does not affect the management.

14. A 45-year-old male receives a cadaveric liver transplant for alcoholic cirrhosis. Postoperatively, the patient is taken to the surgical intensive care unit. There is concern for primary nonfunction of the allograft. Which of the following is a sign of this?

    (A) coagulopathy with an international normalized ratio (INR) of 2
    (B) normalizing albumin level
    (C) hyperglycemia requiring an insulin drip
    (D) initial rise of transaminases
    (E) high urine output

15. Which of the following statements is true about immunosuppressive drugs used in transplant?

    (A) High dose steroids can be used alone to prevent episodes of rejection.
    (B) Cyclosporine's main action is to prevent T-cell activation.
    (C) Cyclosporine's renal toxicity is not dose dependent.
    (D) Tacrolimus mainly affects B-cell activation.
    (E) Mycophenolate mofetil binds to intracellular receptors to block gene transcription.

16. A 50-year-old man undergoes sigmoid colectomy and colostomy for perforated diverticulitis of the midsigmoid colon. The surgeon reports a difficult dissection in the pelvis secondary to adhesions of the sigmoid to the abdominal wall. On postoperative day #1, he reports appropriate abdominal pain. His pulse is 100 and BP 120/60. He has made 400 mL of urine over the past 8 h. The urine in the Foley bag is blood tinged. He reports no problems with his urination preoperatively. What is the appropriate management?

    (A) Remove the Foley catheter. The irritation of the catheter is probably causing the hematuria.
    (B) Increase his IV fluids and add bicarbonate in case this is rhabdomyolysis.
    (C) Start antibiotics for a urinary tract infection.
    (D) Order intravenous pyelogram to assess for ureteral injury.
    (E) Send a prostate-specific antigen (PSA) to screen for a prostatic process.

17. A 75-year-old man undergoes a right colectomy for stage 3 colon cancer. He has a history of emphysema requiring chronic steroid use. He also has diabetes and coronary heart disease. On postoperative day #2, the surgeon is called because the patient acutely began to have a large amount of pinkish, serous drainage from the wound. There is no evidence of infection. Which of the following factors probably contributed to this complication?

(A) The surgeon used a running stitch to close the fascia instead of interrupted sutures.

(B) Coronary artery disease.

(C) Early mobilization of patient.

(D) Aggressive abdominal examination performed on postoperative day #1 by a medical student.

(E) Pulmonary disease.

18. A 22-year-old male presents with a 1-month history of progressive dysphagia. He reports occasional regurgitation of undigested food at night. His past medical history is noncontributory. The condition has worsened to the point that he is on a liquid diet. A contrast swallow study is below (see Fig. 2-2). What is the best treatment for this patient?

(A) proton pump inhibitors

(B) referral to a surgeon for a Nissen fundoplication

(C) calcium channel blockers

(D) serial esophageal sphincter dilations

(E) referral to a surgeon for esophagomyotomy

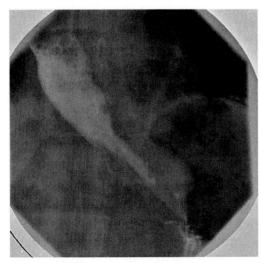

FIG. 2-2 (*Courtesy of H.J. Kim, MD.*)

19. A 45-year-old woman undergoes uncomplicated thyroidectomy for a goiter. Later that night, she becomes agitated and complains of difficulty breathing. The surgeon notices some neck swelling at the incision site, but the dressing is clean. The next step should be:

(A) Start oxygen by nasal cannula.

(B) Check STAT serum calcium level.

(C) Endotracheal intubation to protect her airway.

(D) Open the incision.

(E) Administer propranolol and morphine.

20. A patient presents with a new neck mass. On examination, she has a palpable thyroid nodule and a palpable cervical lymph node on the same side. Needle biopsy of the thyroid nodule shows amyloid in the stroma. The treatment for this patient is:

(A) total thyroidectomy and modified neck dissection

(B) resection of the involved thyroid lobe, isthmusectomy, and removal of the palpable lymph node

(C) total thyroidectomy and radiation therapy

(D) resection of the involved lobe and part of the contralateral lobe, isthmusectomy, and removal of the palpable lymph node

(E) radioactive iodine administration

21. Which of the following statements is true about primary hyperparathyroidism?

(A) It is associated with chronic renal failure and is the result of hypocalcemia caused by hyperphosphatemia.

(B) It is seen most commonly in patients with renal failure who undergo kidney transplantation.

(C) It is commonly a result of a parathyroid adenoma in one of the parathyroid glands.

(D) Most patients with the condition are symptomatic. They usually present with renal stones, bone pain, or mental status changes.

(E) Is more common in men than women.

22. A 50-year-old male with a history of alcohol abuse presents with acute pancreatitis. Which of the following facts about a patient is included in Ranson's criteria?

    (A) age of 65 years old
    (B) elevated amylase
    (C) thrombocytosis
    (D) elevated lipase
    (E) evidence of pancreatic necrosis on CT scan

23. A 45-year-old man presents with suprapubic tenderness, fevers, and nausea. After a thorough evaluation, he is found to have acute cystitis and bladder stones. The organism most likely responsible for this infection is:

    (A) *Staphylococcus aureus*
    (B) *Pseudomonas*
    (C) *Escherichia coli*
    (D) *Proteus mirabilis*
    (E) *Klebsiella* species

24. Curling's ulcers are found in which population of patients?

    (A) alcoholics
    (B) cancer patients
    (C) patients with intracranial pathology
    (D) burn patients
    (E) postoperative patients

25. During laparoscopic abdominal procedures, the abdominal cavity is usually insufflated with carbon dioxide to a pressure of 15 mmHg. Increasing the intraabdominal pressure to these levels produces which of the following physiologic responses?

    (A) decreased afterload
    (B) depressed cardiac output
    (C) hypercarbia
    (D) depressed diaphragm
    (E) alkalosis

26. A 21-year-old male presents to the emergency department after sustaining a gunshot wound to the neck. After evaluation, it is determined that he has C6 quadriplegia. Which of the following activities will be limited by this injury?

    (A) wrist extension
    (B) elbow extension
    (C) elbow flexion
    (D) shoulder flexion
    (E) raising his arms above his shoulders

27. Patients with septic arthritis of the hip joint usually present with which position:

    (A) internal rotation and flexion
    (B) internal rotation and extension
    (C) internal rotation and abduction
    (D) external rotation and flexion
    (E) external rotation and abduction

28. Which of the following structures can be found OUTSIDE of the spermatic cord during a hernia repair?

    (A) direct hernia sac
    (B) indirect hernia sac
    (C) vas deferens
    (D) testicular artery
    (E) ovary

Questions 29 and 30

29. A 30-year-old male is brought to the ED after being hit in the head by a baseball. He is making incomprehensible sounds, but no words. He opens his eyes and withdraws to painful stimuli. His Glasgow Coma Scale score is:

    (A) 10
    (B) 9
    (C) 8
    (D) 7
    (E) 6

30. The most appropriate next step in the treatment of this patient is:

    (A) neurosurgery consult
    (B) intubation and mechanical ventilation
    (C) CT scan of head to evaluate for intra-cranial blood

(D)   administration of mannitol to prevent cerebral herniation

(E)   blood and urine toxicology screens

31.   A severely traumatized patient, who has been receiving prolonged parenteral alimentation, develops diarrhea, mental status depression, alopecia, and perioral and periorbital dermatitis. Administration of which of the following trace elements is most likely to reverse these complications?

(A)   iodine
(B)   zinc
(C)   selenium
(D)   silicon
(E)   tin

32.   A man who underwent total thyroidectomy 24 h ago now complains of a generalized "tingling" sensation and muscle cramps. Appropriate treatment would include:

(A)   intravenous infusion of calcium gluconate
(B)   administration of oxygen by mask
(C)   administration of an anticonvulsant
(D)   administration of a tranquilizer
(E)   neurologic consultation

33.   Vital capacity is best described as the volume of air:

(A)   inhaled during normal respiration
(B)   expelled during passive expiration
(C)   remaining in the lungs after passive expiration
(D)   actively exchanging with pulmonary venous blood
(E)   able to be expelled following maximal inspiration

34.   The most common site of aortic transection in deceleration injuries is:

(A)   the root of the aorta
(B)   at the level of the right innominate artery
(C)   at the level of the left innominate artery

(D)   near the origin of the left subclavian artery

(E)   in the middle portion of the descending thoracic aorta

35.   The most common site of gastrinoma is the:

(A)   gastric antrum
(B)   duodenum
(C)   pancreas
(D)   spleen
(E)   gallbladder

36.   Avascular necrosis is most likely to occur in fracture dislocations involving the:

(A)   femoral head
(B)   shaft of the femur
(C)   shaft of the humerus
(D)   scapula
(E)   clavicle

37.   A 38-year-old man, previously in good health, suddenly develops severe abdominal pain radiating from the left loin to groin and associated with nausea, perspiration, and the need for frequent urination. He is restless and tossing in bed, but has no abnormal findings. The most likely diagnosis is:

(A)   herpes zoster
(B)   left ureteral calculus
(C)   sigmoid diverticulitis
(D)   torsion of the left testicle
(E)   retroperitoneal hemorrhage

Questions 38 through 40

38. A 50-year-old man comes to the emergency room with a history of vomiting of 3 days duration. His past history reveals that for approximately 20 years, he has been getting epigastric pain, lasting for 2–3 weeks, during early spring and autumn. He remembers getting relief from pain by taking milk and antacids. Physical examination showed a fullness in the epigastric area with visible peristalsis, absence of tenderness, and normoactive bowel sounds. The most likely diagnosis is:

    (A) gastric outlet obstruction
    (B) small bowel obstruction
    (C) volvulus of the colon
    (D) incarcerated umbilical hernia
    (E) cholecystitis

39. Which of the following metabolic abnormalities would be typical in the above patient?

    (A) decreased antidiuretic hormone
    (B) hypercalcemia
    (C) hypokalemia
    (D) hyperchloremia
    (E) decreased aldosterone secretion

40. The most important electrolyte to replenish in this patient is:

    (A) sodium
    (B) chloride
    (C) potassium
    (D) bicarbonate
    (E) phosphorus

41. An absolute contraindication for lung resection in a patient with lung cancer is:

    (A) involvement of more than one ipsilateral lobe
    (B) ipsilateral mediastinal node involvement
    (C) chest wall invasion
    (D) liver metastases
    (E) pleural effusion

Questions 42 and 43

42. A 45-year-old woman, mother of four children, comes to the emergency room complaining of the sudden onset of epigastric and right upper quadrant pain, radiating to the back, associated with vomiting. On examination, tenderness is elicited in the right upper quadrant and bowel sounds are decreased. Laboratory data show leukocytosis, normal serum levels of amylase, lipase, and bilirubin. The most likely diagnosis is:

    (A) acute cholecystitis
    (B) perforated peptic ulcer disease
    (C) myocardial infarction
    (D) acute pancreatitis
    (E) sigmoid diverticulitis

43. The most specific test to confirm the diagnosis is:

    (A) a two-way roentgenogram of the abdomen
    (B) ultrasonography of the upper abdomen
    (C) barium swallow
    (D) hydroxyiminodiacetic acid (HIDA) scan
    (E) peritoneal lavage

44. A patient is operated on with the presumptive diagnosis of acute appendicitis. However, at operation, the appendix and cecum are found to be normal. The terminal ileum, for a distance of approximately 30 cm, is red, edematous, and thickened with creeping of the mesenteric fat onto the ileum. There is no dilation of the bowel proximal to the area of involvement. The remainder of the small bowel is normal. The appropriate operative procedure is:

    (A) closure of the abdomen
    (B) appendectomy
    (C) ileostomy proximal to the area of involvement
    (D) side-to-side ileo-transverse colostomy
    (E) right hemicolectomy

45. The most likely testicular tumor in a 25-year-old man is:

(A) Leydig cell tumor

(B) choriocarcinoma

(C) seminoma

(D) teratocarcinoma

(E) androblastoma

46. Which of the following statements is true regarding tracheoesophageal fistula following cuffed tracheostomy tube placement?

(A) Sudden bright red bleeding is a common feature.

(B) The incidence increases with the duration of tracheal intubation.

(C) It is best managed by nonsurgical means.

(D) The presence of a nasogastric tube does not change the risk of developing this complication.

(E) Mortality is greater than 90%.

47. Which of the following is characteristic of Hirschsprung's disease?

(A) Constipation is the most frequent presenting feature.

(B) Severity of the symptoms corresponds with the extent of bowel involvement.

(C) Acetylcholinesterase activity is decreased in the aganglionic segment.

(D) The proximal colon is most commonly affected.

(E) It presents most commonly in young adults.

48. Elevated serum gastrin level is seen in:

(A) Zollinger–Ellison syndrome

(B) patients taking nonsteroidal anti-inflammatory drugs

(C) cirrhotic patients

(D) uncomplicated duodenal ulcer patients

(E) secretin-secreting adenoma

49. A 25-year-old male comes to the emergency room after a motor vehicle collision, complaining of vague left-sided abdominal pain.

After initial evaluation, a CT of the abdomen is obtained (see Fig. 2-3). Which of the following statements is true concerning the injury?

(A) Even hemodynamically unstable patients on initial examination can be managed nonoperatively.

(B) Patients should be vaccinated against tetanus before hospital discharge.

(C) Splenic salvage is contraindicated in the presence of other major abdominal injuries.

(D) *Pseudomonas aeruginosa* is the most frequent organism responsible for postsplenectomy sepsis.

(E) Most patients require operative management.

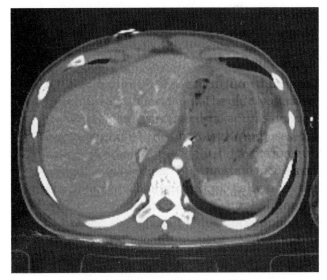

FIG. 2-3 (*Courtesy of H.J. Kim, MD.*)

50. A 50-year-old male presents with difficulty swallowing. Esophageal manometry demonstrates absence of peristaltic waves and a nonrelaxing lower esophageal sphincter. The most likely diagnosis is:

(A) Barrett's esophagus

(B) diffuse esophageal spasm

(C) achalasia

(D) Plummer-Vinson syndrome

(E) esophageal cancer

51. Which of the following statements is true regarding Barrett's esophagus?

(A) It is three times more common in women than men.

(B) Most cases are congenital in origin.

(C) The columnar-lined epithelial changes are always in direct continuity with the gastric epithelium.

(D) Surgical antireflux therapy does not necessarily result in regression of the Barrett's changes.

(E) Once the diagnosis of Barrett's esophagus is established, the patient does not need further biopsies on follow-up endoscopy.

52. A 49-year-old male presents with crushing substernal pain and rules out for a myocardial infarction. He is noted to have "Hamman's crunch" on auscultation. You are concerned for an esophageal perforation. Select the true statement regarding esophageal perforation.

(A) They should never be managed nonoperatively.

(B) The best diagnostic test is cervical and thoracic CT.

(C) Early endoscopy is contraindicated.

(D) Primary repair is the first approach to treatment in perforations diagnosed within 24 h.

(E) Esophageal perforations diagnosed late require esophageal resection.

53. A patient presents with a 24-h history of periumbilical pain, now localized to the right lower quadrant. An abdominal CT scan is obtained in the emergency room, which is shown in Fig. 2-4. Which of the following is a symptom or sign often associated with this diagnosis?

(A) onset of vomiting before the development of abdominal pain

(B) the patient has an increased appetite

(C) flank bruising

(D) pain in the right lower quadrant with palpation of the left lower quadrant

(E) pain in the right upper quadrant while palpating under the right costal margin as the patient takes in a deep breath

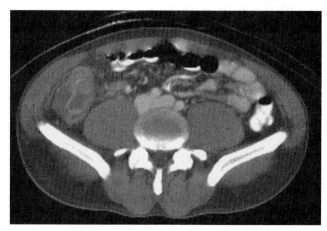

FIG. 2-4 (*Courtesy of H.J. Kim, MD.*)

54. Following an uneventful appendectomy for acute appendicitis, the pathology report reveals the presence of a 1-cm carcinoid at the tip of the appendix. The patient has been otherwise asymptomatic. The most appropriate intervention is:

(A) formal right hemicolectomy

(B) partial cecectomy (excision of the base of the cecum at the appendectomy site)

(C) no further operative intervention required

(D) total abdominal colectomy with ileorectal anastomosis

(E) partial small bowel resection

55. A 52-year-old man suffers a gunshot wound to the left thigh. He received his fourth tetanus booster 3 years ago. What is the most appropriate tetanus prophylaxis for this patient?

(A) no prophylaxis required

(B) tetanus toxoid only

(C) tetanus immunoglobulin and tetanus toxoid

(D) tetanus immunoglobulin only

(E) penicillin and tetanus toxoid

56. A 64-year-old diabetic male undergoes a right hemicolectomy for an adenocarcinoma of the cecum. On the first postoperative night he becomes tachycardic and is noted to have a temperature of 102.8°F. His surgical incision is tender with erythema and murky discharge. Which of the following is the most important intervention?

   (A) Begin broad-spectrum antibiotics, acetaminophen, and cooling blanket.
   (B) Open the wound and begin hyperbaric oxygen treatment.
   (C) Apply sterile warm compress over the incision and replace dressing.
   (D) Open the wound, send for Gram's stain of the fluid, and perform radical debridement.
   (E) Postoperative fever evaluation including sputum, urine, and blood cultures.

57. The treatment of choice for treating patients with *Clostridium difficile* enterocolitis is:

   (A) oral levaquin
   (B) intravenous metronidazole
   (C) oral vancomycin
   (D) oral metronidazole
   (E) intravenous vancomycin

58. A 62-year-old male on total parenteral nutrition (TPN) for 2 weeks following development of a postoperative enterocutaneous fistula has developed high spiking temperatures, up to 102.2°F, over the last 8 h. The only abnormal finding on physical examination is erythema and induration around his central line. The most appropriate management is:

   (A) Begin broad-spectrum antibiotics and observe for 24 h.
   (B) Obtain blood cultures through the central line, begin broad spectrum antibiotics, and await culture results.
   (C) Remove catheter, send tip for culture, and replace with a new central line over the guide wire.

   (D) Remove catheter, send tip for culture, and establish central line at another site.
   (E) Remove catheter, send for culture, and establish peripheral intravenous line.

59. Which of the following is the best initial treatment for bleeding and inflamed second degree internal hemorrhoids?

   (A) high fiber diet, frequent sitz baths, and topical steroid ointment
   (B) rubber band ligation
   (C) sclerotherapy injection
   (D) infrared coagulation
   (E) surgical hemorrhoidectomy

60. Which of the following regarding anorectal abscess and fistula is true?

   (A) The most common cause is a subepithelial extension of a genital infection.
   (B) Conservative management should always be considered for fistula-in-ano as many heal spontaneously.
   (C) Most acute anorectal abscesses require a course of antibiotics.
   (D) The treatment protocol is not altered for patients with valvular heart disease.
   (E) Anal fistula is classified as intersphincteric, transsphincteric, suprasphincteric, or extrasphincteric

61. The most common indication for surgery in a patient with Crohn's disease is:

   (A) carcinoma
   (B) fistula
   (C) bleeding
   (D) obstruction
   (E) abscess

62. A 26-year-old male presents with abdominal pain and bloody diarrhea. On examination he has a low-grade fever and mildly tender abdomen. Lower endoscopy is performed, which reveals edematous mucosa with contiguous involvement from the rectum to the left colon. Random biopsies are performed, which reveal acute and chromic inflammation of the mucosa and submucosa with multiple crypt abscesses. There are no granulomas seen. Which of the following statements is true regarding his diagnosis?

    (A) He will likely require an operation.
    (B) There is no known cure.
    (C) The use of intravenous corticosteroids is contraindicated.
    (D) Perianal fistulas are characteristic.
    (E) There is a substantially increased long-term risk of developing colon cancer.

63. A 46-year-old female presents to your office with rectal bleeding, itching, and irritation. On examination, a 3-cm ulcerating lesion is seen in the anal canal. Biopsy of the lesion reveals squamous cell carcinoma. The most appropriate treatment is:

    (A) chemotherapy and pelvic radiation
    (B) low anterior resection
    (C) abdominal perineal resection
    (D) wide local excision of the lesion
    (E) wide local excision of the lesion and bilateral inguinal lymph node dissection

64. During initial exploration in a patient scheduled to undergo a right hemicolectomy for colon cancer, a deep 4-cm liver mass is seen in the right lobe of the liver. The left lobe appears to be normal. Intraoperative biopsy of the lesion is positive for metastatic colon cancer. The best management of this patient includes which of the following?

    (A) Immediately close the patient and refer for chemotherapy only.
    (B) Perform right hemicolectomy only.
    (C) Perform right hemicolectomy and right hepatic lobectomy.

    (D) Perform right hemicolectomy and wide excision of the liver lesion.
    (E) Perform liver resection only.

65. A mobile mass is found on rectal examination in a 77-year-old male with complaints of blood in his stool. On workup, he is found to have a stage I (Dukes' A), well differentiated adenocarcinoma. The most appropriate intervention is:

    (A) transanal excision
    (B) abdominal perineal resection
    (C) low anterior resection
    (D) placement of endorectal Wallstent
    (E) neoadjuvant chemotherapy followed by transanal resection

66. A 67-year-old man recently had a colonoscopy for rectal bleeding in which a circumferential and nearly obstructing sigmoid adenocarcinoma was found. He was scheduled to undergo a low anterior resection but, during initial exploration, an unexpected 5.5-cm abdominal aortic aneurysm (AAA) was found. The most appropriate management is:

    (A) Abort the procedure and perform a cardiac workup.
    (B) Proceed with low anterior resection and schedule repair of AAA at a later date.
    (C) Proceed with repair of AAA and perform low anterior resection at a later date.
    (D) Proceed with low anterior resection followed by AAA repair.
    (E) Proceed with AAA repair followed by low anterior resection.

67. A 27-year-old female whose father had a colon resection for adenocarcinoma undergoes her first colonoscopy. Over 100 small polyps are seen distributed mainly in her sigmoid and rectum. Multiple polyps are removed and histologic review reveals tubular adenomas with no evidence of atypia or dysplasia. The most appropriate next step in her management is:

    (A) total proctocolectomy with ileoanal J pouch reconstruction
    (B) surveillance colonoscopy in 5 years

(C) surveillance colonoscopy every 2 years until all polyps are removed

(D) flexible sigmoidoscopy with representative biopsy every 6 months for 2 years, then yearly for 3 years, then every 3–5 years

(E) abdominal perineal resection with sigmoid resection and end colostomy

68. Biopsy of a 4-cm sessile polyp of the cecum during colonoscopy reveals it to be a villous adenoma with atypia. Attempt at piecemeal snare polypectomy through the colonoscope is unsuccessful. The most appropriate management is:

(A) right hemicolectomy

(B) colonoscopy with electrocoagulation of the tumor

(C) colonoscopy with repeat biopsy in 1 year

(D) open surgery with colotomy and excision of polyp

(E) external beam radiation

Questions 69 through 71

69. A 56-year-old man comes to the hospital with colicky abdominal pain, vomiting, abdominal distention, and constipation for the past 5 days. The most appropriate measure, after IV hydration and nasogastric decompression, in the initial management of this patient includes:

(A) upper GI endoscopy

(B) supine and erect x-rays of the abdomen

(C) abdominal sonography

(D) antiemetic agents

(E) promotility drugs

70. The man described undergoes barium enema examination. The findings on barium enema (Fig. 2-5) are most compatible with a diagnosis of:

(A) mechanical small-bowel obstruction

(B) intussusception

(C) volvulus

(D) carcinoma of the colon

(E) diverticulitis

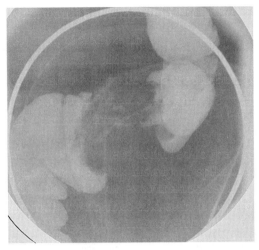

FIG. 2-5 (*Courtesy of H.J. Kim, MD.*)

71. During definitive surgical treatment of the lesion shown on the barium enema, the left ureter is accidentally transected at the level of the pelvic brim. The most appropriate management of this complication is:

(A) ureteroneocystostomy

(B) left to right ureteroureterostomy

(C) anastomosis of the two cut ends over a "double-J" stent

(D) nephrectomy

(E) ligation of the transected ends

72. Which of the following criteria is not considered to be a prognostic factor in the evaluation of a patient with melanoma?

(A) anatomic location of lesion

(B) presence of ulceration

(C) evidence of metastatic disease

(D) histologic type

(E) age of patient

73. A 60-year-old woman presents with an abnormal cluster of microcalcifications on a routine mammogram and undergoes a needle-localized excisional biopsy. The pathology is shown below (see Fig. 2-6). Which of the following statements is true concerning surgical management of this disease?

    (A) Modified radical mastectomy differs from a Halsted mastectomy in that the pectoralis major is spared in the modified radical approach.
    (B) Modified radical mastectomy differs from Halsted mastectomy in that an axillary lymphadenectomy is not performed in the modified radical approach.
    (C) The anatomic limits of the modified radical mastectomy include the sternum medially and the anterior border of the serratus anterior muscle laterally.
    (D) Injury to the thoracodorsal nerve during mastectomy results in a "winged scapula."
    (E) Lymphedema occurs mainly as a complication of the Halsted radical mastectomy and should not be seen after modified radical mastectomy.

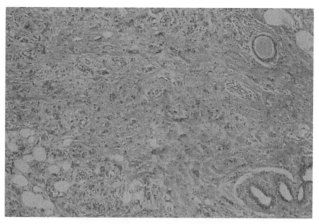

FIG. 2-6 (*Courtesy of H.J. Kim, MD.*)

74. A 45-year-old man undergoes a distal esophagectomy for Barrett's esophagus. During his hospital course, a left chest tube is placed for an effusion. Milky white fluid is found to come out through the tube. Which of the following statements is most accurate about this condition?

    (A) Diagnosis can be confirmed by checking the lymphocyte count and triglyceride level in the fluid.
    (B) This condition requires immediate surgical intervention to repair.
    (C) The chest tube should be removed due to the possibility of an iatrogenic source of infection.
    (D) This condition is usually found on the right if due to a traumatic source.
    (E) Early oral refeeding postoperatively helps to speed recovery.

75. Which of the following vessels is an appropriate conduit for coronary artery bypass graft?

    (A) left axillary artery
    (B) internal mammary arteries
    (C) ulnar artery
    (D) common femoral vein
    (E) femoral artery

76. A 60-year-old male presents with vague symptoms of abdominal pain. He is afebrile with a normal white blood cell (WBC) count. The emergency physician orders a CT scan which reveals an enlarged appendix. He is taken to the operating room for an appendectomy. Intraoperative findings include a 1-cm firm mass at the tip of the appendix concerning for a malignant process. There are no other abnormalities seen in the abdomen. Which of the following statements is true?

    (A) The most common appendiceal malignancy is adenocarcinoma.
    (B) The most appropriate management is an appendectomy.
    (C) The most appropriate management is a right hemicolectomy.
    (D) The therapy for this is not surgical, it is chemoradiation.
    (E) Carcinoid syndrome is usually seen with this condition.

77. Which of the following statements regarding esophageal cancer is true?

   (A) The incidence of squamous cell carcinoma (SCC) of the esophagus is rising more rapidly than adenocarcinoma.
   (B) Premalignant conditions include caustic esophageal burns, Plummer-Vinson syndrome, and tylosis.
   (C) It is more common in women than men.
   (D) Smoking is not a risk factor for esophageal cancer.
   (E) Barrett's esophagus increases the risk for esophageal SCC.

78. A 70-year-old male presents with dysphagia, regurgitation of undigested food, and halitosis. Which of the following statements is true?

   (A) Diagnosis is made by upper endoscopy as the first test of choice.
   (B) The diverticulum is situated posteriorly, just proximal to the cricopharyngeal muscle.
   (C) The diverticulum will involve all layers of the esophageal wall.
   (D) Treatment requires a diverticulectomy and cricopharyngeal myotomy.
   (E) Vocal cord paralysis is most likely secondary to a traumatic endotracheal intubation at the time of surgery.

79. A 40-year-old woman presents with epigastric pain and is found on upper endoscopy to have a duodenal ulcer. Select the true statement regarding her clinical management.

   (A) The ulcer is most likely secondary to a malignancy and requires further workup to rule out distant metastases.
   (B) Surgery is the most effective first-line therapy.
   (C) Recurrence rate of a duodenal ulcer 15 years after vagotomy and a drainage procedure is less than 5%.

   (D) Patients operated on for intractability are more prone to developing postgastrectomy symptoms.
   (E) Incidence of dumping syndrome is lower after a highly selective vagotomy than after a truncal vagotomy.

80. Select the true statement regarding GI hormones:

   (A) Vagal activation, antral distension, and antral protein are all stimuli for gastrin release.
   (B) Secretin stimulates gastrin.
   (C) Secretin is released from the antrum of the stomach.
   (D) Cholecystokinin (CCK) release is stimulated by fat in the duodenum and results in release of insulin by the pancreas.
   (E) CCK is released by the pancreas and relaxes the sphincter of Oddi.

81. A 65-year-old woman complains that she has become increasingly light-headed after playing golf. She also has had some cramping type pain in her left arm, which coincides with the episodes. She undergoes arteriogram and is found to have a stenotic lesion of her subclavian artery. Which of the following is true?

   (A) The stenotic lesion is proximal to the take off of the vertebral artery.
   (B) It is unusual for these patients to have coronary artery disease as well.
   (C) The patient's light-headedness is caused by an incomplete circle of Willis.
   (D) The operation of choice for this patient is a carotid-subclavian bypass.
   (E) Radial pulses in this patient will be equal bilaterally.

82. A patient presents to the ED complaining of abdominal pain out of proportion to examination. Initial vital signs are BP 70/30, heart rate (HR) 120. He reports a prior history of abdominal pain after eating. Which of the following is true with regard to this patient's condition?

(A) A CT scan which shows any type of superior mesenteric artery (SMA) thrombosis or gas in the bowel wall requires an immediate operation.

(B) The most common site of embolic event is the SMA.

(C) Nonocclusive mesenteric ischemia is treated with arterial bypass.

(D) Patients with cardiac arrhythmias are not at increased risk for mesenteric ischemia.

(E) After volume resuscitation, the initial diagnostic study for this patient is upper GI endoscopy.

83. A 64-year-old male is referred to your office for evaluation of a pulsatile abdominal mass. His primary care physician orders a CT scan of the abdomen and pelvis (shown in Fig. 2-7). Which of the following statements is true regarding the finding illustrated on the CT?

(A) 75% of patients with the above finding have a positive family history of aneurysmal disease.

(B) This finding is not associated with aneurysms of peripheral vessels.

(C) Type II diabetes is a risk factor for this condition.

(D) Risk of rupture when reaching >5 cm in diameter is approximately 10% per year.

(E) Standard of care is currently endovascular repair.

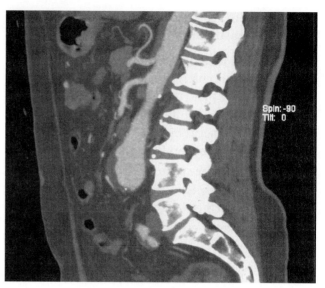

FIG. 2-7 (*Courtesy of H.J. Kim, MD.*)

84. A 59-year-old White male with a 40-pack-year history of smoking presents to your clinic complaining of three prior episodes, over the last 2 months, of a "shade passing over his left eye." Last week, he reports that he experienced some weakness in his right arm, which resolved after 5 min. Which of the following statements is true?

(A) Initial management of this patient should include bilateral cerebral vessel duplex Doppler ultrasonography.

(B) Reversible ischemic neurologic deficit (RIND) lasts several minutes, transient ischemia attacks (TIA) resolves after 24 h and a stroke describes symptoms that persist longer than 24 h.

(C) The most common cause of strokes in these patients is related to decreased blood flow.

(D) Carotid bruit is a hallmark finding in these patients.

(E) Asymptomatic patients with >25% stenosis should undergo operative repair.

Questions 85 and 86

85. You have been asked to see a patient of one of your colleagues. He is a 67-year-old Black male who has been having left foot pain at night. He tells you that the pain is relieved by

dependent positioning. After a thorough history and physical examination, your next step in diagnostic workup would be:

(A) three view x-rays of his left foot and ankle

(B) left lower extremity arterial duplex Doppler ultrasonography

(C) lower extremity angiogram with runoff

(D) trial of pentoxifylline with 3-month follow-up

(E) magnetic resonance imaging (MRI) of sacral nerves

86. When will conservative measures, like antiplatelet therapy, be considered rather than surgical intervention?

(A) complaints of rest pain

(B) presence of tissue necrosis

(C) complaints of intermittent claudication

(D) presence of a nonhealing wound

(E) failure of conservative therapy with severe inhibition of lifestyle

87. A patient with a known family history of multiple endocrine neoplasia (MEN) I now presents with intractable ulcer disease. Which of the following statements about his care is correct?

(A) Diarrhea is a frequent complaint.

(B) Tumors are rarely multiple.

(C) Tumors are rarely malignant.

(D) An elevated fasting gastrin level is diagnostic for the Zollinger-Ellison syndrome.

(E) Computed tomography is useful in localizing the tumor in greater than 75% of patients.

Questions 88 and 89

88. A 60-year-old Asian male presents with early satiety and 40-lb weight loss over 3 months. Upper endoscopy shows an irregular mass in the antrum of the stomach. Which of the following statements is true?

(A) Weight loss indicates distant metastases and surgical resection is not indicated.

(B) Antral tumors have a worse prognosis than tumors at other sites in the stomach.

(C) CT is the most effective imaging modality for determining TNM stage.

(D) Five-year survival for patients with gastric adenocarcinoma confined to the mucosa with no nodal metastasis approaches 90%.

(E) Chemotherapy is an effective treatment modality in stage IV gastric adenocarcinoma, with significant benefit in overall survival.

89. This patient's endoscopic biopsies are suggestive of a gastric lymphoma. Which of the following is true?

(A) The incidence of gastric lymphoma is increasing.

(B) Obstruction, perforation, and bleeding are common presenting symptoms.

(C) Upper endoscopy with biopsy is highly accurate for diagnosis.

(D) Gastric involvement of systemic lymphoma is best treated with gastric resection.

(E) Survival rates are dismal, with overall prognosis similar to that seen in gastric adenocarcinoma.

90. Which of the following statements is true about Barrett's esophagus?

(A) Is a condition where the esophagus is lined by columnar epithelium.

(B) Is a condition where the esophagus is lined by dysplastic squamous cells.

(C) Needs two biopsies with histologic changes to confirm the diagnosis.

(D) The main risk is bleeding.

(E) Is related to peptic ulcer disease.

91. The classic radiologic abnormality seen on contrast esophagram in patients with diffuse esophageal spasm is:

(A) "Bird's beak" pattern.

(B) "Corkscrew" pattern.

(C) No abnormality is usually seen. Manometry is the diagnostic tool of choice.

(D) Pulsion diverticula.

(E) "Punch out" appearance.

92. The stomach has a rich vascular supply. Which of the following is a true statement about the blood supply to the stomach?

(A) Right gastric artery arises from the celiac axis.

(B) Left gastric artery arises from the common hepatic artery.

(C) Right gastroepiploic arises from the right hepatic artery.

(D) Short gastric arteries arise from the splenic artery.

(E) Left gastroepiploic arises from the left gastric artery.

93. Which of the following statements is true concerning Zenker's diverticulum?

(A) Found within 2 ft of the ileocecal valve.

(B) Does not change in size over time.

(C) Can cause painless gastrointestinal bleeding.

(D) Symptoms include regurgitation of undigested food.

(E) Endoscopy should be the first procedure performed when the diagnosis is suspected.

94. Which of the following statements about ulcer disease is true?

(A) Gastric ulcers are usually caused by hypersecretion of acid.

(B) Type III gastric ulcer is caused by a duodenal ulcer and the resulting pyloric obstruction.

(C) *Helicobacter pylori* is associated with both gastric and duodenal ulcers.

(D) Most patients with *H. pylori* have ulcers.

(E) Duodenal ulcer patients tend to be older than gastric ulcer patients.

95. The liver is divided into how many segments?

(A) 2

(B) 3

(C) 7

(D) 8

(E) 9

96. In comparing ileostomies to colostomies, which of the following statements is true?

(A) improved hydration status with ileostomies

(B) decreased risk for electrolyte disturbances with ileostomies

(C) decreased risk for malnutrition with ileostomies

(D) increased risk of malignancy with ileostomies

(E) higher rate of peristomal skin irritation if the ostomy is flush with the skin

97. Which of the following statements is true in regard to carcinoid syndrome?

(A) Common symptoms include jaundice and liver failure.

(B) Symptoms include left heart failure without right heart failure.

(C) Most patients with metastatic carcinoid disease display symptoms of carcinoid syndrome.

(D) Diagnosis can be established by urinary vanillymandelic acid (VMA).

(E) Patients with symptoms have hepatic disease, or disease in sites such as the retroperitoneum or ovaries, that bypass hepatic processing.

98. Which of the following statements is true about postgastrectomy syndromes?

(A) Most patients tolerate gastrectomy without a change in their digestive habits.

(B) Dumping syndromes can be treated with high carbohydrate liquid diets.

(C) Cholestyramine is a treatment for postvagotomy diarrhea.

(D) Most patients with these syndromes require surgical intervention.

(E) Proton pump inhibitors are effective against alkaline reflux syndrome.

99. A 19-year-old female presents to the ED complaining of swelling in her left lower extremity. She reports that she had undergone arthroscopy of the right knee about a week ago. The swelling started last night and is uncomfortable. Which of the following is true?

(A) This patient is at decreased risk for this complication of surgery because she is female.

(B) The patient should be put on strict bed rest with leg elevation until her swelling resolves.

(C) Postoperative use of a sequential compression device is not useful in preventing this problem.

(D) If a D-dimer test ordered by the ED physician is positive, no further diagnostic testing needs to be performed.

(E) Directed lytic therapy is indicated for this patient if her lower extremity becomes bluish and has evidence of vascular compromise.

100. Which of the following is correct with regard to surgical wound infections?

(A) Infections remote from the site of surgical incision can increase rates of wound infection.

(B) Hand washing by health care practitioners in the postoperative setting has not been shown to have a significant effect on the transmission of infectious pathogens between patients.

(C) The most common flora found in the large bowel is *E. coli.*

(D) In order for preoperative antibiotics to be effective, they should be administered just after skin incision.

(E) The treatment of an infected wound consists solely of antibiotic therapy.

101. A patient is found to have right-sided abdominal pain and undergoes a CT scan of the abdomen looking for renal calculi. The CT scan is remarkable for an unexpected finding, as shown in Fig. 2-8. She has never been symptomatic from this disease, and all of her serum laboratory examinations are within normal limits. Which of the following is an indication for surgery?

(A) age >45

(B) stone size <2 cm

(C) evidence of "porcelain" features seen on CT

(D) type II diabetes mellitus

(E) finding of "sludge" on ultrasound

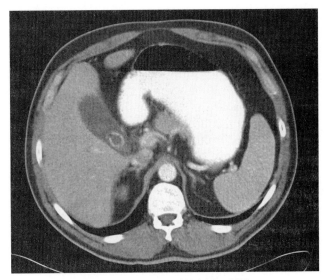

FIG. 2-8 (*Courtesy of H.J. Kim, MD.*)

102. Which of the following is a boundary of the triangle of Calot?

(A) falciform ligament

(B) common hepatic duct

(C) pancreatic duct

(D) infundibulum of the gallbladder

(E) cystic artery

103. Which of the following is true with regard to the diagnosis of acute cholecystitis?

(A) Pain is similar to cholelithiasis, but does not last as long (usually <3 h).

(B) Findings on ultrasound include thickened gallbladder wall and pericholecystic fluid.

(C) A patient with a normal WBC can not have cholecystitis.

(D) A HIDA scan in a patient with cholecystitis will usually show uptake of radiotracer by the gallbladder within 1 h.

(E) A negative Murphy's sign rules out the diagnosis of acute cholecystitis.

104. A 40-year-old man presents with chronic diarrhea and peptic ulcer disease refractory to medical management with proton pump inhibitors. An octreotide scan is shown in Fig. 2-9, which demonstrates an abnormal area of increased uptake of radionuclide in the region of the head of the pancreas. Which of the following factors directly results in the release of the hormone produced by this tumor?

(A) secretin

(B) glucagon

(C) antral pH <2.0

(D) vagus nerve

(E) somatostatin

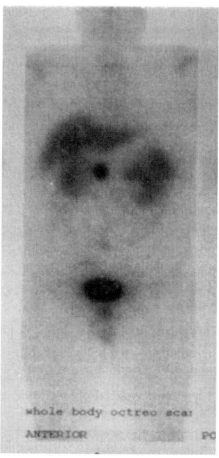

FIG. 2-9 (*Courtesy of H.J. Kim, MD.*)

105. Which of the following is true regarding the development of the large intestine?

(A) The embryonic origin of the large bowel is the foregut.

(B) The blood supply to the large bowel is solely from the SMA.

(C) During development, the midgut rotates 270° clockwise around the axis of the SMA.

(D) Distal anus is derived from ectoderm.

(E) The gut is derived from mesoderm.

Answers and Explanations

1. **(B)** Spontaneous pneumothorax is usually found in young males. A tall, thin habitus is common. Eighty-five percent of patients are found to have pulmonary blebs on the affected side. The correct management is placement of a chest tube, pain control, oxygen supplementation, and serial chest x-rays to monitor resolution. Thoracotomy is required if the pneumothorax does not resolve with a chest tube or if there is persistent air leak. Bleb resection and pleurodesis is usually performed at time of operation to prevent future bleb rupture and to promote adhesions of the lung to the chest wall. Thoracotomy is also offered to patients after a recurrence to prevent future episodes. Fifty percent of patients will have a recurrence on the ipsilateral side after a spontaneous pneumothorax. *(Schwartz, p. 711)*

2. **(B)** Intussusception is usually seen in children 8–12 months of age. They present with paroxysmal, crampy abdominal pain, and sometimes emesis. "Currant-jelly" stools are sometimes seen. They usually report a history of gastrointestinal viral infection in the recent past. Enlarged Peyer's patches are usually the lead point of the intussusception. Polyps, tumors, and Meckel's diverticula are less frequent causes. On examination, these children may have a mass in the epigastrium or right upper quadrant with an absence of intestines in the right lower quadrant. This is referred to as Dance's sign. The diagnostic tool of choice is air contrast enema. This is also therapeutic in 60–90% of cases. If the intussusception cannot be reduced by the enema, laparotomy is required to prevent bowel ischemia. Compromised bowel is resected at that time. Only 5% of children have a recurrence after successful reduction. *(Schwartz, pp. 1733–34)*

3. **(D)** Pyloric stenosis usually presents in the first 4–8 weeks of life. Parents usually report nonbilious emesis after feeds which progressively worsen to a projectile nature. Untreated, this will become a complete obstruction. On examination, an "olive sign" or mass in the right upper quadrant is often found. Ultrasound is the best radiologic test. These infants may present with dehydration and metabolic abnormalities from the emesis. The most common abnormality is hypokalemic, hypochloremic metabolic alkalosis. While surgical correction is urgent, it is not emergent. These infants should be resuscitated with IV fluids and their metabolic derangements corrected before an operation. Pyloromyotomy is the surgical therapy and involves splitting the hypertrophic muscles of the pylorus while keeping the mucosa intact. Patients are usually allowed to feed within hours of their operation. *(Schwartz, pp. 1731, 1732)*

4. **(A)** Any infant or child that presents with bilious emesis should be evaluated immediately for malrotation with midgut volvulus. This is a surgical emergency since the volvulus can compromise the vascular supply to the intestine. These patients are born with malrotation. In malrotation, the normal prenatal rotation of the midgut is incomplete and results in the cecum staying in the epigastrium with a narrow SMA pedicle. When this happens, bands form between the cecum and the abdominal wall (Ladd's bands). A volvulus may result around the shortened mesentery, cutting off the vascular supply to the midgut and causing obstruction. In volvulus, patients present with acute onset of bilious emesis and, later, with bloody stools or hemodynamic instability. The diagnosis of malrotation can be best made with an upper GI contrast study, which will show the duodenojejunal junction displaced to the right of midline. Sometimes this can also reveal volvulus. Patients with volvulus must be taken emergently to the operating room to reduce

the volvulus. If intestinal ischemia is advanced, a significant portion of small bowel may have to be removed, resulting in "short gut" syndrome.

In this patient presenting with bilious emesis, malrotation with volvulus must be considered and addressed early. The correct answer is to get an upper GI contrast study to evaluate for malrotation and obtain a surgical consult. Observation (answer C) may result in intestinal ischemia or death. Pyloric stenosis (answer B) presents with nonbilious emesis. Answer D refers to intussusception. While this abnormality often presents with bloody stools, bilious emesis is unlikely. Necrotizing enterocolitis (answer E) can also present with bloody stools, but usually occurs in premature infants as they approach full enteral feeds. (Schwartz, pp. 1731, 1732)

5. **(B)** Meckel's diverticula are usually found incidentally, although they can present with painless lower GI bleeding or inflammation (often confused with acute appendicitis). They are usually found within 2 ft of the ileocecal valve. They represent a remnant of the vitelline (or omphalomesenteric) duct and are found on the antimesenteric side of the ileum. They often contain ectopic gastric mucosa. Acid secretion from this leads to ileal ulceration and bleeding. They can be diagnosed using nuclear medicine scans (technetium pertechnetate). The treatment is surgical resection. (Schwartz, p. 1735)

6. **(D)**

7. **(C)**

Explanations 6 and 7

In patients with liver failure, the source of an upper GI bleed is esophageal varices in 50%, gastritis in 30%, and duodenal ulcers in only about 10%. Esophageal variceal bleeding is a potentially fatal complication of portal hypertension. The initial management should include fluid resuscitation and replacement of blood and clotting factors as needed. The second step is to control the source of bleeding. Medical management may include vasopressin or octreotide. Once the patient is stabilized, endoscopic

evaluation of the bleeding is crucial. Once the diagnosis is made, endoscopic attempts to stop bleeding can include sclerotherapy, banding, or balloon tamponade. If these methods are ineffective or the bleeding continues to recur, portal shunting options can be performed. TIPS have increased in popularity as a method for portal decompression. This can be performed in the acute setting. Surgical shunts are also an option, but are primarily used in patients with recurrent bleeding, not in the acute setting. Mesocaval shunts connect the SMV to the IVC in a variety of manners. Splenorenal shunts are actually the most common type of shunt. Nonselective shunts that completely divert portal blood flow from the liver can actually increase hepatic encephalopathy. Most surgeons prefer selective shunts which preserve a component of hepatic blood flow and, thus, function. Synthetic graft material can be safely used to create the shunts. Postoperative mortality is directly related to the patient's preprocedure medical condition and degree of hepatic failure (i.e., Child's class). (Schwartz, pp. 1417, 1418)

8. **(E)** Breast cancer usually presents as a nontender palpable mass. Mammography is helpful in the evaluation but a tissue biopsy is mandatory (i.e., core biopsy, stereotactic biopsy, or excisional biopsy). Mammography is helpful in detecting DCIS. The upper outer quadrant is a common site for breast cancer because of the amount of tissue contained there, including the tail of Spence. In the TNM classification, T1 refers to tumors <2 cm, T2 is >2 cm but <5 cm, T3 is >5 cm, and T4 denotes any size with extension into the chest wall. (Schwartz, pp. 554–562)

9. **(B)** Sentinel lymph node biopsy offers an alternative to full axillary dissection as a diagnostic tool in breast cancer with clinically negative axillary lymph nodes. Patients are injected with technetium-labeled sulfur colloid and isosulfan blue dye. A gamma probe is used along with the visual cues of the blue dye to identify the "sentinel node." The theory is that if this node is negative for malignancy, then the rest of the axilla will be negative as well. This spares these patients from an unnecessary axillary lymph node dissection and morbidity that it entails.

Patients with a positive sentinel lymph node require further therapy. Contraindications to the procedure include palpable axillary lymph nodes (because the diagnosis of axillary metastasis is apparent), multicentric disease, and a history of reaction to the blue dye (anaphylaxis and urticaria have been reported). If the lesion is very close to the axilla, there may be too much background radiotracer activity to discern the sentinel node. Lesions under the nipple are quite amenable to this procedure. There are several studies showing that the accuracy and success of this technique is related to surgeon experience. Surgeons are required to perform 20–30 procedures with some supervision or confirmation of results before relying completely on sentinel node biopsy. (*Cameron, pp. 708, 709*)

10. **(C)** The first step in any trauma assessment is the primary survey. This entails:

    A - Airway maintenance
    B - Breathing and ventilation
    C - Circulation
    D - Disability/neurologic status
    E - Exposure/environment

    The first thing done should be to establish an airway (intubation) and ventilation. While facial lacerations may indicate fractures, these patients can often be successfully intubated. This should be attempted first with a cricothyroidotomy done if an adequate airway cannot be established. The patient has two large-bore IVs which should be sufficient for the initial resuscitation, although central intravenous access is sometimes indicated if adequate peripheral access cannot be established. Once the primary survey is complete, the patient can be assessed for evidence of pneumothorax or abdominal injury requiring further intervention. (*Advanced Trauma Life Support Program for Doctors, pp. 21–46*)

11. **(B)** One in every four trauma deaths in North America is due to thoracic trauma. Many deaths from thoracic trauma can be prevented with prompt diagnosis and treatment of their injuries. The first step is the primary survey, which has already been completed by the transport team, with intubation and fluid/blood

resuscitation. Since hemothorax and pneumothorax are possibilities in this unstable patient with a chest injury, a chest tube should be placed immediately. This should be performed without the delay of a chest x-ray. A hypovolemic patient with cardiac tamponade may not have neck vein distension. ED thoracotomies should only be performed in a pulseless patient. All other patients requiring thoracotomy should go to the operating room. This patient is too unstable for the delay of an angiogram. (*Advanced Trauma Life Support Program for Doctors, pp. 125–141*)

12. **(D)** A compartment syndrome can occur in any extremity. It is caused by an increase of pressure in a closed space, often by blood or swelling, which impedes blood flow into the area. One of the first signs is paresthesias between the first and second toe, as the deep peroneal nerve is compressed. As the pressure increases, all of the answers listed can be found. In any extremity injury, the diagnosis of a compartment syndrome must be considered. If there is suspicion, the pressures can be checked with a manometer. Pressures over 30 mmHg should be addressed immediately. The treatment is decompression of the fascial spaces which can be performed at the bedside or in the operating room. The best prognosis is related to early fasciotomy before tissue perfusion is compromised. (*Schwartz, p. 206*)

13. **(D)** Like other trauma patients, the initial management of burn patients is crucial in improving survival and function. Inhalation injury should be suspected in anyone with a history of confinement in smoke, facial burns, singed eyebrows or nasal hairs, carbonaceous sputum, or carboxyhemoglobin levels greater than 10%. These patients sometimes look stable initially but soon develop airway edema. These patients should be placed on high-flow oxygen and observed closely. There should be a very low threshold for endotracheal intubation to protect the airway. Burn patients require large volume fluid resuscitation that should begin immediately. If patients develop pulmonary edema, they should be intubated. Fluid resuscitation should not be withheld to prevent intubation.

Heat loss is also a major concern in burn patients who have lost their thermoprotective skin covering. They should be wrapped in warm, moist dressings. Depth of burn affects management in resuscitation efforts, as well as need for debridement or escharotomy, and should be evaluated in every patient. The American Burn Association recommends transfer to a burn center for patients with:

> Partial thickness and full thickness burns of >10% of total body surface area (TBSA) in patients with age <10-years or >50-years
> Partial or full thickness burns of >20% in patients of any other age
> Partial or full thickness burns involving face, hands, feet, genitalia, or perineum
> Full thickness burns of >5% TBSA in any age group
> Significant electrical or chemical burns
> Inhalation injury

(*Advanced Trauma Life Support Program for Doctors, pp. 273–288*)

14. **(A)** Early clinical decline in a transplant patient is concerning for primary organ failure. This can be related to donor issues, technical issues, or donor organ ischemia. Signs of liver dysfunction include hypoglycemia (since liver unable to perform gluconeogenesis), coagulopathy with elevated prothrombin times, elevated ammonia levels, acid-base changes (unable to clear lactate via the Cori cycle), hyperkalemia, and oliguria. All liver transplant patients have an initial rise in transaminases which should decrease over the first 48 h. (*Schwartz, p. 394*)

15. **(B)** Steroids alone do not prevent rejection, although they can be used in high doses to treat acute cellular rejection. They work by binding intracellular receptors that act to block transcription. Cyclosporine binds to the calcineurin-calmodulin complex which acts to block activation of T cells. Its nephrotoxic effects are dose dependent. Tacrolimus acts in a similar fashion to cyclosporine to block T-cell activation. Mycophenolate mofetil interferes with purine metabolism, thus affecting T- and B-cell proliferative responses. (*Schwartz, pp. 376, 377*)

16. **(D)** Ureteral injuries are a well-known complication of pelvic surgery. The risk is greatly increased in the setting of inflammation, which can make the ureters difficult to identify. Intravenous pyelogram is a sensitive test for injury. CT scan and retrograde pyelogram are also diagnostic options. Injuries identified early are usually amenable to primary surgical repair, making early diagnosis essential. Delayed recognition usually results in a staged repair requiring urinary diversion with percutaneous nephrostomy tubes. (*Schwartz, pp. 1800, 1801*)

17. **(E)** Dehiscence refers to a separation of the fascial layer. Evisceration is when peritoneal contents extrude through the fascial separation. Malnutrition, obesity, diabetes, uremia, malignancy, immunologic abnormalities, steroid use, infection, and coughing, which increase abdominal pressures, are all factors that increase the risk of this complication. Technical factors are also very important in the risk of dehiscence, although there is no proof that running versus interrupted sutures is more successful in preventing this. (*Schwartz, p. 451*)

18. **(E)** This patient has achalasia, which is a disorder with nonrelaxing (LES) and decreased peristalsis of the esophageal body. The bird's beak deformity is a classic sign with a dilated esophagus which tapers to a small area at the LES. Esophagomyotomy is the best long-term treatment. Serial Botox injections and dilations can be used as well; however, their long-term results are inferior to myotomy. Proton pump inhibitors can be used for gastroesophageal reflux disease (GERD). A Nissen fundoplication is also a treatment for GERD. Calcium channel blockers are sometimes used in esophageal spasm disorders. (*Schwartz, pp. 1127–1129*)

19. **(D)** One of the most feared complications of neck surgery is postoperative hemorrhage causing airway compromise. Any patient with neck swelling and dyspnea must be assessed for this emergently. The treatment is to immediately open up the neck wound to release the hematoma. (*Schwartz, p. 1692*)

20. **(A)** The needle biopsy revealing amyloid makes the diagnosis of medullary thyroid

cancer. Patients often present with a neck mass and palpable lymph nodes (15–20%). Because of the aggressive nature of the malignancy, and the fact that it is often multicentric, total thyroidectomy is the treatment of choice. Modified radical neck dissection is indicated in patients with palpable lymphadenopathy and in patients with nodules larger than 2 cm, because 60% of these patients will have lymph node involvement. Because medullary carcinomas originate from the thyroid C cells, they do not respond to thyroxine or radioactive iodine therapy. (Schwartz, pp. 1687–1688.)

21. **(C)** Primary hyperparathyroidism is usually the result of a parathyroid adenoma. It can also be associated with multiglandular hyperplasia. Secondary hyperparathyroidism is associated with the hyperphosphatemia, and resultant hypocalcemia, in chronic renal disease. Tertiary hyperparathyroidism is seen after kidney transplant. Most patients (about 80%) with primary hyperparathyroidism are asymptomatic. Symptoms can include renal stones, bone abnormalities, peptic ulcer disease and mental status changes. It is more common in females and the incidence increases with age. (Schwartz, pp. 1698–1708)

22. **(A)** Ranson's criteria is a way to estimate mortality of acute pancreatitis. Patients get one point for each of the following that they develop:

Present on admission:

> Age >55 years
> WBC count >16,000
> Blood glucose >200 mg/mL
> Serum lactate dehydrogenase >350 IU/L
> SGOT (AST) > 250 IU/dL

Developing during the first 48 h:

> Hematocrit fall >10%
> Blood urea nitrogen increase >8 mg/dL
> Serum calcium <8 mg/dL
> Arterial PO_2 <60 mmHg
> Base deficit <4 meq/L
> Estimated fluid sequestration >600 mL

Mortality for any given point score is:

0–2	2%
3–4	15%
5–6	40%
7–8	100%

Amylase, lipase, and platelet counts are not considered in this equation although they are often elevated. (Schwartz, p. 1475)

23. **(D)** *E. coli* is the most common culprit for acute cystitis, although it is often caused by enterococci, *S. aureus*, *Klebsiella*, *Pseudomonas*, and streptococci. *P. mirabilis* can split urea, which results in alkaline urine and precipitation of calcium. Patients with this organism often present with bladder calculi. (Schwartz, p. 1770)

24. **(D)** Curling's ulcers are found in burn patients. They occur in 12% of burn patients and may be multiple. The risk of developing Curling's ulcers increases with the amount of TBSA covered by a burn. Cushing's ulcers are found in postoperative patients. (Schwartz, p. 1063)

25. **(C)** Increasing abdominal pressure for laparoscopic procedures has several systemic effects. By increasing the carbon dioxide, patients become hypercarbic and acidotic. There is decreased venous return and increased afterload. The peritoneum is distended and the diaphragm elevated. In patients with normal cardiac function, cardiac output is not affected until the abdominal pressures reach about 20 mmHg. (Schwartz, p. 2147)

26. **(B)** This patient should be able to perform any activity that requires innervation from C6 or above. The biceps and deltoid are innervated by C5, so he should be able to lift his arms above his head, have shoulder flexion, and elbow flexion. C6 innervates the extensor carpi radialis, so wrist extension should be preserved. The triceps rely on C7; therefore, he would not be able to perform elbow extension. (Schwartz, p. 1913)

27. (D) The joint space is most relaxed when the hip is flexed and externally rotated. This tends to be the least painful position for patients with septic arthritis. *(Schwartz, pp. 1991–1996)*

28. (A) A direct hernia comes through the medial inguinal canal floor and is found behind the spermatic cord. An indirect hernia passes through the internal inguinal ring, and thus can be found within the spermatic cord. The spermatic cord also contains the vas deferens, the testicular artery lymphatics, and nerve fibers. *(Schwartz, pp. 1586–1592)*

29. (C)

30. (B)

Explanations 29 and 30

The Glasgow Coma Scale (Table 2-1) is used to quantify a neurologic examination in patients with a head injury. It is based on three elements: eye opening, best motor response, and verbal response. The total score ranges from 3 (worst) to 15 (best) with a score of eight or lower generally considered as coma. The scale is shown below. This patient has a score of 2(E) + 4(M) + 2(V) = 8. Thus, this patient has evidence of a severe head injury. The initial step should be to protect his airway and prevent hypoxia which could adversely affect his head injury. Therefore, the initial step should be endotracheal intubation. Neurosurgical expertise, imaging to define the injury and screens to rule out drugs or alcohol as contributions are all important, but should be performed after airway, breathing, and circulation are addressed. Mannitol is indicated in patients with evidence of herniation, such as those with pupillary dilatation. *(Advanced Trauma Life Support Program for Doctors, pp. 181–206)*

31. (B) Symptoms of zinc deficiency include diarrhea, mental status changes, alopecia, and periorbital, perinasal, and perioral dermatitis. Persons who have cirrhosis, who are receiving steroids, who have excessive loss of gastrointestinal secretions or who are severely traumatized are at risk for zinc deficiency. Deficiency

TABLE 2-1   GLASGOW COMA SCALE

	Score
Eye opening (E)	
Spontaneous	4
To speech	3
To pain	2
None	1
Motor response (M)	
Obeys commands	6
Localizes pain	5
Withdraws to pain	4
Abnormal flexion (decorticate)	3
Extension (decerebrate)	2
None (flaccid)	1
Verbal response (V)	
Oriented	5
Confused conversation	4
Inappropriate words	3
Incomprehensible sounds	2
None	1

states resulting from inadequate ingestion of selenium, silicon, and tin have not been described. Deficiency of iodine produces hypothyroidism. *(Sabiston Textbook of Surgery: The Biological Basis of Modern Surgical Practice, p. 164)*

32. (A) During total thyroidectomy, parathyroid glands may inadvertently be removed or their vascular supply interrupted. Hypoparathyroidism may then develop, the manifestations of which include tingling, muscle cramps, convulsions, and a positive Chvostek's sign. These symptoms are dramatically relieved by intravenous administration of calcium. Oral calcium and vitamin D are administered for long-term correction of hypocalcemia. *(Sabiston Textbook of Surgery: The Biological Basis of Modern Surgical Practice, p. 164)*

33. (E) Vital capacity is an important measure of respiratory function. It is defined as the maximum volume of air a person can expel following a maximum inspiratory effort. When vital capacity is normal, significant restrictive pulmonary disease is not present. Acutely decreased vital capacity indicates decreased ventilatory reserve. *(Sabiston Textbook of Surgery: The Biological Basis of Modern Surgical Practice, p. 1787)*

34. (D) In deceleration injuries, laceration involving the aorta most frequently occurs just distal to the left subclavian artery. This is where the aorta is fixed and, thus, more susceptible to shear forces. The tear may be complete or partial. Diagnosis is difficult; aortography is helpful in establishing the diagnosis. (*Sabiston Textbook of Surgery: The Biological Basis of Modern Surgical Practice, pp. 310, 311*)

35. **(C)** Gastrinoma produces Zollinger-Ellison syndrome, which is associated with markedly elevated gastric acid secretion and ulcer disease of the upper gastrointestinal tract. The most common site of occurrence is the pancreas.

However, gastrinoma has been known to occur in the gastric antrum, duodenum, spleen, and ovary. Removal of the gastrinoma can result in a cure. A thorough search must be made at surgical exploration to locate the tumor, which in early stages will be small. The gastrinoma triangle is defined as the junction of the cystic and common bile ducts, second and third portion of the duodenum, and the division of the pancreatic neck and body. Ninety percent of gastrinomas are located here. (*Sabiston Textbook of Surgery: The Biological Basis of Modern Surgical Practice, pp. 1177–1180*)

36. **(A)** Avascular necrosis results when, following a fracture, the blood supply to a bone fragment is disrupted. The femoral head, humeral head, scaphoid, and talus, because of their precarious blood supplies, are particularly vulnerable to this complication. A dense appearance of the bone on x-ray is a diagnostic clue. Radioisotope scanning can detect avascular necrosis at an earlier stage than is possible with roentgenography. (*Sabiston Textbook of Surgery: The Biological Basis of Modern Surgical Practice, p. 1400*)

37. **(B)** Contraction of hollow organs against obstruction or excessive contraction causes colic. Typical ureteral colic is severe, sudden in onset, radiates from loin to groin, and is associated with an urge to urinate. Blood clots and calculi in the ureter can cause colic, the latter being more frequent. Urine examination demonstrates macroscopic or microscopic hematuria. (*Sabiston Textbook of Surgery: The Biological Basis of Modern Surgical Practice, pp. 1526, 1527*)

38. **(A)**

39. **(C)**

40. **(B)**

Explanations 38 through 40

In a patient who is known to have had symptoms of peptic ulcer disease for many years and who presents with nausea and vomiting, one should consider gastric outlet obstruction. This can be due to exacerbation of the ulcer and edema or scar tissue formation. Usually in these patients, epigastric fullness, with visible peristalsis going from the left side to the right, will be seen. The history of periodicity and pain relief by taking antacids also favors a diagnosis of previous peptic ulcer disease. Patients with umbilical hernia will have a mass in the region of the umbilicus. Patients with acute cholecystitis usually present with the sudden onset of pain, radiating to the back, with fever and chills. Volvulus of the sigmoid colon presents with constipation and abdominal distention. Vomiting is a late feature. Small-bowel obstruction would be associated with a history of colicky abdominal pain, nausea, and vomiting. Patients will usually have hyperactive high-pitched bowel sounds.

With persistent vomiting, the patient loses fluid, resulting in dehydration (hypovolemia). Loss of hydrogen ions, potassium, and chloride in the vomited gastric contents leads to alkalosis, hypokalemia, and hypochloremia. Because of hypovolemia, adrenocortical and renal mechanisms are stimulated to conserve sodium at the expense of potassium and hydrogen ions. Excretion of potassium in the urine further aggravates hypokalemia. The kidneys then compensate for the loss of potassium by conserving potassium and excreting more hydrogen ions, which results in a paradoxical aciduria and self-perpetuating metabolic alkalosis.

The treatment of hypochloremic, hypokalemic metabolic alkalosis involves replenishing the extracellular volume with isotonic sodium chloride (normal saline) and potassium.

Chloride is the most important electrolyte to replace, as it facilitates increased reabsorption of sodium in the proximal tubule that begins to reverse the alkalosis. In refractory cases, hydrochloric acid may be required. *(Sabiston Textbook of Surgery: The Biological Basis of Modern Surgical Practice, pp. 100–104; 858, 859)*

41. **(D)** Vocal cord paralysis indicates involvement of recurrent laryngeal nerve. Tumor invasion of the left recurrent laryngeal nerve in the aortopulmonary window is generally considered an indication of nonresectability. However, recurrent laryngeal nerve may be involved above the level of the aortic arch by direct tumor extension in which case resection is not contraindicated. Some patients with chest wall invasion are cured following enbloc resection, and it, therefore, is not an absolute contraindication for resection. Tumors with ipsilateral mediastinal node involvement could be resected with a reasonable chance for cure. Malignant cells in pleural effusion indicate noncurability, but before a patient is denied a chance for cure, the presence of malignant cells in the effusion has to be proved beyond doubt. Involvement of more than one lobe has no bearing on prognosis as long as the patient's preoperative ventilation parameters will allow for safe resection. Metastasis to the liver is an absolute contraindication for resection since lung cancer in this circumstance is not curable. *(Sabiston Textbook of Surgery: The Biological Basis of Modern Surgical Practice, pp. 1865–1875)*

42. **(A)**

43. **(D)**

Explanations 42 and 43

Women are more often affected by gallstones than men. Pregnancy predisposes for the occurrence of gallstones. Gallstones may remain asymptomatic or may cause symptoms when they cause obstruction to the cystic duct. The usual presenting symptom is biliary colic, which is experienced as epigastric pain radiating to the back, associated with nausea and vomiting. The presence of tenderness in the right upper quadrant and leukocytosis, under these circumstances, are very indicative of acute cholecystitis. The diagnosis of gallstones is best confirmed by ultrasonography. Ultrasonography also provides details about the presence of gallstones, the wall of the gallbladder, and the presence or absence of tenderness over the gallbladder during the examination. Gallstones are seen on a two-way roentgenogram of the abdomen in only 20% of cases. Barium swallow in this instance is of no help. Failure to visualize the gallbladder with HIDA scan indicates cystic duct obstruction. In a majority of patients, acute cholecystitis is secondary to cystic duct obstruction. Lack of visualization may also occur in patients who have had a previous cholecystectomy (history is helpful) or agenesis of the gallbladder (rare). Peritoneal lavage in this instance will be of no help, except in detecting fluid, which may contain leukocytes. *(Sabiston Textbook of Surgery: The Biological Basis of Modern Surgical Practice, pp. 837, 838)*

44. **(B)** From the description, the diagnosis in this patient is acute regional enteritis. Incidental findings of regional enteritis in patients operated on for presumed diagnosis of acute appendicitis are medically treated unless there is proximal obstruction. The risk of operating on patients with regional enteritis is formation of fistula and abscess, especially if the area to be resected is involved with the disease process. However, if the cecum and the appendix are not involved, it is advisable to perform appendectomy. In this instance, it would be safe and if the patient were to have a recurrence in the future, acute appendicitis would no longer be a possible diagnosis and the patient could be treated for an exacerbation of regional enteritis. *(Sabiston Textbook of Surgery: The Biological Basis of Modern Surgical Practice, pp. 923–932)*

45. **(C)** The majority of testicular tumors occurring in young adults are malignant tumors. The tumors may originate from germinal or nongerminal cells. Those that arise from germinal cells include seminoma (the most common), embryonal cell carcinoma, choriocarcinoma, and teratocarcinoma. Leydig cell tumors and androblastoma originate from nongerminal cells and may produce excess testosterone. Benign tumors, such as fibroma, can occur but are rare. (*Sabiston Textbook of Surgery: The Biological Basis of Modern Surgical Practice, p. 1558*)

46. **(B)** Tracheoesophageal fistula is a serious complication of tracheostomy and tracheal intubation. The presence of a nasogastric tube, positive-pressure ventilation, and prolonged periods of intubation are predisposing factors. The complication should be suspected when an intubated patient develops violent coughing after swallowing food or saliva. The recommended treatment is primary closure of the fistulous opening in the trachea and the esophagus with a transposed regional muscle flap interposed between the trachea and esophagus. Nonsurgical corrective measures are associated with a higher rate of mortality. Sudden bright red bleeding is a symptom of tracheoinominate artery fistula. Surgical repair of tracheoesophageal fistula has a low mortality rate. (*Sabiston Textbook of Surgery: The Biological Basis of Modern Surgical Practice, pp. 1816–1820*)

47. **(A)** Although constipation is the most common presenting feature of Hirschsprung's disease, some patients suffer from diarrhea. The severity of symptoms does not correlate well with the extent of bowel involvement. Enterocolitis, a major cause of death, requires vigorous treatment. This complication can occur even after removal of the aganglionic segment of the bowel. Increased acetylcholinesterase activity has been noted in the serum, affected aganglionic bowel and erythrocytes of afflicted persons. Eighty percent of affected infants are boys. (*Sabiston Textbook of Surgery: The Biological Basis of Modern Surgical Practice, pp. 1243, 1244*)

48. **(A)** Elevated serum gastrin is found in patients with and without peptic ulcer disease. Hypergastrinemia affects patients with gastrinoma, G-cell hyperplasia, gastric stasis, retained antrum, renal failure, and massive small-bowel resection. Most studies have shown no difference in gastrin level between uncomplicated duodenal ulcer patients and those persons in a control group. Pernicious anemia is commonly associated with loss of intrinsic factor secondary to atrophic gastritis. The atrophic gastritis and loss of acid secretion is what stimulates the hypergastrinemic state. Nonsteroidal anti-inflammatory drugs disrupt the mucosal barrier of the stomach. Secretin decreases gastrin levels. (*Sabiston Textbook of Surgery: The Biological Basis of Modern Surgical Practice, pp. 848–866*)

49. **(C)** Because of the risk of postsplenectomy sepsis, attempts should be made for splenic salvage when possible. Most patients are managed nonoperatively. Nonoperative management is contraindicated in the presence of hypotension or persistent bleeding. If patients are treated operatively, attempts are still made at splenic salvage if possible instead of splenectomy. Attempts at splenic salvage are contraindicated in hemodynamically unstable patients or patients with multiple concomitant injuries, as it prolongs the operation and increases blood loss. The CT scan provided shows a traumatic laceration through the hilum of the spleen, which is usually not amenable to conservative management and almost always requires a splenectomy. The risk of postsplenectomy sepsis persists throughout life, the highest incidence being in the first 2 years following splenectomy. This is caused by encapsulated organisms. Patients should be vaccinated against *Pneumococcus*, *Meningococcus*, and *Haemophilus influenzae*. (*Cameron, pp. 963, 964*)

50. **(C)** Esophageal achalasia is characterized by the findings of aperistalsis/atony and a failure of the LES to relax normally, resulting in esophageal dilatation proximally with a functional obstruction at the LES. Long-standing achalasia results in the characteristic barium swallow finding of a bird's beak. Iatrogenic or tumor-related elevation of LES pressure can result in a "pseudoachalasia," but should have normal peristaltic patterns on manometry. Patients with Barrett's esophagus may have a "cobblestone" appearance on barium swallow with normal peristalsis and do not characteristically demonstrate

esophageal dilatation; LES pressures may be normal or low. Finally, patients with Plummer-Vinson syndrome develop cervical dysphagia due to iron deficiency anemia. They often present with cervical esophageal webs and can be at higher risk for developing esophageal squamous cell carcinoma. *(Cameron, pp. 15–17)*

51. **(D)** Barrett's esophagus is a condition often related to chronic GERD, in which the normal stratified squamous esophageal mucosa is replaced by a columnar-lined epithelium. If left untreated, patients can develop dysplasia and esophageal adenocarcinoma. Persons with Barrett's esophagus require lifelong endoscopic surveillance with repeated biopsies. Barrett's esophagus is more common in men than women and in whites more than Blacks. The prevalence increases with age. Although effective medical and surgical antireflux therapies can cause regression of symptoms, the Barrett's esophagus segment rarely regresses and the potential for dysplasia or adenocarcinoma is not eliminated. *(Cameron, pp. 47–48)*

52. **(D)** Hamman's crunch on auscultation results from the heart sounds in the setting of mediastinal emphysema and is suggestive of esophageal perforation. The most common cause of esophageal perforation is iatrogenic, but it may occur spontaneously (Boerhaave's syndrome) or secondary to a malignancy or stricture. Diagnosis is often made after clinical suspicion by endoscopy or plain films with water-soluble contrast study. If diagnosed early (within 24 h), a primary repair is the first approach to treatment. Closure is dependent on the amount of infected or necrotic tissue, tension on the anastomosis, etiology of the perforation, and the ability to adequately drain the contaminated areas. Late perforations may be complicated in their management, requiring several procedures or a diversion to provide for adequate healing. *(Cameron, pp. 8–15)*

53. **(D)** The diagnosis of acute appendicitis can often be made based on the history and physical findings. The sequence of symptoms classically begins with anorexia followed by periumbilical pain which localizes to the right lower quadrant after 6–12 h. The onset of nausea and emesis occurs after the development of abdominal pain. If the patient has an appetite or if bouts of vomiting begin before the onset of abdominal pain, the diagnosis should be reconsidered. In this patient, the acute appendicitis has progressed to a rupture, resulting in a localized right lower quadrant abscess (marked with arrow in Fig. 2-10).

The signs of acute appendicitis are also characteristic. On examination, tenderness is often maximal at McBurney's point, approximately one-third the distance on a line drawn from the anterior spinous process of the ileum to the umbilicus. Other physical signs include the Rovsing sign (pain initiated in the right lower quadrant on palpation in the left lower quadrant), Dunphy sign (increased pain with coughing), obturator sign (pain on internal rotation of the hip), and the psoas sign (pain during extension of the right hip). Grey Turner's sign is bruising of the flanks which may occur in severe, acute pancreatitis due to subcutaneous tracking of inflammatory peripancreatic exudate from the pancreatic area of the retroperitoneum. Murphy's sign is right upper quadrant (RUQ) pain with inspiration while palpating under the right costal margin associated with acute cholecystitis. *(Schwartz, pp. 1384, 1385)*

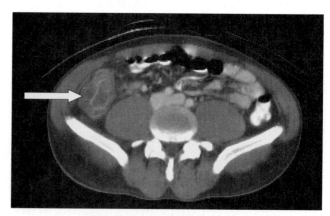

FIG. 2-10 *(Courtesy of H.J. Kim, MD.)*

54. **(C)** Carcinoids are the most common neoplasm of the appendix and arise from Kulchitsky cells, a type of enterochromaffin cell. Aside from the appendix, the next most frequent site of involvement is the small bowel followed by the rectum. Appendiceal and rectal carcinoids are almost never associated with carcinoid syndrome unless metastatic disease is present. Small bowel carcinoids are more commonly multifocal, metastatic, and associated with carcinoid syndrome.

The majority of appendiceal carcinoids are located at the tip, and the extent of surgical resection depends on the size and resulting malignant potential. Lesions less than 1 cm rarely metastasize and therefore require only simple appendectomy, as in this question. Lesions greater than 2 cm require a right hemicolectomy due to the high potential for metastasis. Partial small bowel resection is indicated for a carcinoid of the small intestine. Partial cecectomy and total abdominal colectomy are not appropriate options. (*Schwartz, pp. 1244–1246*)

55. **(A)** Tetanus is caused by the release of toxins from *Clostridium tetani* and may result in life-threatening convulsions with ensuing respiratory depression. Trauma and burn wounds are tetanus prone. These require appropriate immunization as well as surgical debridement of devitalized tissue.

The need for tetanus prophylaxis depends on the patient's current immunization status. For tetanus-prone wounds, patients with three or more tetanus toxoid boosters require no further prophylaxis as long as the last booster was within 5 years. Patients with unknown immunization history, or fewer than three toxoid boosters, require both tetanus toxoid and immune globulin. The role of antibiotics for prophylaxis has not been determined. (*Sabiston Textbook of Surgery: The Biological Basis of Modern Surgical Practice, pp. 331, 332*)

56. **(D)** Postoperative wound infections usually occur between the fifth and eighth postoperative day. Evidence of a wound infection within the first 24 h after surgery should alert the physician to the possibility of necrotizing fasciitis. Necrotizing fasciitis is a life-threatening infection most commonly caused by clostridial myositis and hemolytic streptococcus. In addition to spiking temperature, the patient may be septic with tachycardia, leukocytosis, and hemodynamic instability. On examination of the wound, crepitus (gas in the soft tissue) and a dishwater-appearing effluent may be apparent.

Early diagnosis by opening the wound and sending a Gram's stain is life saving. The Gram's stain will reveal a mixed flora of gram-negative rods and gram-positive cocci. Although broad spectrum antibiotics are indicated, definitive treatment requires aggressive debridement of the affected tissues on an emergent basis. Hyperbaric oxygen treatment has no role.

Diabetic patients are especially prone to necrotizing fasciitis. Fournier's gangrene is a type of necrotizing fasciitis that affects the groin and perineum. The mortality rate can be as high as 75%. (*Schwartz, p. 451*)

57. **(D)** Nearly all broad-spectrum antibiotics may result in superinfection of the colon with *C. difficile*. This anaerobic enteric pathogen produces a toxin that causes necrosis of the colonic mucous membrane resulting in enterocolitis (pseudomembranous colitis). The infection can occur several weeks after the discontinuation of the inciting antibiotic. The presentation varies from mild diarrhea to systemic illness with abdominal pain, fever, and leukocytosis. Severe cases may progress to colonic dilatation and perforation.

Lower endoscopy reveals the characteristic yellow pseudomembranes which represent ulceration and necrosis. The diagnosis is confirmed with either colonic wall biopsy for the organism or, more commonly, stool studies with identification of the toxin.

Orally administered metronidazole is the treatment of choice. Vancomycin is also effective but, due to its side-effect profile and expense, it is reserved for refractory cases. (*Sabiston Textbook of Surgery: The Biological Basis of Modern Surgical Practice, p. 279*)

58. **(D)** A high index of suspicion is warranted for catheter sepsis in any patient who has had a central line for several days and suddenly

spikes high fever. The catheter site may have erythema, induration, tenderness, and pus extruding from the skin. Often, however, the skin appears normal. A thorough search for other possible sources of fever including pulmonary, intraabdominal, urinary, and wound infections is always prudent.

Catheter sepsis can be life threatening and early intervention is essential. Peripheral and central blood cultures should be obtained, and the catheter must be removed promptly. It is contraindicated to replace the catheter over a guide wire because the infected skin tract is still present. When the infected catheter is removed, it is not mandatory to treat with antibiotics unless the fever persists or signs of sepsis are present. TPN cannot be administered through a peripheral intravenous line. (*Sabiston Textbook of Surgery: The Biological Basis of Modern Surgical Practice, pp. 165, 166*)

59. **(A)** Internal hemorrhoids are highly vascularized submucosal cushions located in the anal canal. They are classified as first degree if no prolapse is present, second degree if prolapse occurs with spontaneous reduction, third degree if they require manual reduction, and fourth degree if they are irreducible. Treatment is based on the symptoms and degree of prolapse.

Nearly all patients with first and second degree hemorrhoids should initially be placed on a trial of conservative measures including a bowel management program with high fiber diet to avoid straining and constipation, frequent warm tub baths, and an anti-inflammatory topical cream. If symptoms continue, both rubber band ligation (a small rubber band is placed at the neck of the hemorrhoid resulting in eventual death and detachment of tissue) and infrared coagulation (controlled burn of the vessels at the neck of the hemorrhoid) are good alternatives to surgical therapy. For refractory first and second degree hemorrhoids, most third degree and all fourth degree hemorrhoids, surgical hemorrhoidectomy is the treatment of choice.

A thrombosed external hemorrhoid is a blood clot resulting in painful swelling of the tightly held anoderm. In most cases conservative management is indicated. Excision is

reserved for patients with debilitating pain or signs of necrosis. (*Sabiston Textbook of Surgery: The Biological Basis of Modern Surgical Practice, pp. 1036, 1037*)

60. **(E)** The most common cause of anorectal fistula and abscess is infection of the anal glands which empty into the anal canal at the level of the dentate line. Classification of anal fistula is based on the relationship of the epithelialized tract to the anal sphincter muscle and can be intersphincteric (most common), transsphincteric, suprasphincteric, and extrasphincteric (least common). A symptomatic fistula is an indication for surgery because it rarely heals spontaneously.

Despite popular teaching, there is little use for antibiotics in the primary treatment of anal abscess. As a rule, surgical drainage is required, and antibiotics are only indicated if cellulitis is present. However, those patients who are immunocompromised have valvular heart disease or poorly controlled diabetes should always be considered for antibiotics. (*Gordon, pp. 242, 249, 255*)

61. **(D)** Crohn's disease is a chronic inflammatory disease of the gastrointestinal tract of unknown etiology. Both medical and surgical treatments are palliative in nature—there is no known cure. Approximately 70% of patients with Crohn's disease will require an operation during their lifetime. The most common indication for surgery is recurrent bowel obstruction, followed by perforation with abscess and fistula formation. (*Sabiston Textbook of Surgery: The Biological Basis of Modern Surgical Practice, pp. 923, 925–926*)

62. **(E)** Ulcerative colitis is a diffuse inflammatory disease of the colon and rectum with unknown etiology. Unlike Crohn's disease, surgical removal of the entire colon and rectum provides a complete cure. Nonetheless many patients are treated successfully with medical therapy including corticosteroids and can avoid the potential complications of surgery and life-long ileostomy.

Ulcerative colitis usually presents as bloody diarrhea, fever, and abdominal pain. The disease process begins in the rectum, advances proximally in a contiguous fashion, and affects the superficial layers of the colon wall. Crohn's disease is located anywhere from the mouth to anus, has skip lesions, and is transmural in nature. Histologically, superficial inflammation with crypt abscesses is more indicative of ulcerative colitis, whereas deeper involvement with granulomas and fissures is more characteristic of Crohn's disease. Both diseases may present with extraintestinal manifestations, such as arthritis, skin lesions, and hepatic dysfunction. Perianal disease with fistula formation is characteristic of Crohn's disease.

Patients with ulcerative colitis have a 10–20% risk of developing colon cancer within 20 years of diagnosis. The incidence is also increased in those with Crohn's disease, but to a lesser extent. Surveillance colonoscopy is essential in patients with long-standing disease. (*Sabiston Textbook of Surgery: The Biological Basis of Modern Surgical Practice, pp. 1001–1005*)

63. **(A)** Anal carcinoma can arise from several epithelial cell types in the anal canal, including squamous, basaloid, cloacogenic, and mucoepidermoid. For early, superficial lesions less than 2 cm, an attempt can be made to excise the lesion completely with negative margins. Otherwise, the standard of care is a multimodality chemoradiation protocol which classically includes mitomycin C and 5-fluorouracil. The long-term survival rate after chemoradiation alone compares favorably with radical surgery. Abdominal perineal resection is reserved for persistent or recurrent disease. Low anterior resection refers to resection of the upper and middle rectum and plays no role in the treatment of anal cancer

Inguinal lymph node dissection is not indicated. Any clinically suspicious node should be biopsied and, if positive, treated with radiation. Thus, even a small anal cancer with a positive lymph node should be treated with chemotherapy instead of surgery. (*Sabiston Textbook of Surgery: The Biological Basis of Modern Surgical Practice, p. 1042*)

64. **(B)** Colon cancer is the most common metastatic lesion of the gastrointestinal tract to the liver. In approximately 25% of the cases, liver metastases are present at the time of initial diagnosis of the colon cancer. Generally, synchronous liver metastasis should not be resected during the initial operation for the primary tumor. Only a solitary, small, peripherally located lesion in a hemodynamically stable patient would be an acceptable indication for a wedge resection. Otherwise, the planned colon resection should be completed. A second procedure can be planned after a thorough metastatic evaluation using various diagnostic modalities such as intraoperative ultrasound, CT, MRI, and/or positron emission tomography (PET) scan.

A delay of weeks to months between surgeries has not been shown to have a negative impact on long-term survival. The delay may help select patients who may benefit the most and exclude those who develop widespread metastatic disease during the interval.

Chemotherapy alone is inappropriate because, even in the presence of metastatic disease, the primary colon carcinoma should be resected to prevent later complications such as bleeding, perforation, or obstruction.

The 5-year survival rate following hepatic resection for colorectal metastases ranges from 25–40%. (*The M.D. Anderson Surgical Oncology Handbook, pp. 277–279*)

65. **(A)** Local treatment of rectal cancer is the treatment of choice in selected individuals with low-lying rectal cancers. The lesion must be mobile, nonulcerated, within 10 cm of the anal verge, less than 3 cm in diameter, less than one-fourth the circumference of the rectal wall, and stage T1 or T2 on endorectal ultrasound.

Transanal excision is the most straightforward technique of local treatment. It entails full thickness excision of the lesion into the perirectal fat with 1-cm margins. For early lesions into the submucosa only (T1), no adjuvant therapy is required unless poor prognostic features are present on final pathology (poorly differentiated or lymphatic/vascular invasion). If the lesion penetrates the muscular wall (T2), adjuvant radiation therapy with or without chemotherapy is indicated following surgical removal. Overall, the disease free survival rate is 80%.

Dukes originally proposed a staging classification for colon cancer. Dukes' A lesions are confined to the bowel wall, Dukes' B lesions extend beyond the wall involving the serosa or fat, and Dukes' C lesions have accompanying regional lymph node involvement. TNM staging is now probably the most widely used system for staging.

STAGING OF COLORECTAL CANCER

Stage I	T1 – invades submucosa
	T2 – invades muscularis propria
Stage II	T3 – invades through muscularis propria into subserosa
	T4 – invades into contiguous organs
Stage III	Any T with presence of positive lymph nodes
Stage IV	Distant metastatic disease present

(M.D. Anderson Handbook, pp. 224, 239–240)

66. **(B)** In this situation the surgeon must decide which lesion poses the most threat. Since the cancer is nearly obstructing and the AAA is less than 6 cm, the best option is to proceed with the planned colon resection and perform the AAA repair at a later date. If the AAA is known to be symptomatic or is larger than 7 cm, then it carries a significant risk of postoperative rupture and should be repaired in the same setting. In such a scenario, the AAA should be repaired first, the graft reperitonealized and the area protected with laparotomy sponges before colon surgery begins. *(Gordon, pp. 1327, 1328)*

67. **(A)** The patient described has familial adenomatous polyposis (FAP). FAP is a rare autosomal dominant inherited form of colorectal cancer that results from a germline mutation in the APC gene. The disease is characterized by over 100 polyps in the large intestine, as well as extraintestinal manifestations such as epidermoid cysts, desmoid tumors, and osteomas. All patients with FAP will develop colorectal cancer if left untreated. The average age of diagnosis is 29, and the average age of development of cancer is 39.

Once diagnosed, the most definitive treatment requires complete removal of the entire colon and rectum in a timely fashion. Surveillance colonoscopy is not protective

against the development of cancer, regardless of the frequency. The surgical procedure of choice is a proctocolectomy with permanent ileostomy or creation of an ileoanal anastomosis with ileal reservoir such as a J-pouch. Abdominal perineal resection with sigmoid colectomy leaves a significant portion of colon in situ, with subsequent risk of developing colon cancer. *(Schwartz, pp. 309, 1330–1332)*

68. **(A)** Villous adenoma is a premalignant condition. The incidence of carcinoma in a polyp depends on the histologic type and size of the polyp. Tubular adenomas are the most common type of polyps (60–80%), but are the least likely to harbor carcinoma (less than 5%). Villous adenomas are the least common type, but overall the most likely to contain malignant foci (35–40%). In terms of size, polyps less that 1 cm have a 1–10% risk of containing carcinoma. Those larger than 2 cm have a 35–50% risk.

In this patient, a formal right hemicolectomy is indicated due to the high probability of finding cancer in the specimen. A lesser operation, such as open or laparoscopic polypectomy, would then require a second operative procedure if cancer is present.

Colonoscopic fulguration of such a large lesion carries a high risk for perforation and would not allow histologic examination. Observation with repeat colonoscopy in 1 year is also inappropriate. *(Sabiston Textbook of Surgery: The Biological Basis of Modern Surgical Practice, pp. 995, 996)*

69. **(B)**

70. **(D)**

71. **(C)**

Explanations 69 through 71

Abdominal ultrasonography has a limited role in the diagnosis or management of intestinal obstruction. Serum electrolyte determination helps in identifying the electrolyte disturbances that have taken place. Fluid loss needs to be corrected with rehydration and nasogastric suction helps in decreasing abdominal distention.

Upper GI endoscopy would increase distention and is, therefore, contraindicated. Antiemetics should not be given until a definitive diagnosis is made and then only if indicated. Promotility agents have little to no role in the management of a patient with bowel obstruction and may even be contraindicated. (*Sabiston Textbook of Surgery: The Biological Basis of Modern Surgical Practice, pp. 915–923*)

An annular, constricting lesion with overhanging edges is typical of annular carcinoma of the colon. Mechanical small-bowel obstruction results in multiple air-fluid levels in distended small-bowel loops. Intussusception produces a corkscrew appearance on barium enema and sigmoid volvulus produces a bird's beak appearance. In diverticulitis, extravasation of barium outside the lumen of the colon is typically seen. (*Greenfield, pp. 1014–1031*)

The ureters may be injured during pelvic operations. The principles of ureteral repair include early recognition, debridement of nonviable tissue, and tension-free anastomosis over an internal ureteral stent. The type of repair largely depends on the location of injury.

If the injury occurs above the pelvic brim, the best option is primary end-to-end repair over a double-J stent. If there is a large defect precluding a tension-free anastomosis, ureteroureterostomy (anastomosis to the opposite ureter) should be considered. However, this may result in injury to the uninvolved kidney and is reserved as a second-line option.

When the injury occurs below the pelvic brim, ureteroneocystostomy (ureteral reimplantation into the bladder) is the procedure of choice. Ligating the transected ends should be reserved for unstable patients. In this scenario, a nephrostomy tube is required as a temporizing measure until definitive repair. (*Schwartz, pp. 202, 1801, 1875*)

72. **(E)** Several independent prognostic factors for melanoma have been identified. Patients with lesions on extremities have a better prognosis than those with lesions on the face or trunk. Ulceration points to a worse prognosis. Females have a higher survival rate. Nodular and superficial spreading melanomas have similar survival patterns when matched for depth. However, lentigo maligna types have a better prognosis while acral lentiginous lesions have a worse prognosis. (*Schwartz, pp. 524, 525*)

73. **(A)** The pathology slide provided shows invasive ductal carcinoma of the breast. The Halsted radical mastectomy involves removal of all breast tissue, lymphadenectomy, and removal of the pectoralis major. The modified radical mastectomy preserves the pectoralis major muscle, thus decreasing the morbidity of the surgery with the same survival. The modified radical mastectomy does include a lymph node dissection. The anatomic limits of the modified radical mastectomy include the sternum medially, the subclavius muscle superiorly, the inframammary fold inferiorly, and the latissimus muscle laterally. The surgeon must identify the thoracodorsal nerve, which innervates the latissimus dorsi muscle, as well as the long thoracic nerve, which innervates the serratus muscle. Damage to the long thoracic nerve results in a winged scapula. After a complete dissection of level I, II, and III lymph nodes, regardless of the mastectomy, the use of radiation therapy needs to be critically evaluated because of the long-term morbidity of lymphedema. (*Schwartz, pp. 576, 577*)

74. **(A)** Damage to the thoracic duct can be seen as a complication following distal esophagectomy or any procedure that involves dissection into the cervical region. It is most commonly seen on the left if iatrogenic. Aspiration of an odorless, milky fluid from the chest cavity is diagnostic, although increased lymphocyte counts and triglyceride levels in the fluid help confirm the diagnosis. Normal chyle flow is around 2 L a day. Therefore a chylous leak can result in nutritional depletion as well as decreased systemic lymphocytes to fight infection. The first therapy is placement of a chest tube to drain the chyle and to allow for approximation of the lung against the mediastinum. Stopping oral intake and starting total parenteral nutrition is usually tried for 7–10 days to see if there is spontaneous resolution of the leak. If conservative measures fail, ligation of the thoracic duct can be performed. (*Schwartz, pp. 707, 708*)

75. (B) Finding a conduit for use in coronary artery bypass grafting can sometimes be a challenge as these patients often have diffuse atherosclerotic disease. The left internal mammary artery is most commonly used. Bilateral internal mammary arteries can be used; however, this increases the chances of sternal healing problems. Saphenous vein grafts are used in patients with multivessel disease, although this may not be an option in patients with deep venous thrombosis (DVT), venous insufficiency, or arterial insufficiency to the legs (because they will not heal the harvest wound). Radial arteries, the right gastroepiploic artery, and inferior epigastric arteries have also been used. *(Schwartz, pp. 863–865)*

76. (B) Carcinoid is the most common malignancy found in the appendix. Most are located in the tip of the appendix. If it is less than 2 cm and is located in the tip, appendectomy is the only therapy required. Larger tumors or those with extension into the mesoappendix should be treated by right hemicolectomy. Carcinoid syndrome is only seen in 3% of cases. *(Schwartz, p. 1392)*

77. (B) Esophageal cancer is increasing in incidence in North America, largely due to the rise in incidence of esophageal adenocarcinoma. Premalignant lesions for esophageal cancer include Barrett's changes, radiation esophagitis, caustic esophageal burns, Plummer-Vinson syndrome, leukoplakia, esophageal diverticula, ectopic gastric mucosa, and tylosis. It is more common in men. Smoking, along with alcohol use, is clearly a risk factor. Barrett's esophagus requires frequent surveillance examinations with biopsies and increases the risk for adenocarcinoma of the esophagus at the GE junction. *(Cameron, pp. 58, 59)*

78. (B) Pharyngoesophageal (Zenker's) diverticulum is the most common diverticulum of the esophagus and is an example of a pulsion diverticulum. It is not made up of all layers of the esophageal wall like a traction diverticulum. It is situated posteriorly, just proximal to the cricopharyngeal muscle, at a weak point in the esophagus. Symptoms include dysphagia, spontaneous regurgitation of undigested food/pills, noisy swallowing, halitosis, aspiration, bronchospasm, and frequent pneumonias. The first test of choice is a barium swallow. Endoscopy may be complicated by perforation. Treatment includes cricopharyngeal myotomy, with or without a diverticulectomy, depending on the size of the diverticulum. Complications of surgery include infection, recurrence, vocal cord paralysis secondary to injury to the recurrent laryngeal nerve, and esophagocutaneous fistulas. *(Cameron, pp. 28–30)*

79. (E) The indications for surgery for duodenal ulcers include intractability, hemorrhage, obstruction, and perforation. Initial management includes dietary and behavior modification, H2 blockade, proton pump inhibitors and treatment for *H. pylori*. Unlike gastric ulcers, which have a higher incidence of association with malignant processes, duodenal ulcers are rarely secondary to a malignancy and are related to acid production. Surgical approaches include vagotomy (truncal, selective, highly selective), vagotomy combined with antrectomy, or subtotal gastrectomy. There are varying rates of perioperative morbidity and effectiveness reported in the literature. Recurrence rates after vagotomy and pyloroplasty alone approach 30% in long-term follow-up. The complication of dumping after a highly selective vagotomy is significantly lower than truncal vagotomy. A drainage procedure after highly selective vagotomy is unnecessary, and vagal denervation of the proximal stomach reduces receptive relaxation. *(Cameron, pp. 78–81)*

80. (A) Gastrin is the humoral mediator of the gastric phase of secretion. The release of gastrin is stimulated by antral distension, antral protein/amino acids, and by the vagus itself. Gastrin stimulates gastric acid secretion, promotes gut motility, and is a trophic factor for gut mucosa. Secretin is released by duodenal mucosal S cells in response to acid and promotes water and bicarbonate secretion from the pancreas. CCK is released in the gut by intestinal mucosal I cells and stimulates emptying of the gallbladder, increases bile flow, and relaxes the sphincter of Oddi. CCK has a structure very similar to gastrin. (*Sabiston Textbook of Surgery: The Biological Basis of Modern Surgical Practice, pp. 762–764, 834*)

81. **(D)** This patient is presenting with subclavian steal syndrome, which is caused by subclavian stenosis distal to the takeoff of the vertebral artery. Exertion of the extremity causes blood to be shunted away from the brain to the arm, resulting in vertigo or even syncope. These patients usually have diminished radial pulses on the affected side and have other evidence of atherosclerotic disease. A carotid-subclavian bypass is the operation of choice for these patients. (*Current: Diagnosis and Treatment in Vascular Surgery, pp. 105–107*)

82. **(B)** Severe abdominal pain is the hallmark presentation of acute mesenteric ischemia. The pain is often described as being out of proportion to examination. It is most often caused by an embolic event to the SMA. Patients with cardiac arrhythmias are at greater risk for having an embolic event. Nonocclusive mesenteric ischemia is thought to be due to reactive arterial vasoconstriction and is not a surgically correctible disease. CT scan findings of *acute* SMA thrombosis or gas in the bowel wall would necessitate emergency surgery. Option A is incorrect because *chronic* SMA thrombosis may not require an emergency operative intervention. (*Current: Diagnosis and Treatment in Vascular Surgery, pp. 263–272*)

83. **(D)** AAA is most common in the infrarenal aorta (shown by the arrow in Fig. 2-11). Fifteen to twenty-five percent of patients with an AAA have a first degree relative with an AAA. Fifteen percent of patients with an AAA will have an aneurysm of a peripheral vessel. Risk factors include smoking, hypertension, family history, and collagen vascular diseases such as Marfan's syndrome, but it has not been found to be associated with diabetes. The risk of rupture of an AAA > 5 cm is approximately 10% per year. The current standard of care for repair is open surgical repair; however, newer endovascular techniques are emerging. (*Current: Diagnosis and Treatment in Vascular Surgery, pp. 220–229*)

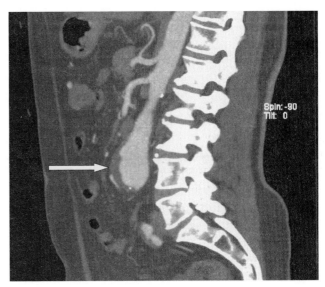

FIG. 2-11 (*Courtesy of H.J. Kim, MD.*)

84. **(A)** This patient is experiencing multiple TIAs associated with carotid artery disease. TIAs last only a few minutes, while RINDs typically resolve after 24 h and strokes result in long-term deficit. The symptoms are typically related to embolic events rather than reduced blood flow. The finding of carotid bruit on examination is more sensitive for coronary artery disease than it is for carotid disease. The initial work-up for these patients should be bilateral carotid duplex ultrasound. Operative repair is indicated for asymptomatic patients with >60% stenosis or symptomatic patients. (*Current: Diagnosis and Treatment in Vascular Surgery, pp. 88–94*)

85. **(B)**

86. **(C)**

Explanations 85 and 86

The patient is experiencing rest pain which is caused by atherosclerosis of the arteries of the leg. Relief with dependent positioning is frequently described by these patients. Initially, work-up of this should include an arterial duplex study of the vessels of the affected leg. Patients with severe disease indicated by rest pain, tissue necrosis, and nonhealing wounds should be considered for arterial bypass. Intermittent claudication is pain with walking or exertion, usually described as an "ache" in the region of the calf. These patients are typically started on a trial of pentoxifylline, which decreases platelet aggregation and increases red cell deformation, and a gradual exercise regimen. They are considered for operative repair when their symptoms severely inhibit their lifestyle. *(Current: Diagnosis and Treatment in Vascular Surgery, pp. 333–341)*

87. **(A)** The Zollinger-Ellison syndrome was described in 1955 in two patients with the triad of gastroduodenal ulcerations, gastric hypersecretion, and non-beta islet cell tumors of the pancreas. Gastrinomas arise from neuroendocrine cells and represent the third most common neuroendocrine tumors (after carcinoids and insulinomas). These tumors are associated with the MEN I. These tumors occur predominantly in the pancreas, duodenum, antrum, and peripancreatic lymph nodes, but can also occur at distant sites like the ovary. Isolated gastrinomas are found in 50% of cases and multiple tumors in 50%; however, when gastrinomas are found in association with MEN I, there is a higher incidence of multiple tumors. Tumors are malignant in 50%, with metastases to the regional lymph nodes and the liver. Once the diagnosis has been established, tumor localization can be achieved with Indium-labeled octreotide scan, CT with fine cuts through the pancreas, ultrasound, MRI, or selective angiography. None of these tests are highly sensitive. Often the tumors are not localized until the time of exploration and intraoperative directed ultrasonography. *(Cameron, pp. 83–87)*

88. **(D)**

89. **(A)**

Explanations 88 and 89

Gastric adenocarcinoma is associated with a dismal overall prognosis, with long-term survival seen only in patients with early stage disease. Surgical resection remains the mainstay of potentially curative therapy, with poor responses to chemotherapy in the majority of clinical trials. Patients often present with vague epigastric discomfort, occult GI bleeding/anemia, anorexia, weight loss, and even hematemesis/vomiting. Patients are staged with endoscopic ultrasound, which is the most effective imaging modality for determining T and N stage. CT may also be useful for determining nodal metastases but is more accurate for determining distant metastases (liver). Antral tumors may have a better prognosis than more proximal gastric tumors, with a decreased incidence of nodal metastases. Five-year survival rates for stage I disease is excellent, approaching 80–90% in both the Western countries and in Asia. However, 5-year survival rates are dismal for stage III and stage IV disease. Most Western series report overall 5-year survival rates for gastric cancer of 10–21%.

In contrast to gastric adenocarcinoma in the United States, the incidence of gastric lymphoma is rising. Gastric lymphoma accounts for two-thirds of gastrointestinal lymphomas. Symptoms are similar to gastric adenocarcinoma, but obstruction, perforation, and massive bleeding are very uncommon symptoms. Because gastric lymphoma spreads by submucosal infiltration, mucosal biopsies at the time of upper endoscopy can often be nondiagnostic. Repeated biopsies to obtain submucosal tissue are needed to establish a diagnosis. Treatment protocols vary among institutions, but most often center on chemotherapy; surgical resection of isolated or localized gastric lymphoma can be curative, but is rarely seen. Fortunately, survival rates for gastric lymphoma is much better than those seen in gastric adenocarcinoma, with cure rates of 70% seen in patients with stage IE and IIE disease treated with chemotherapy alone. *(The M.D. Anderson Surgical Oncology Handbook, pp. 120–131, 137–139)*

90. **(A)** Barrett's esophagus is related to GERD. It is found proximal to the (LES) and is thought to be a result of constant acidic exposure. It is a condition where the normal esophageal squamous cell epithelium is replaced by columnar epithelium, similar to intestinal metaplasia. A single biopsy is all that is needed to confirm diagnosis. In fact, many biopsies should be taken during endoscopy, if the diagnosis is suspected, in an effort to find dysplasia. The risk

of malignant degeneration is the most important risk associated with Barrett's esophagus. *(Schwartz, pp. 1116, 1117)*

91. **(B)** Diffuse esophageal spasm is diagnosed by the characteristic corkscrew appearance on contrast esophagram. The bird's beak pattern is found in achalasia. Leiomyosarcomas usually appear as punch out abnormalities on contrast studies. *(Schwartz, p. 1127)*

92. **(D)** The main blood supply to the stomach comes from the right gastric artery (from the hepatic artery), the left gastric artery (from the celiac axis), the right gastroepiploic artery (from the gastroduodenal artery), the left gastroepiploic (from the splenic artery), and the short gastric arteries from the splenic artery. *(Schwartz, p. 1182)*

93. **(D)** Zenker's diverticulum is a cricopharyngeal diverticulum. Patients often present with dysphagia and regurgitation of undigested food. It tends to enlarge over time as the muscle compliance decreases. The diagnosis is established by a contrast study. Endoscopy in these patients is often difficult and carries a significant risk of perforation. *(Schwartz, p. 1125)*

94. **(C)** Duodenal ulcers are usually associated with hypersecretion of acid, whereas gastric ulcers may be related to breakdown of the mucosal protective mechanisms or to malignancy. Type I gastric ulcers are the most common. They are usually associated with altered mucosal defense and not hypersecretion of acid. Type II gastric ulcers are caused by a duodenal ulcer and the resulting pyloric obstruction. Type III gastric ulcers are found proximal to the pylorus and are associated with hypersecretion and duodenal ulcers. *H. pylori* is found in 95% of duodenal and 80% of gastric ulcer patients. However, only 10% of people who carry the bacteria actually manifest ulcer disease. Gastric ulcer patients tend to be older than duodenal ulcer patients. *(Schwartz, pp. 1191–1193)*

95. **(D)** The liver is divided into eight segments based on functional units according to Couinaud's nomenclature (see Fig. 2-12). Segment I is the caudate lobe. Segments II, III,

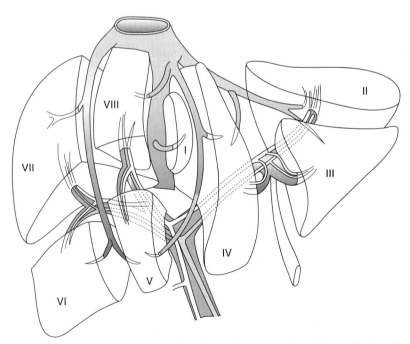

FIG. 2-12 The functional division of the liver and segments according to Courinaud's nomenclature. (*Reproduced, with permission, from Zinner MJ, Schwartz SI, Ellis H, Ashley SW, McFadded DW. "Maingot s Abdominal Operations, 10th ed." Stamford, CT: Appleton & Lange, 1997.*)

and IV are in the left lobe while segments V–VIII are in the right lobe. *(Schwartz, pp. 1395, 1396)*

96. **(E)** Because the small bowel is responsible for a large amount of enteral absorption, patients with ileostomies often have problems with dehydration, electrolyte disturbances, and malnutrition. They should actively try to maintain their hydration with adequate oral intake as well as the use of antidiarrheal medications to slow transit times. There is no increase in malignant risk with either a colostomy or an ileostomy. A properly created ileostomy should be protruding from the abdominal wall to help decrease the amount of ileal contents that actually touch the skin. *(Schwartz, p. 1328)*

97. **(E)** Carcinoid syndrome is seen in fewer than 10% of patients with metastatic carcinoid disease. It is seen in patients with elevated serotonin levels, which is metabolized by the liver. Thus, only patients with massive hepatic metastasis or with tumors that bypass the hepatic filter show symptoms. 5-hydroxyindoleacetic acid (5-HIAA) levels can be tested in the urine to give the diagnosis (urinary VMA is indicative of a pheochromocytoma). Symptoms include flushing, diarrhea, right heart failure, and asthma. Weight loss and liver failure are uncommon symptoms. *(Schwartz, p. 1246)*

98. **(C)** Most patients have a change in their digestive habits after gastrectomy. These symptoms are actually related to the vagotomy done with the operation. The majority of patients learn to manage their symptoms, with only a small amount requiring surgical intervention. Dumping syndrome is associated with abdominal pain, nausea, vomiting, dizziness, and palpitations related to the quick hyperosmolar emptying into the small intestine. These symptoms can be managed by eating small, low carbohydrate meals throughout the day. Postvagotomy diarrhea is related to the rapid transit of unconjugated bile salts and is effectively treated with cholestyramine. Proton pump inhibitors are not a useful therapy for alkaline reflux. *(Schwartz, pp. 1211, 1212)*

99. **(E)** This patient has developed a DVT of her left leg. This is a complication following surgery that can be prevented, in part, by the use of subcutaneous heparin and sequential compression devices. Risk factors for developing DVTs include female gender, obesity, orthopedic surgery, use of oral contraceptives, smoking, and long periods of being sedentary. Diagnosis can be made by, among other techniques, venous duplex Doppler ultrasonography and contrast venography. D-dimer testing has a high negative predictive value. A negative D-dimer test helps to rule out the diagnosis of DVT, but a positive D-dimer should lead to further definitive testing. *(Current: Diagnosis and Treatment in Vascular Surgery, pp. 375–381; Sabiston Textbook of Surgery: The Biological Basis of Modern Surgical Practice, pp. 1421–1435)*

100. **(A)** Wound infection is a complication of surgery that can lead to a great deal of morbidity and longer hospital stays. Prevention of wound infection includes perioperative antibiotics, which should be at their peak tissue concentration at the time of skin incision. This means they should be given at least 30 min prior to incision. Patients who have other infections, such as urinary tract infections, are at increased risk for wound infection. Bowel surgery exposes the wound to normal intestinal flora, the most common being *Bacteroides*. Washing hands between patients is an essential part of preventing spread of infectious pathogens between patients. Once a wound is infected, it must be opened and drained. Antibiotic therapy alone is not adequate. *(Greenfield, pp. 79–81)*

101. **(C)** The patient presents with asymptomatic cholelithiasis (shown by the arrow in Fig. 2-13). In the absence of symptoms or findings of ductal obstruction on ultrasound, a cholecystectomy is not routinely performed. However, certain patients are at greater risk for developing complications. Patients with stones greater than 2 cm in size are at greater risk for obstruction. Also, the finding of a porcelain gallbladder on CT should raise the suspicion of carcinoma and a cholecystectomy should be recommended. *(Greenfield, pp. 1004–1059)*

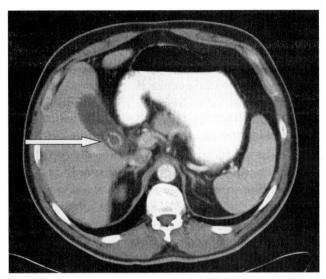

FIG. 2-13 (*Courtesy of H.J. Kim, MD.*)

102. **(B)** Knowledge of gallbladder anatomy is essential during laparoscopic cholecystectomy. Careful identification of the structures that define the triangle of Calot helps ensure that the cystic duct and artery are properly ligated and divided and that the common bile and common hepatic ducts are spared. The borders of the triangle of Calot are the cystic duct, the common hepatic duct, and the inferior border of the liver. The cystic artery and the right hepatic artery are anatomic features found within this triangle. (*Greenfield, pp. 1004–1059*)

103. **(B)** Acute cholecystitis necessitates prompt operation. Diagnosis is essential in proper management and prevention of progression to ascending cholangitis. Patients with acute cholecystitis often have pain similar to that of cholelithiasis, but longer in duration. Patients usually have a normal WBC; however, those who are immunocompromised or early along in the course of disease may not. Ultrasound findings include a thickened gallbladder wall, presence of cholecystic fluid and, often, stones, sludge, or dilated ducts. A positive sonographic Murphy's sign can help confirm the diagnosis, but the absence of one does not negate the diagnosis. In the presence of acute cholecystitis, a HIDA scan usually shows very slow uptake by the gallbladder. (*Greenfield, pp. 1004–1059*)

104. **(D)** This patient has a gastrinoma, seen in Zollinger-Ellison syndrome and should also be evaluated for possible multiple endocrine neoplasia I. Gastrin is a gastrointestinal hormone that is released from the antral G cells of the stomach to regulate acid secretion by the gastric parietal cells. It is released when the stomach gets the signal that it is needed to initiate the digestion process. It also acts to stimulate chief cells to secrete pepsinogen and to increase gastric mucosal blood flow. Known stimulants for the release of gastrin include vagal stimulation, calcium, alcohols in the stomach, proteins/amino acids in the stomach, antral distension, and gastric pH greater than three. Antral pH less than 2.0 and somatostatin inhibit gastrin release. Secretin has no effect or decreases gastrin levels in healthy patients, but increases gastrin release in patients with Zollinger-Ellison syndrome. Glucagon has little to no effect on gastrin release. (*Greenfield, pp. 745–747*)

105. **(D)** The primitive gut begins to form during the fourth week of gestation. The gut is derived from the endoderm. The distal anus is derived from ectoderm. For embryologic purposes, the gastrointestinal tract is divided into the foregut, midgut, and hindgut. This question focuses on the colon, which is derived partially from the midgut (which gets its blood supply from the SMA) and the hindgut (which is supplied by the inferior mesenteric artery, IMA). During development, the bowel herniates into the extraembryonic space during which time it elongates and develops. It also undergoes a 270° counterclockwise rotation around the SMA. Around the 10th week of gestation the structure returns to the abdomen. (*Greenfield, pp. 1063–1069*)

BIBLIOGRAPHY

American College of Surgeons. *Advanced Trauma Life Support Program for Doctors,* 6th ed. Chicago, IL: American College of Surgeons, 1997.

Cameron, JL (ed). *Current Surgical Therapy,* 8th ed. St. Louis, MO: C. V. Mosby, 2004.

Greenfield LJ, Mulholland MW, Oldham KT, et al. (eds). *Surgery: Scientific Principles and Practice,* 3d ed. Philadelphia, PA: Lippincott, Williams & Wilkins, 2001.

Feig, BW, Berger DH, Fuhrman GM (eds). *The M.D. Anderson Surgical Oncology Handbook,* 3d ed. Philadelphia, PA: Lippincott, Williams & Wilkins, 2002.

Gordon PH, Nivatvongs S (eds). *Principles and Practice of Surgery for the Colon, Rectum, and Anus,* 2d ed. St. Louis, MO: Quality Medical Publishing, 1999.

Townsend CM, Beauchamp RD, Evers BM, et al. (eds). *Sabiston Textbook of Surgery: The Biological Basis of Modern Surgical Practice,* 17th ed. Philadelphia, PA: W.B. Saunders, 2004.

Dean RH, Yao JS, Brewster DC (eds). *Current Diagnosis and Treatment in Vascular Surgery,* New York, NY: McGraw-Hill, 1995.

Schwartz SI, Shires GT, Spencer FC, et al. (eds). *Principles of Surgery,* 7th ed. New York, NY: McGraw-Hill, 1999.

Mann CV, Russell RCG, Williams NS. *Bailey & Love's Short Practice of Surgery,* 22d ed. London: Chapman & Hall, 1995.

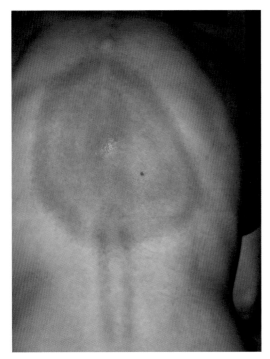

FIG. 1-7 (Question 95)

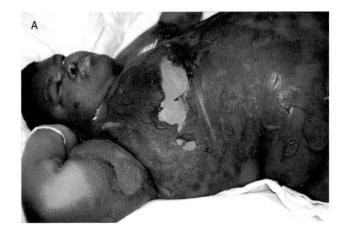

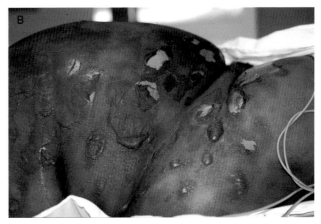

FIG. 1-8 (Question 122)

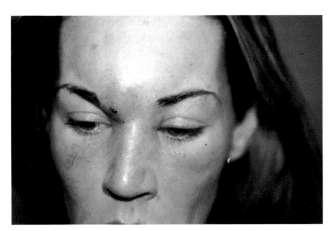

FIG. 1-10 (Question 126)

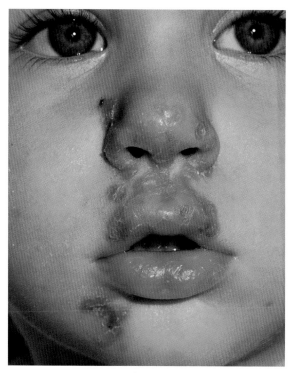

FIG. 3-2 (Question 30 and 31)

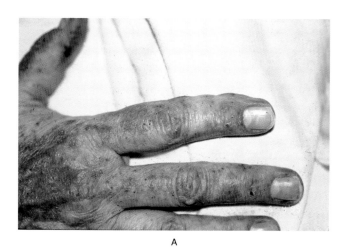

A

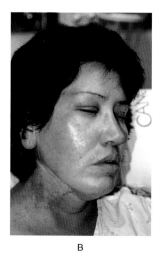

B

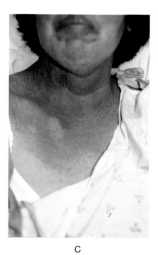

C

FIG. 9-3 (Question 28 and 29)

CHAPTER 3

Pediatrics
Questions

1. A newborn male is brought to you in the neonatal intensive care unit (NICU). On physical examination, you notice that the infant has deficient abdominal musculature and undescended testes. Your suspicion is high for a certain condition. You order a voiding cystourethrogram that shows posterior urethral valves. You diagnose the child with:

   (A) VATER association
   (B) Cushing's triad
   (C) Potter syndrome
   (D) Jones criteria
   (E) Eagle-Barrett syndrome

2. What is the most sensitive indicator of pneumonia in a child?

   (A) tachycardia
   (B) tachypnea
   (C) hypotonia
   (D) vomiting
   (E) coughing

3. A 12-month-old male child is brought to your office for a well child examination and immunizations. You have been following the child since delivery and are aware that he has acquired immune deficiency syndrome (AIDS) and a markedly reduced T-cell count. Which of the following vaccinations should not be given?

   (A) diphtheria, tetanus, and acellular pertussis (DTaP)
   (B) diphtheria tetanus (dT)
   (C) hepatitis B
   (D) injectable polio vaccine (IPV)
   (E) varicella

Questions 4 and 5

While working in the emergency room you see a 14-month-old boy brought in with apparent leg pain. His parents tell you that he has recently been learning to walk and that this injury is the result of a fall. You obtain the following x-ray (see Fig. 3-1).

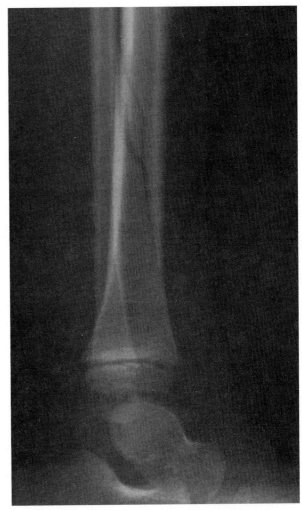

FIG. 3-1 (*Source: Schwartz DT, Reisdorff EJ.* Emergency Radiology. *New York, NY, p.181.*)

4. What is your interpretation of the x-ray?

   (A) dislocation of the ankle
   (B) a "chip" fracture of the proximal tibia
   (C) a spiral fracture of the distal tibia
   (D) a buckle fracture involving the distal tibia and fibula
   (E) a transverse fracture of the distal tibia

5. What is the mechanism that likely resulted in this injury?

   (A) twisting on a planted leg while learning to walk
   (B) forced rotation of the leg by another person (child abuse)
   (C) fall from a piece of furniture or stairs
   (D) inversion of the ankle
   (E) motor vehicle accident while not restrained in a car seat

Questions 6 and 7

A 16-year-old sexually active woman is being seen in the emergency department. She is complaining of vaginal discharge. She has a temperature of 99.5°F, but is otherwise well. On pelvic examination you see a mucopurulent cervical discharge with scant blood. Samples of the discharge are sent to the lab for culture. There are no cervical ulcers noted. She does not have any medical allergies.

6. Which of the following is the most common sexually transmitted disease in adolescents?

   (A) herpes simplex virus (HSV)
   (B) chlamydia
   (C) gonorrhea
   (D) human immunodeficiency virus (HIV)
   (E) syphilis

7. For this patient, what is the most appropriate regimen for initial therapy?

   (A) azithromycin (Zithromax) 1 g orally once and ceftriaxone (Rocephin) 125-mg intramuscular (IM) once
   (B) amoxicillin/clavulanic acid (Augmentin) 500 mg orally twice a day for 7 days and ceftriaxone 125-mg IM once

   (C) metronidazole (Flagyl) 500 mg orally twice a day for 7 days and amoxicillin/clavulanic acid 500 mg orally twice a day for 7 days
   (D) ceftriaxone 125-mg IM once
   (E) azithromycin 1 g orally once and metronidazole 500 mg orally for 7 days

8. What is the most common cause of injury in the first year of life?

   (A) falls down stairs
   (B) child abuse
   (C) motor vehicle collisions
   (D) dog bites
   (E) other children

Questions 9 through 13

You are called to see a newborn in the nursery because the nurse is concerned that the baby may have Down syndrome.

9. Which of the following signs is associated with Down syndrome?

   (A) café-au-lait spots
   (B) high arched palate
   (C) ambiguous genitalia
   (D) hypotonia
   (E) club feet

10. After confirming that the child does indeed have Down syndrome, the parents ask you what problems their baby may have in the future. With which of the following is the infant most likely to have problems?

   (A) renal failure
   (B) hypothyroidism
   (C) osteoporosis
   (D) hemophilia
   (E) lens dislocation

11. The infant begins to have progressively large amounts of bilious emesis. The infant feeds well and has only a small amount of abdominal distension. What is the most likely diagnosis?

(A) pyloric stenosis

(B) Hirschsprung disease

(C) biliary atresia

(D) duodenal atresia

(E) milk protein allergy

12. If you were to perform an abdominal x-ray, what is the most likely finding that would be seen?

(A) "double-bubble" sign

(B) scimitar sign

(C) normal gas patterns

(D) free fluid in the abdomen

(E) pneumatosis intestinalis

13. What is the most common central nervous system (CNS) complication of Down syndrome?

(A) seizures

(B) hydrocephalus

(C) microcalcifications

(D) berry aneurysms

(E) mental retardation

Questions 14 and 15

A father and son come to your office because of persistent diarrhea. They relate the presence of watery diarrhea for over 2 weeks. They noted that the diarrhea began after returning from a Boy Scout camping trip in the Rocky Mountains. The diarrhea has waxed and waned for 2 weeks. It is nonbloody and foul smelling. They have had increased flatulence and mild abdominal cramping.

14. What is the most likely etiology of their diarrhea?

(A) Enterotoxigenic *Escherichia coli*

(B) *Giardia lamblia*

(C) *Rickettsia rickettsii* (Rocky Mountain spotted fever [RMSF])

(D) rotavirus

(E) Norwalk virus

15. What would be the most appropriate treatment?

(A) oral ciprofloxacin

(B) oral metronidazole

(C) bismuth subsalicylate (Pepto-Bismol)

(D) an antidiarrheal agent only

(E) oral rehydration only

16. A 5-year-old male is admitted to the hospital following a 3-week history of spiking fevers and fatigue. Your examination reveals pale mucous membranes and skin. You also find splenomegaly. You are concerned about a possible malignancy. What is the most common malignancy of childhood?

(A) medulloblastoma

(B) Wilms tumor

(C) leukemia

(D) neuroblastoma

(E) rhabdomyosarcoma

17. While in the emergency department you see a 3-week-old infant. The mother says that the child felt warm earlier in the day and has not been eating very well. The infant has a temperature of 100.9°F and has mildly decreased tone.

What is the most appropriate initial management?

(A) Give acetaminophen and reassess in a few hours.

(B) Draw a blood culture, recommend increased fluid intake, and follow-up for reexamination in 24 h in the primary pediatrician's office.

(C) Admit to the hospital and perform a full "sepsis workup."

(D) Draw a blood culture, give a shot of ceftriaxone (Rocephin) to cover for any infections and follow-up in 24–48 h.

(E) Get a urine culture and begin trimethoprim/sulfamethoxazole (Septra).

Questions 18 and 19

You see a 2-month-old infant in the emergency department for vomiting. The mother says that the baby has been spitting up more over the past few days and has become more irritable. She denies any fever, diarrhea, or change in formula. The mother tells you that there is a family history of "heartburn" and that her other children have all spit up. The infant has some emesis in the emergency department that seems to be formula mixed with some bile. The infant is intermittently irritable and sleepy.

18. What is the most concerning diagnosis that this could be?

    (A) biliary atresia
    (B) malrotation
    (C) pyloric stenosis
    (D) imperforate anus
    (E) diaphragmatic hernia

19. Which of the following would be the most appropriate initial test?

    (A) abdominal computed tomography (CT)
    (B) barium enema
    (C) abdominal ultrasound
    (D) upper GI series with small-bowel follow through
    (E) radionuclide scan

20. An 8-year-old male presents to your office complaining of a 1-week history of painful knee and elbow joints. On examination, you find a painful, hot, and swollen knee. He also has multiple erythematous macules with pale centers on his trunk and extremities. The lab work you order reveals elevated antistreptococcal antibodies. You diagnose the child with acute rheumatic fever (ARF). Which of the following is true regarding ARF?

    (A) The child must currently have a fever.
    (B) The child must have arthritis.
    (C) The presence of a group A streptococcal (GAS) infection must be documented.
    (D) The child may have chorea alone.
    (E) The child is contagious.

Questions 21 and 22

On a Monday morning you see a 12-year-old otherwise healthy boy in the emergency department. The parents brought the boy in because they noticed that he started to have an abnormal gait in the past few days. He seems to be shuffling his feet. The boy complains that his legs feel heavy and are tingling. He relates that his arms feel fine. His past history is significant for attention deficit/hyperactivity disorder (ADHD) for which he is taking methylphenidate. He denies trauma or taking any other medicines or drugs. On examination, he is afebrile with normal vital signs. His entire physical examination is normal with the exception of the examination of his lower extremities. He has 3/5 strength throughout both of his lower extremities with a normal muscle mass. His joints all have a full range of motion, without any pain or swelling. His reflexes are absent and he describes some paresthesias of his feet and ankles.

21. What is the most likely diagnosis?

    (A) methylphenidate toxicity
    (B) acute inflammatory demyelinating polyneuropathy (Guillain-Barré syndrome)
    (C) acute poliomyelitis
    (D) malingering (school avoidance)
    (E) polymyositis

22. Which of the following is the most appropriate initial management plan?

    (A) hospitalization and close observation for progression of his weakness
    (B) high dose corticosteroids
    (C) gastric lavage and activated charcoal
    (D) outpatient family counseling
    (E) plasmaphoresis

23. You are called to see a 12-h-old male infant who was born to a 19-year-old G_1 woman with no prenatal care. She presented to the emergency room completely dilated and crowning. The baby was born minutes later. On examination, the baby is febrile and tachypneic. A chest

x-ray (CXR) confirms the presence of pneumonia. What is the most likely infectious agent?

(A) group B *Streptococcus* (GBS)
(B) HSV
(C) *E. coli*
(D) respiratory syncytial virus
(E) *Streptococcus pneumoniae*

Questions 24 and 25

A 4-year-old is brought to your office by his mother for evaluation. She is concerned because the child has been spiking fevers and pulling on his left ear. Your examination reveals a bulging and erythematous tympanic membrane.

24. What is the most common bacterial cause of otitis media in childhood?

(A) *Hemophilus influenza*, type B (HIB)
(B) *Moraxella catarrhalis*
(C) *mycoplasma pneumonia*
(D) group A *Streptococcus*
(E) *S. pneumoniae*

25. You determine that the child should receive antibiotics. The initial antibiotic of choice should be?

(A) amoxicillin
(B) azithromycin (Zithromax)
(C) erythromycin
(D) trimethoprim/sulfamethoxazole (Septra)
(E) tetracycline

26. Which of the following has a carrier state that is not considered contagious?

(A) *E. coli*
(B) HSV
(C) *Chlamydia trachomatis*
(D) group A *Streptococcus*
(E) respiratory syncitial virus

27. What is the most common cause of aseptic meningitis in childhood?

(A) mycobacterium tuberculosis
(B) HSV
(C) *C. trachomatis*
(D) respiratory syncitial virus
(E) nonpolio enteroviruses

28. You are working in the emergency department and are called to the bedside of a 3-month-old male infant to assist with a lumbar puncture. The infant presented with increasing lethargy and fever. Meningitis is suspected. Which of the following is the most common cause of meningitis in a 3-month-old infant?

(A) GBS
(B) HSV
(C) group A *Streptococcus*
(D) *S. pneumoniae*
(E) *E. coli*

29. You are working in a community clinic on a Native American reservation. A mother brings in her 8-year-old son for an ophthalmic evaluation. On examination, you find bilateral corneal ulceration and decreased visual acuity. What is the most common infectious cause of blindness in the world?

(A) HSV
(B) *C. trachomatis*
(C) group A *Streptococcus*
(D) *S. pneumoniae*
(E) *E. coli*

Questions 30 and 31

A 4-year-old girl is brought in to the office by her mother. She developed chicken pox about 6 days ago. She appeared to be recovering well but mother became concerned because she was persistently scratching at several of the lesions and they were not healing. On examination the child is afebrile and generally well appearing. On examination of her skin you see the following image (see Fig. 3-2).

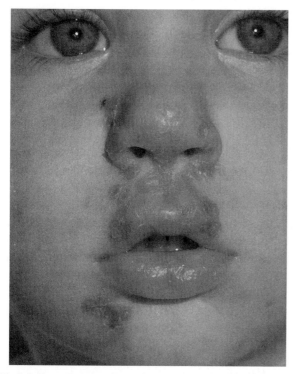

FIG. 3-2 Also see color plate. (*Source: Fitzpatrick TB, Johnson RA, Wolff K, et al.* Color Atlas and Synopsis of Clinical Dermatology, *4th ed. New York, NY: McGraw-Hill, 2001, p. 587.*)

30. What is the most likely current diagnosis?

    (A) tinea corporis
    (B) impetigo
    (C) warts
    (D) contact dermatitis
    (E) reactivated chicken pox

31. What is the most likely responsible agent?

    (A) *Trichophyton rubrum*
    (B) poison ivy

    (C) human papilloma virus
    (D) group A *Streptococcus*
    (E) varicella virus

Questions 32 through 34

32. A well appearing 6-year-old presents to your office with a chief complaint of bruising. The parents report that the child had a cold 2 weeks ago but completely recovered. The child is sitting on the examining table, in no distress, discussing her favorite cartoons. On examination, you find mucosal bleeding and bruises on the child's arms and chest. You order a complete blood count (CBC) that has the following results: WBC 12,000, hemoglobin 11 G/DL and a platelet count of 45,000. What is the most likely cause of this child's bleeding and bruising?

    (A) immune thrombocytopenic purpura (ITP)
    (B) Henoch-Schönlein purpura (HSP)
    (C) Evans syndrome
    (D) meningococcemia
    (E) hemolytic uremic syndrome (HUS)

33. After discussing various options with a regional pediatric hematologist and the patient's parents, your most appropriate initial management would be:

    (A) a platelet transfusion at the regional children's hospital
    (B) an IM dose of methylprednisolone as an outpatient
    (C) reassurance to the parents with close outpatient follow-up
    (D) intravenous immunoglobulin (IVIG) at the regional children's hospital
    (E) bone marrow biopsy at the regional children's hospital

34. Following your initial evaluation and treatment, you see the child for follow-up in 1 week. She continues to appear well but still has obvious purpura and her platelet count is now 17,000. All other cell lines are normal. Of the options listed below, what is your most appropriate management at this time?

(A) admission to the regional children's hospital for a platelet transfusion

(B) admission to the children's hospital for a splenectomy

(C) reassurance to the parents and close outpatient follow-up

(D) admission to the children's hospital for IVIG and steroids

(E) whole-blood transfusion with several hours of observation to ensure that there is no transfusion reaction

35. A 4-year-old child is brought to your office because of a sudden onset of irritability, weakness, and pallor. The mother tells you that both of her children have been experiencing episodes of vomiting and diarrhea. Your physical examination reveals a blood pressure (BP) of 115/80, dry mucus membranes, petechia, and diffuse abdominal pain. The following lab work is obtained:

Urinalysis: microscopic hematuria and proteinuria
Blood urea nitrogen (BUN)/Cr: 20/1.0 mg/dL
Hemoglobin: 7 g/dL
Peripheral blood smear: fragmented red blood cells
Prothrombin time, partial thromboplastin time: normal
Coombs: negative

What is the most likely diagnosis?

(A) ITP
(B) Henoch-Schönlein purpura
(C) Evans syndrome
(D) meningococcemia
(E) HUS

36. A mildly mentally retarded 9-year-old girl is brought to your office for acne. On examination, she does not actually have acne but has small flesh colored papules along her nasolabial fold. Her past history is significant for having had a seizure last year. Which condition would she most likely have?

(A) Sturge-Weber syndrome
(B) neurofibromatosis, type 1 (von Recklinghausen disease)
(C) tuberous sclerosis
(D) CHARGE association
(E) Beckwith-Wiedemann syndrome

37. Which of the following conditions usually causes hypoglycemia at birth?

(A) Sturge-Weber syndrome
(B) neurofibromatosis, type 1 (von Recklinghausen disease)
(C) tuberous sclerosis
(D) CHARGE association
(E) Beckwith-Wiedemann syndrome

38. A 10-month-old infant has a dysplastic right external ear, some preauricular tags, and a small notch (coloboma) in the iris and lower lid. Which condition does he likely have?

(A) Sturge-Weber syndrome
(B) neurofibromatosis, type 1 (von Recklinghausen disease)
(C) tuberous sclerosis
(D) CHARGE association
(E) Beckwith-Wiedemann syndrome

Questions 39 and 40

A term infant male is born after an uncomplicated vaginal delivery. The mother's prenatal labs were negative with the exception of being GBS positive at 36 weeks gestation. The mother received two doses of ampicillin prior to delivery and did not have a fever. The infant had APGAR scores of 9 at 1 min and 9 at 5 min. The infant was brought to the newborn nursery and appears well.

39. The most appropriate management of the infant would be which of the following:

(A) Draw a CBC and blood culture, but do not start empiric antibiotics.

(B) Give the baby a prophylactic dose of ampicillin.

(C) Routine care.

(D) Cultures of blood, urine, and spinal fluid and wait for culture results before starting antibiotics.

(E) Cultures of blood, urine, and spinal fluid and begin empiric antibiotics before getting culture results.

40. The father tells you that he has hemophilia. His wife neither has hemophilia nor is a carrier. What does this mean for the baby?

(A) The baby has a 50% chance of having hemophilia.

(B) The baby neither has hemophilia nor is a carrier of the hemophilia gene.

(C) The baby is a carrier of the hemophilia gene but does not have the disease.

(D) The baby has a 25% chance of being a carrier for hemophilia.

(E) The baby has a 50% chance of being a carrier for hemophilia.

41. A mother brings her 4-year-old son to your office, relating that he fell earlier that morning while at the playground. She says that the boy tripped over another child and landed on his outstretched hands. On examination the boy has some mild swelling around his left wrist, and he says that it hurts when you palpate it. What is the most appropriate next step?

(A) Call the department of Children's Protective Services to investigate the accident.

(B) Attempt a nursemaid's elbow reduction.

(C) Perform anterior-posterior (AP) and lateral x-rays of the left wrist and elbow.

(D) Wrap the wrist in an ACE wrap, and put the arm in a sling.

(E) Order an MRI of the wrist looking for a growth plate injury.

Questions 42 through 45

You see a $3^1/_2$-year-old child in the emergency department who has had fever for the past week. The parents relate that their son has some swollen glands, fever, and now seems to be getting a rash on his arms. On examination, you find an uncomfortable appearing young boy whose vital signs are normal with the exception of a temperature of 104°F. You note that he has a red posterior oropharynx with dry, cracked lips. His tympanic membranes are normal. He has mild conjunctival injection bilaterally without any discharge. His chest is clear, and his heart sounds are normal. He does not have any hepatosplenomegaly. His has a lacy, confluent macular rash on his chest and upper arms, with mild peeling of the tips of his fingers.

42. What is the most likely diagnosis?

(A) group A β-hemolytic streptococcal pharyngitis

(B) hand-foot-mouth disease (coxsackie viral infection)

(C) Kawasaki disease

(D) ITP

(E) erythema infectiosum (parvovirus B-19 infection)

43. Which laboratory result would be most consistent with the diagnosis?

(A) an elevated platelet count

(B) a positive rapid strep test

(C) a low platelet count

(D) elevated viral IgM titers

(E) a low erythrocyte sedimentation rate (ESR)

44. What is the most appropriate treatment at this point?

(A) no medicine is needed, only supportive care.

(B) an IM dose of long acting penicillin (LA-Bicillin)

(C) oral Acyclovir

(D) IVIG

(E) topical lidocaine gel 1%

45. What is the most worrisome complication of this disease?

    (A) encephalitis
    (B) coronary artery aneurysm
    (C) cardiac valve dysfunction
    (D) intracerebral hemorrhage
    (E) hemorrhagic stroke

Questions 46 and 47

You see a 3-week-old infant in your office for an acute visit. She was born via spontaneous vaginal delivery following a term, uncomplicated prenatal course. The parents are concerned because they have seen some streaks of blood in her diaper over the past few days. The infant's stools have been soft and not difficult to pass. The parents relate that she is eating 2 oz every 2 h of a cow's milk based formula.

46. What is the carbohydrate source in most infant formula?

    (A) casein
    (B) lactose
    (C) human milk fortifier
    (D) coconut oil
    (E) soy oil

47. What is the most likely cause of the blood in her stool?

    (A) Meckel diverticulum
    (B) group B streptococcal colitis
    (C) cow's milk protein intolerance
    (D) pseudomembranous colitis
    (E) lactose intolerance

Questions 48 through 50

In January, you see an 18-month-old boy in the middle of the night in the pediatric emergency department. The father relates that 1 h ago his son started coughing. The father describes the cough as barking ("seal" like). The child has mild stridor at rest, but otherwise is not in respiratory distress. His respiratory rate is 45 breaths per minute. He has a temperature of 103.4°F.

48. What is the most likely diagnosis?

    (A) epiglottitis
    (B) croup
    (C) pneumonia
    (D) sinusitis
    (E) bronchiolitis

49. What is the most common etiology of this illness in children?

    (A) *H. influenza*, type B
    (B) respiratory syncitial virus
    (C) influenza, type B
    (D) parainfluenza, types 1 and 2
    (E) *S. pneumoniae*

50. What is the most common x-ray finding in this illness?

    (A) swollen adenoids
    (B) the "thumb" sign
    (C) a lobar pulmonary infiltrate
    (D) a deviated tracheal air column
    (E) the "steeple" sign

Questions 51 and 52

51. Parents bring their 12-year-old son to your clinic for evaluation. The child states that he gets teased a lot in school because of his short stature. His weight and height are below the 10th percentile for his age. His parents are of average height. Following your physical examination, you determine that he has tanner stage 1 development and his bone age is that of a 9-year-old male. His examination is otherwise normal. What is the most likely diagnosis?

    (A) familial short stature
    (B) constitutional growth delay
    (C) deficiency in growth hormone
    (D) chronic renal failure
    (E) vitamin D deficiency

52. Which of the following is a true statement regarding the assessment of a child with short stature?

(A) An advanced bone age indicates that the child's final height will be greater than his peers.

(B) A slower growth velocity means the child will have more time to "catch up."

(C) A spot growth hormone (GH) level is a good test in screening for growth hormone deficiency.

(D) somatomedin-C (insulin-like growth factor-1) will be low in a child with growth hormone deficiency.

(E) The most common cause of short stature in children is chronic renal disease.

Questions 53 and 54

A mother brings her 15-year-old son in for a preparticipation sports physical examination. She feels that her son has not yet undergone pubertal changes and that makes her concerned.

53. Which of the following is a true statement regarding puberty delay?

(A) The onset of puberty in males is earlier than that in females.

(B) A puberty delay is not considered pathologic unless accompanied by short stature.

(C) Hypothyroidism can be a cause of pubertal delay.

(D) Males do not have a true adrenarche as females do.

(E) The most common cause for pubertal delay is pan-hypopituitarism.

54. Which of the following physical examination findings is usually the first sign of the onset of puberty in males?

(A) increased testicular volume

(B) increased skeletal muscle mass

(C) deepening of the voice

(D) increased facial hair

(E) physiologic gynecomastia

Questions 55 and 56

A mother brings her 2½-year-old daughter to your office for evaluation of frequent urination. The mother relates that the daughter seems to be urinating more frequently, up to 8–10 times in a day, over the past week. The girl complains of pain when she urinates, but the urine does not have any different odor to it. The mother says that the girl otherwise seems fine and still loves to take her bubble bath at night. The girl does not have a fever, weight loss, diarrhea, or vomiting.

55. What is the most appropriate next step in evaluating this girl?

(A) fingerstick blood sample for random serum glucose

(B) plain abdominal x-ray

(C) clean urine sample for urinalysis and urine culture

(D) vaginal examination for discharge and cultures

(E) synchronized serum and urine osmolality

56. What is the most likely diagnosis?

(A) pyelonephritis

(B) chemical urethritis

(C) retained vaginal foreign body

(D) type 1 diabetes mellitus

(E) diabetes insipidus

57. A mother relates seeing worms in her 3-year-old's stool. She describes them as 1-cm long white threads that seemed to be moving. What is the most likely infectious etiology for this finding?

(A) *Ascaris lumbricoides*

(B) *Diphyllobothrium latum*

(C) *Taenia Solium*

(D) *Toxocara canis*

(E) *Enterobius vermicularis*

58. Deficiency of which of the following is the most common nutritional cause of anemia?

(A) calcium

(B) vitamin B$_{12}$ deficiency

(C) iodine

(D) iron

(E) vitamin C

59. A 9-month-old male infant is brought to your office for evaluation of new skin lesions. The mother tells you that she recently had to return back to work, and the child is now in day care. He has since developed new erythematous facial plaques (see Fig. 3-3). She also reports that the child has been irritable with chronic diarrhea. On examination, the child has dry scaly plaques symmetrically distributed in the perianal and perioral areas. Which deficiency does this child likely have?

(A) calcium

(B) zinc

(C) iodine

(D) iron

(E) vitamin C

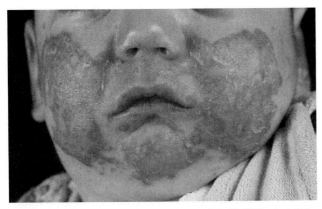

FIG. 3-3 (*Source: Fitzpatrick TB, Johnson RA, Wolff K, et al.* Color Atlas and Synopsis of Clinical Dermatology, *4th ed. New York, NY: McGraw-Hill, 2001, p. 432.*)

60. Which of the following is regulated by the parathyroid gland?

(A) calcium

(B) zinc

(C) iodine

(D) iron

(E) vitamin B$_{12}$

Questions 61 and 62

A 6-month-old male infant presents to your clinic because the mother is concerned that he is not eating well. The mother tells you that her prenatal course and delivery were uneventful. On physical examination, the infant has a puffy face, large tongue, and persistent nasal drainage.

61. Which of the following conditions is most likely to present with these findings?

(A) rickets

(B) scurvy

(C) hypothyroidism

(D) microcytic anemia

(E) adrenocortical insufficiency

62. The above condition can be caused by a deficiency of:

(A) iron

(B) vitamin C

(C) vitamin D

(D) iodine

(E) cortisol

Questions 63 through 65

A 4-year-old child is seen in the emergency department after having a seizure at home. This is the first time that this has happened. The mother says that the child was sitting on the couch watching television when she suddenly became limp, started drooling, and having generalized tonic-clonic movements of her arms and legs. The mother relates that the child felt like she was "burning up" and that the tonic-clonic activity stopped after a few minutes. The mother says that the child is otherwise healthy, does not take any medicines, and has never been hospitalized. The child's immunizations are up to date, and she has no known drug allergies. On examination the vital signs are temperature of 104°F, BP 97/49, heart rate (HR) 112, and respiratory rate (RR) 26. The child is sitting on the examination table playing with stickers and drawing. She has a mild amount of clear nasal congestion but her examination is otherwise normal. When asked, the child replies that she feels fine.

63. What is the most likely diagnosis?

 (A) bacterial meningitis
 (B) first seizure in an epilepsy syndrome
 (C) viral encephalitis
 (D) typical febrile seizure
 (E) hypocalcemic tetany

64. Which test(s) should be performed while the child is in the emergency department to evaluate the cause of these seizures?

 (A) electroencephalogram (EEG)
 (B) no testing is needed
 (C) noncontrast head CT
 (D) lumbar puncture
 (E) blood and urine cultures

65. Which of the following medications would be most appropriate to be given to the child while in the emergency department?

 (A) acetaminophen (Tylenol) for fever as needed
 (B) phenytoin (Dilantin)
 (C) phenobarbital
 (D) diazepam (Valium)
 (E) ceftriaxone (Rocephin)

66. A 2-week-old infant is brought to the office for a check-up. The father relates that they have no concerns except that the baby seems to have tearing from his left eye. They also point out some swelling at the edge of his left eye. The infant is eating, sleeping, stooling, and voiding well. On examination you find a $1/2 \times 1/2$ cm firm nodule inferior to the medial canthus of the left eye. What does this most likely represent?

 (A) dermoid cyst
 (B) nasolacrimal duct obstruction
 (C) mucocele
 (D) accessory lacrimal gland
 (E) frontal encephalocele

Questions 67 through 69

A 14-year-old boy is brought to the emergency department for evaluation of fever and headache. The mother relates that her son has had a worsening headache for 5–6 days. She says that she took him to a walk-in clinic, and he was put on amoxicillin for a sinus infection. His headaches have been getting worse and that he is now having fevers as high as 103.6°F. The mother says that he normally is very active and that he currently has a summer job at a local park clearing out underbrush. Since he has become ill, he has had such a decrease in energy that he cannot go to work. He has had a decrease in his appetite and has been sleeping more. He denies any sore throat, abdominal pain, chest pain, dysuria, vomiting, or diarrhea. On examination he is an uncomfortable young man whose vital signs are temp 101.9°F, RR 26, HR 124, and BP 79/56. His head, ear, eye, nose, and throat examination reveals normal tympanic membranes (TMs,) a mildly erythematous hypopharynx, and some shotty cervical lymphadenopathy. His lungs are clear. His cardiac examination is normal. His liver edge is palpable just below the right costal margin and is mildly tender. His spleen is not palpable. His skin examination is normal with the exception of scattered petechiae around his ankles and wrists. A CBC reveals WBC 13,000 with 65% segs and 22% lymphs, hematocrit of 35, and platelet count of 95,000. His electrolytes reveal a Na 125, K 5.1, Cl 102, and bicarbonate 21. His BUN and Creatinine are normal.

67. What is his most likely diagnosis?

 (A) enteroviral encephalitis
 (B) measles
 (C) Still disease
 (D) RMSF
 (E) Kawasaki syndrome

68. The best treatment course would include which of the following?

 (A) continue amoxicillin only
 (B) begin oral doxycycline
 (C) add acyclovir to the amoxicillin
 (D) begin oral corticosteroids
 (E) stop all antimicrobials

69. What additional testing would be warranted at this point?

 (A) serum rickettsial titers
 (B) ESR

(C) C-reactive protein (CRP)

(D) enteroviral polymerase chain reaction (PCR) on cerebrospinal fluid

(E) head CT without contrast

70. A 4¹/₂-year-old girl is brought to your office during summertime hours for ear pain. She has been swimming at camp for the past few days and now has copious cloudy discharge from her left external auditory canal with pain on movement of the pinna. You diagnose otitis externa. What organism is the most common cause of this infection?

(A) methicillin resistant *Staphylococcus aureus* (MRSA)

(B) *Streptococcus pneumoniae*

(C) *Pseudomonas* species

(D) Nontypable *H. influenzae*

(E) group A *Streptococcus*

Questions 71 through 73

Parents bring you a 9-month-old boy they recently have adopted from western Russia. They have sparse medical records of the child's past. They do know that the boy was the result of a sexual assault on the mother and was given up at birth. The child has been in a "baby home" for 5 months. The records which accompanied the boy indicate that there had been some testing done. These tests include HIV, hepatitis B and C serologies, and a rapid plasma reagin (RPR), all of which are negative at 8 months of age. There is what appears to be a Russian immunization record as well. It seems to indicate that the child has had three diphtheria, tetanus, pertussis (DTP), three oral polio, and three hepatitis B vaccinations. There is also an indication that BCG was given.

71. The parents are interested in having the boy tested for infections. What is the most appropriate evaluation at this time?

(A) No need to repeat the serologies because they have been done within the past month.

(B) Collect stool for ova and parasites only.

(C) Repeat all serologies (HIV, hepatitis B, hepatitis C, RPR) now.

(D) Perform a full sepsis workup (blood culture, urine culture, cerebrospinal fluid [CSF] culture).

(E) Screen for infections using CBC.

72. The parents are concerned about fetal alcohol syndrome (FAS). Which physical feature is most consistent with FAS?

(A) smooth philtrum

(B) single palmar crease

(C) hypertelorism

(D) synophrys (confluent eye brows)

(E) low set ears

73. You place a purified protein derivative (PPD) and the parents come back in 48 h to have it read. The response is 15 mm of induration. The boy does not have any respiratory symptoms at this time. What is the most appropriate response to this information?

(A) Collect three morning sputum and send for acid fast stain and TB culture.

(B) Give a repeat BCG vaccine.

(C) Do nothing as the PPD is considered negative given the prior BCG vaccination.

(D) Perform a CXR and begin isoniazid (INH) for 9 months if the x-ray is negative.

(E) Perform a CXR and begin "triples" (INH, rifampin, pyrazinamide) even if the x-ray is negative.

Questions 74 and 75

A 9-year-old boy comes to clinic for evaluation of a rash. The boy says that he began developing some blisters on his cheek the night prior. He says that over the past few days he has spent time outside with his friends "down by the creek." The rash appears to be a linear crop of vesicles beginning in front of his left ear and extending to the corner of his mouth. There is no erythema, and he describes them as quite pruritic. He has not had any fever, vomiting, or changes in his hearing.

74. What does this rash most likely represent?

  (A) HSV infection of the facial nerve (Ramsey-Hunt syndrome)
  (B) bullous impetigo
  (C) allergic contact dermatitis (rhus dermatitis)
  (D) erythema chronica migrans
  (E) cutaneous larval migrans

75. Along with good skin hygiene, which of the following is the best treatment plan for this child?

  (A) topical diphenhydramine for comfort
  (B) oral diphenhydramine for pruritus
  (C) topical and oral antibiotics which would cover *Staphylococcus* and *Streptococcus*
  (D) topical high-potency fluorinated steroid
  (E) oral acyclovir

Questions 76 through 78

A 16-year-old woman comes to see you for a yearly physical examination. Her only concern is that her periods are very irregular, and she desires oral contraceptives to regulate them. She relates that menarche was at 12 year of age and that her periods have always been irregular. On examination she is a markedly obese woman with a body mass index of 35 and with normal linear growth. She has some coarse facial hair down both of her cheeks as well as cystic acne along her hair line. On the nape of her neck she is noted to have acanthosis nigricans. She has tanner 4 breast development as well as tanner 4 pubic hair. Her urinalysis in the office is normal.

76. What is the most likely cause of her irregular periods?

  (A) hypothyroidism
  (B) polycystic ovarian syndrome (PCOS)
  (C) late-onset congenital adrenal hyperplasia
  (D) Cushing's syndrome
  (E) testosterone insensitivity

77. Which of the following would confirm your diagnosis?

  (A) ultrasound of the pelvis showing multiple ovarian follicles ("string of pearls" sign)
  (B) a low serum thyroid stimulating hormone (TSH) level
  (C) an elevated serum prolactin level
  (D) elevated high-density lipoprotein (HDL) with low triglycerides
  (E) normal glucose tolerance test

78. What would be the best intervention to achieve the best long-term outcome in this woman?

  (A) Begin low-dose subcutaneous insulin to prevent diabetes mellitus.
  (B) Begin daily corticosteroid therapy to suppress testosterone secretion.
  (C) Begin a regimen of lifestyle changes, including dietary and exercise alterations.
  (D) Begin levothyroxine (Synthroid) for control of weight gain.
  (E) Oophorectomy to decrease hormone levels.

79. What is the major mode of transmission of HIV infection in young children today?

  (A) biting
  (B) blood transfusion
  (C) vertical transmission
  (D) horizontal transmission
  (E) sexual abuse

80. Prolonged use of which medication can result in gingival hyperplasia?

  (A) theophylline
  (B) aspirin
  (C) vancomycin
  (D) phenytoin (Dilantin)
  (E) cefaclor (Ceclor)

81. Parents bring their 6-year-old son to the emergency room following an acute onset of vomiting and combative behavior. The parents state that the child has recently had chickenpox. They have been giving him medication to reduce his fever, which has been as high as 102°F. Which medication is the likely cause of his current condition?

(A) acetaminophen
(B) aspirin
(C) amoxicillin
(D) ibuprofen
(E) diphenhydramine

82. Use of which medication can result in enamel staining of primary teeth?

(A) erythromycin
(B) ciprofloxacin (Cipro)
(C) cephalexin
(D) trimethoprim/sulfamethoxazole (Septra)
(E) tetracycline

83. A 10-year male has a history of seizures which are controlled with dilantin. The child also has asthma and often uses an albuterol inhaler. Which of the following asthma medications can lower the seizure threshold in children?

(A) theophylline
(B) salmeterol
(C) beclomethasone
(D) montelukast
(E) nedocromil

Answers and Explanations

1. **(E)** The constellation of cryptorchidism, posterior urethral valves, and abnormal abdominal musculature is called Eagle-Barrett syndrome. Another name is prune belly syndrome. The greatest morbidity comes from the poor amniotic fluid production, due to bladder outlet obstruction, with a resulting pulmonary hypoplasia. VATER association has multiple anomalies, none of which are the three mentioned. VATER is a mnemonic which stands for **V**ertebral anomalies, **A**nal atresia (imperforate), **T**racheo-**E**sophageal fistula and **R**enal anomalies (the R also indicated **R**adial anomalies). It is sometimes referred to as VACTERL association in which the C indicated **C**ardiac anomalies with the L indicating **L**imb anomalies. Potter syndrome is bilateral renal agenesis. This condition is fatal, due to marked pulmonary hypoplasia. The Jones criteria are used in the diagnosis of ARF. (*Rudolph's Pediatrics, pp. 1737–1738*)

2. **(B)** Tachypnea is the most sensitive clinical parameter for diagnosing a lower respiratory tract infection. The child may have tachycardia from a fever or anxiety but, typically, not simply from pneumonia. Coughing is common in children with pneumonia but it is not specific for lower respiratory tract infections, as it can also be seen in upper and lower respiratory tract infections. (*Rudolph's Pediatrics, pp. 1980*)

3. **(E)** All of the vaccines mentioned, except varicella, are killed or synthetic vaccines. Varivax is an attenuated varicella strain (OKA) from Japan. Live virus vaccines are contraindicated in the case of AIDS with a markedly reduced T-cell count. The IPV is the inactivated version of the live polio vaccine, oral polio vaccine (OPV). (*The Red Book, pp. 11–14*)

4. **(C)**

5. **(A)**

Explanations 4 and 5

The x-ray provided shows a nondisplaced spiral fracture of the distal tibia. This is also known as a toddler's fracture. This fracture can occur when the toddler begins to walk and twists on a planted leg. This torque can result in a spiral fracture of the planted tibia. There usually is no dislocation of the ankle joint and minimal displacement of the fracture. A chip fracture of the metaphysis is a common fracture seen in abused infants and is commonly termed as a "bucket-handle" or "corner" fracture. A buckle fracture is a common accidental fracture seen in falls from a height. (*Rudolph's Pediatrics, p. 2451*)

6. **(B)**

7. **(A)**

Explanations 6 and 7

This young woman has cervicitis, but without evidence of pelvic inflammatory disease (PID). Chlamydia is the most common bacterial cause of sexually transmitted diseases in the United States and the most likely etiology of this patient's infection. Gonorrhea would be the next most likely cause and, frequently, there will be coinfection with the two pathogens. The simplest outpatient treatment for these two would be a single 1-g oral dose of azithromycin and a 125-mg IM dose of ceftriaxone. This regimen will ensure complete compliance, which is crucial. Treatment of her sexual partners would also be recommended. Another cause of cervicitis is trichomoniasis, for which metronidazole, either for 1 week of 500 mg BID or a single 2-g oral dose, would be recommended therapy. Of the suggested answers option A is the only one which would cover the two most common infectious agents. (*Centers for Disease Control and Prevention. Sexually transmitted diseases treatment guidelines 2002. MMWR 2002;51 (No. RR-6):32–34)*

8. **(B)** There are nearly 900,000 victims of child abuse in the United States each year. An inflicted injury is the most common cause of injury in the first year of life. As a child becomes more mobile, falls and motor vehicle accidents become increasingly more common. Other children are a very rare cause of serious injury in childhood. *(Child Maltreatment 2002, Department of Health and Human Services, Administration on Children, Youth and Families, Washington, DC)*

9. **(D)**

10. **(B)**

11. **(D)**

12. **(A)**

13. **(E)**

Explanations 9 through 13

The most common finding in a newborn with Down syndrome is hypotonia. Other common findings include single palmar crease, flat facial profile, macroglossia, and wide space between the first and second toes. Hypotonia in the newborn period should prompt close evaluation and followup. Café au lait spots are associated with neurofibromatosis. High arched palates are associated with fragile X syndrome. Ambiguous genitalia are commonly seen in congenital adrenal hyperplasia (CAH). *(Smith's Recognizable Pattern of Human Malformations, pp. 8–13)*

Children with Down syndrome are at an increased risk for hypothyroidism. It may be hard to detect without routine laboratory screening as they will commonly have mental retardation and developmental delay as part of their syndrome. Hypothyroidism may not be present in the immediate newborn period and requires, at a minimum, annual testing throughout the child's life. The other findings listed are not specifically associated with Down syndrome. Lens dislocation is commonly found with Marfan syndrome or homocysteinuria. *(Smith's Recognizable Pattern of Human Malformations, pp. 8–13)*

Children with Down syndrome have an increased prevalence of duodenal atresia. Pyloric stenosis is uncommon to see in the newborn period. It tends to present with nonbilious vomiting usually after 2–4 weeks of age. Hirschsprung disease (aganglionosis coli) presents with constipation and failure to pass stool. Infants with Hirschsprung disease commonly will not pass stool in the first days of life. Biliary atresia is a progressive cause of jaundice in an infant. It is the most common cause of a cholestatic jaundice in the newborn period. Emesis is not typically associated with biliary atresia. Milk protein allergy is a common cause of bloody stools in the first few months of life, but does not have bilious emesis associated with it. *(Smith's Recognizable Pattern of Human Malformations, pp. 8–13).*

The double bubble sign is typically seen in duodenal atresia. It represents gas in the stomach and the first part of the duodenum. This finding can also be seen in children with malrotation with a midgut volvulus. A midgut volvulus may also have bilious emesis as well, but malrotation is not specifically associated with Down syndrome. Pneumatosis intestinalis is the radiographic appearance of dissected air in the intestinal wall. It is seen in necrotizing enterocolitis (NEC). Scimitar sign is seen on CXR and is indicative of anomalous pulmonary veins. *(Rudolph's Pediatrics, pp. 203)*

The mean IQ of children with Down syndrome is 50 (the average is 20–85). Children with Down syndrome are not at greater risk of CNS malformations. There is not an increased presence of calcifications or of aneurysms. Five percent of children with Down syndrome can have a seizure disorder, making it a less common finding than mental retardation. Hydrocephalus is not increased in children with Down syndrome. *(Smith's Recognizable Pattern of Human Malformations, pp. 8–13)*

14. **(B)**

15. **(B)**

Explanations 14 and 15

G. lamblia is a common protozoan which can be acquired by ingesting unfiltered water. It is seen frequently in people who drink fresh stream water. It is a cause of chronic, non-bloody diarrhea. There is typically a large amount of gas and cramping associated with *Giardia* infections. RMSF does not typically cause a gastroenteritis. Children with RMSF will commonly have fevers, headaches, and a petechial rash. Rotavirus and Norwalk viruses typically cause acute, self-limited gastroenteritis. The diarrhea is nonbloody, nonmucousy, and typically lasts a few days. *(The Red Book, pp. 283–285).*

The most appropriate treatment for giardiasis is oral metronidazole. Oral rehydration is an important mainstay in the treatment of diarrhea of any cause but is not a specific treatment for giardiasis. Ciprofloxacin is commonly used for traveler's diarrhea caused by *E. coli*.

16. **(C)** The most common malignancy in childhood is leukemia/lymphoma. The most common solid tumors of childhood are CNS tumors, followed by neuroblastoma and Wilm tumors. *(Rudolph's Pediatrics, pp. 1583)*

17. **(C)** A fever in the first 4–6 weeks of life needs to be treated very aggressively. There are no reliable clinical or laboratory findings currently available that can discriminate between a nominal viral illness and a serious bacterial infection. In the newborn period, fever may be the only indicator of bacteremia or meningitis. Any rectal temperature greater than 100.5°F should trigger a full sepsis workup. This should include cultures of the blood, urine, and spinal fluid. In this age range, empiric antimicrobials should be initiated that should cover for GBS, *E. coli*, and *Listeria monocytogenes*. A commonly used regimen is ampicillin and gentamicin. Many would also include empiric acyclovir in this age range. In infants, the routine use of antipyretics should be discouraged. A blood culture alone is not an adequate screening tool for meningitis. While a urinary tract infection (UTI) is a common cause of infection in infants,

a more complete evaluation would be warranted. *(Fleisher and Ludwig, pp. 725–736)*

18. **(B)**

19. **(D)**

Explanations 18 and 19

Bilious emesis in an infant is malrotation until proven otherwise. Malrotation can lead to a midgut volvulus. The volvulus can result in bowel ischemia and necrosis. This makes bilious emesis in a newborn a concerning finding. Pyloric stenosis would cause nonbilious emesis. Imperforate anus would present with the failure of stool passage. Diaphragmatic hernia will present with poor feeding, drooling, and respiratory embarrassment.

The best radiographic test in the diagnosis of malrotation is an upper GI contrast study with small bowel follow through. This will identify the duodenum and its location relative to the ligament of Treitz. The characteristic finding in a midgut volvulus is the "corkscrew" sign, which is seen as contrast media traverses the kinked intestine. An abdominal CT may show malrotation but is less specific for it. Barium enema and radionuclide scans have no role in the diagnosis of malrotation. *(Rudolph's Pediatrics, p. 203)*

20. **(D)** ARF is clinically diagnosed by using the Jones criteria. The Jones criteria are separated into major and minor findings. The major criteria are arthritis (not simply arthralgia), carditis, Sydenham chorea, erythema marginatum, and subcutaneous nodules. The minor criteria include the presence of a fever, arthralgias, documentation of a GAS infection (either currently or in the past), or laboratory evidence of inflammation (increased ESR). Two major criteria, or one major and two minors, are required for the diagnosis of ARF. The only exception to this rule is that the presence of Sydenham chorea alone will make the diagnosis. While the documentation of a prior, or current, GAS infection is compelling, it is not a requirement for the diagnosis of ARF. Children

with rheumatic fever are not considered contagious. *(Rudolph's Pediatrics, pp. 1901–1904)*

21. (B)

22. (A)

Explanations 21 and 22

Acute inflammatory demyelinating polyneuropathy, commonly called Guillain-Barré syndrome, is an ascending paralysis with a hallmark of absent reflexes. There may also be some nominal sensory deficits as well, but they are not as striking as the paresis. Methylphenidate toxicity usually results in seizures and tachycardia. In children with malingering, reflexes are usually present, as they are not under cognitive control. Reflexes are also present in children with polymyositis. Children with polymyositis will usually have fever and muscle pain with weakness, as well. With the use of the polio vaccines (OPV or IPV), poliomyelitis is no longer present in wild type in the United States.

Guillain-Barré is usually a self-limited disease. The most common complication is respiratory failure. The paresis usually advances for 48–72 h and then will slowly recede. The use of corticosteroids is not recommended. Plasmaphoresis is used in the following situations: progressive paresis, nonambulatory patients, or bulbar or respiratory involvement. As this child's disease has plateaued at the time of evaluation, plasmaphoresis would be of little benefit. *(Fenichel, pp. 176–202; Rudolph's Pediatrics, pp. 2281–2283)*

23. (A) GBS is the most common cause of infection in the newborn infant, followed by *E. coli* and *L. monocytogenes*. GBS is the most common cause of pneumonia, septicemia, UTI, and meningitis. The risk of early onset (within the first 7 days of life) GBS infection can be reduced with the antenatal administration of appropriate antimicrobials. The use of perinatal antimicrobials has no effect on the occurrence of late-onset (after 7 days of life) GBS disease. *(The Red Book, pp. 584–591)*

24. (E)

25. (A)

Explanations 24 and 25

The most common cause of otitis media in children is pneumococcus *(S. pneumoniae)*. This is also the most common cause of sinusitis and pneumonia. Otitis media is usually seen in conjunction with an upper respiratory tract infection. *(The Red Book, pp. 490–500)*

Pressure from extensive use of antimicrobials has resulted in a dramatic increase in penicillin resistance in pneumococcus. Amoxicillin remains the recommended initial antibiotic of choice for the treatment of otitis media in children. In an effort to reduce the incidence of antibiotic resistance, and because of the high spontaneous cure rate of otitis media, many authorities are advocating withholding antimicrobial treatment unless symptoms persist for several days in spite of symptomatic treatment.

26. (D) GAS pharyngitis ("strep throat") is a common cause of tonsillitis requiring antibiotics. GAS continues to be very susceptible to penicillin, which still remains the treatment of choice. Occasionally, children will have a persistently positive throat culture for GAS and are considered carriers. This carrier state is not a risk for rheumatic disease and is felt not to be contagious to others. The presence of *E. coli* in the intestinal tract is considered colonization and not carrier state. An example of an enteric bacteria which does have a carrier state would be *Salmonella typhi* (typhoid fever). *(The Red Book, pp. 573–84)*

27. (E) Nonpolio enteroviruses are the most common causes of aseptic meningitis in childhood. There are approximately 65 nonpolio enteroviruses, including the coxsackieviruses, echoviruses, and enteroviruses. Children are the main susceptible population and transmission is from child to child, via fecal-oral or oral-oral (respiratory) contact. Meningitis may result from viremic spread of the virus. Treatment of this is supportive. *(Oski's Pediatrics: Principles and Practice, Chap. 199)*

28. **(D)** In children over 1 month of age, the most common causes of bacterial meningitis are *Streptococcus pneumoniae* and *Neisseria meningitidis*. *H. influenza* type B was also a frequent cause of this disease prior to the widespread use of the HIB vaccine. GBS, *E. coli*, and HSV would be more common causes of CNS infections in neonates. *(Oski's Pediatrics: Principles and Practice, Chap. 142)*

29. **(B)** The most common infectious cause of blindness in the world is trachoma. Trachoma is the chronic effect of a *C. trachomatis* infection acquired in the perinatal period. The most common cause of blindness in the world is noninfectious (glaucoma and diabetic retinopathy). *(The Red Book, pp. 238–243)*

30. **(B)**

31. **(D)**

Explanations 30 and 31

The image provided shows a classic case of impetigo. This is a common skin infection of childhood. It frequently occurs following a case of chickenpox and is due to the child picking or scratching at the varicella lesions, resulting in a secondary bacterial infection. Group A *Streptococcus* (GAS) infection is the most common cause of impetigo associated with varicella infections. It is markedly more prevalent than the next most common infectious agent, *Staphylococcus aureus* (*The Red Book*). Tinea corporis, often due to *T. rubrum*, is also known as ringworm. It classically is a circular lesion with a red, raised border, and central clearing. Contact dermatitis, from exposure to an irritant such as poison ivy, often causes plaques of erythema and edema with superimposed vesicles. This is also frequently secondarily infected with GAS from scratching. Warts, caused by the human papilloma virus, do not typically appear as the lesions in the image. *(The Red Book, pp. 573–584; Fitzpatrick, pp. 18, 696)*

32. **(A)**

33. **(C)**

34. **(D)**

Explanations 32 through 34

The hallmark of immune (also known as idiopathic) thrombocytopenia purpura (ITP) is the otherwise healthy appearing child with isolated thrombocytopenia. ITP is the most common cause of isolated thrombocytopenia in childhood. It occurs with equal frequency in both boys and girls. The presence of thrombocytopenia in a patient with otherwise normal cell lines, and a normal physical examination is enough to make the diagnosis, so further evaluation, such as a bone marrow biopsy, is unnecessary. Which children to treat and which treatment to use are areas of controversy in the management of ITP. Most acute ITP will resolve spontaneously, so many will recommend observation for children who appear well, are asymptomatic and have platelet counts above 30,000. Platelet transfusions should be reserved only in the instance of ongoing or imminent bleeding.

When a decision is made to treat, usually when the platelet count falls below 20,000, there are several options available. Treatment involves using IVIG, steroids, anti-D immunoglobulins, or combinations thereof. Combinations of medications may work synergistically. Prednisone is often used initially, as it can be given orally and is inexpensive. Typically it will be tapered over 2 weeks to 3 months. By using combination therapy when needed, splenectomy can be avoided in the vast majority of cases. When it is necessary, it should be delayed, if at all possible, for at least a year after diagnosis. *(Hoffman, pp. 2102–2104)*

35. **(E)** HUS is, as the name implies, the combination of a microangiopathic hemolytic anemia and acute renal failure. It is commonly associated with *E. coli* 0157/H7 gastroenteritis. HUS is one of the most common causes of acquired renal failure in children. *(Rudolph's Pediatrics, pp. 1696–1698)*

36. **(C)** Children with tuberous sclerosis can develop nasolabial fold angiofibromas (commonly referred to adenoma sebaceum). These can be mistaken for acne in an adolescent. Other cutaneous findings include peri- and subungual fibromas, ash leaf spots (hypomelanocytic macules), and shagreen patches. Tuberous sclerosis can also have CNS cortical defects and "tubers," which may be foci of seizure activity. Skin findings are seen in 75% of cases of tuberous sclerosis. (*Smith's Recognizable Pattern of Human Malformations, pp. 506–507*)

37. **(E)** Of the listed syndromes, only Beckwith-Wiedemann syndrome has neonatal hypoglycemia as part of its clinical spectrum. The constellation of macroglossia, hypoglycemia, and visceral organomegaly (hepatosplenomegaly) is a common finding in children with Beckwith-Wiedemann syndrome. The presence of an omphalocele in a newborn would also be concerning for BWS. (*Smith's Recognizable Pattern of Human Malformations, pp. 164–165*)

38. **(D)** The term CHARGE is a mnemonic standing for **C**oloboma, **H**eart malformations, **A**tresia choanae, **R**etarded (growth and mental), **G**enital anomalies, and **E**ar anomalies. The colobomas are usually seen in the iris, but can be seen in the eyelids and the nasolabial folds as well. The heart anomalies of CHARGE association are usually ventricular septal defects and tetralogy of Fallot. (*Smith's Recognizable Pattern of Human Malformations, pp. 668–669*)

39. **(C)**

40. **(B)**

Explanations 39 and 40

The most common bacterial infection in the newborn period is GBS. GBS is commonly cultured in the adult vaginal tract, and its vertical transmission can be interrupted with maternal antimicrobial treatment prior to delivery of the infant. Mothers are commonly treated in labor with penicillin, ampicillin, clindamycin, or azithromycin in an attempt to interrupt transmission to the infant while passing through the birth canal. If antimicrobial prophylaxis is initiated greater than 4 h prior to delivery, the rate of early onset GBS disease is dramatically decreased. The current recommendation for term infants of GBS-positive women who have received antibiotics in labor (at least two doses or ≥4 h prior to delivery) is observation without testing or antibiotics. (*The Red Book, pp. 584–591*)

Classic hemophilia is an X-linked recessive bleeding diathesis. Hemophilia is inherited on the maternal lineage from carrier (or affected) mothers. This infant, being a male, would receive his X chromosome from his mother. He is, therefore, not at risk for having hemophilia. Further, being an X-linked trait, there cannot be a male "carrier" state. (*Rudolph's Pediatrics, pp. 1570–1573*)

41. **(C)** Falling on outstretched arms is one of the most common injuries among school-aged children. This can result in a buckle, or torus, fracture of the distal radius and/or ulna. This is a common accidental mechanism and should not, by itself, raise suspicions for an inflicted injury. AP and lateral x-rays of the wrist and elbow would be diagnostic of this type of injury. Nursemaid's elbows occur from a pulling or twisting mechanism to the upper extremity and are not the result of falls. An MRI of this injury would be overkill. (*Fleisher and Ludwig, pp. 1455*)

42. **(C)**

43. **(A)**

44. **(D)**

45. **(B)**

Explanations 42 through 45

Kawasaki disease (mucocutaneous lymph node syndrome) is a disease of unclear etiology. The salient diagnostic features include fever for >5 days, cervical lymph node greater than 1 cm, nonpurulent conjunctivitis, oral changes (cracking lips or "strawberry tongue"), polymorphous rash to the trunk, and changes to the hands and feet (peeling of the fingers or toes or edema of the hands or feet). This may be confused with group A β-hemolytic strep pharyngitis, which usually is not associated with conjunctivitis. Coxsackie viral infection is commonly seen as the "hand-foot-mouth" disease, with shallow ulcers on the palms, soles, and in the mouth. There is nominal fever associated, and conjunctivitis is uncommon. Parvovirus B-19 (erythema infectiosum, "fifth disease") is commonly called "slapped cheek" disease because of the exanthem of bright red cheeks. Adenopathy and conjunctivitis are not features of this infection.

Acute phase reactions are often elevated late in the course of Kawasaki disease. The most common blood test result would be a dramatically elevated platelet count. It is usually >750,000 and can be greater than 1,000,000. An ESR is also likely to be elevated, not low. A positive rapid strep test would lead one more toward acute group A strep disease.

The treatment of choice for Kawasaki disease is IVIG and aspirin. IVIG infusion is usually over 12 h and will commonly result in rapid defervescence and clinical improvement. Treatment of Kawasaki disease is important as it will prevent long-term sequelae. A common side effect of IVIG is aseptic meningitis.

Nearly a quarter of untreated children will develop coronary artery dilatation. This is most common cause of acquired heart disease in children younger than 5 years of age. The coronary artery dilatation can result in aneurysm formation and myocardial infarction. (*Rudolph's Pediatrics, pp. 844–845*)

46. (B)

47. (C)

Explanations 46 and 47

Most infant formulas are cow's milk based. The most common form of carbohydrate in these infant formulas is lactose. Soy formulas use corn syrup and/or sucrose as their source of carbohydrate. Casein is a form of protein. Human milk fortifier is a supplement added to breast milk for the premature infant and is a

combination of protein and carbohydrate. (*Rudolph's Pediatrics, pp. 1329–1333*)

GBS colitis is an uncommon disease in infants. Cow's milk protein intolerance is a common cause of blood streaked stool in an infant on cow's milk based formulas. Lactose intolerance is very uncommon in an infant and usually causes chronic, nonbloody diarrhea. Pseudomembranous colitis would be a consideration in a child with diarrhea who recently had been on antibiotics. (*Fleisher and Ludwig, pp. 1445*)

48. (B)

49. (D)

50. (E)

Explanations 48 through 50

This case is a common presentation for viral croup, with the symptoms of a seal-barking cough, stridor, tachypnea, and fever in the winter. Pneumonia must also be considered with tachypnea, cough, and fever, but it is less likely to cause stridor and may not have the seal-bark type of cough. Sinusitis may cause cough and fever, but would be more likely to have a purulent nasal discharge and less likely to have the typical croupy cough. Bronchiolitis due to respiratory syncytial virus (RSV) is a common cause of wintertime cough and fever. It is less likely to have stridor and more likely to have wheezing. Children with epiglottitis are typically found in the "tripod position" and may be drooling. It is, fortunately, becoming rare with the widespread use of the *H. influenzae* vaccine.

Parainfluenza types 1 and 2 account for 60–70% of all viral croup. HIB was a common cause of epiglottitis, but is now rare because of widespread vaccinations. Influenza B and RSV can cause croup, but not as commonly as parainfluenza types 1 and 2. *Streptococcus pneumoniae* would be the most common bacterial cause of pneumonia or sinusitis. (*The Red Book, pp. 454–455*)

The steeple sign is subglottic narrowing of the trachea seen on an AP view of the trachea or a CXR. The trachea is seen to narrow, almost to a point, like the steeple of a church. Swollen adenoids are difficult to identify in lateral neck x-rays. The presence of swollen adenoids is unrelated to the airway narrowing seen in croup. The thumb sign is a swollen epiglottis seen with epiglottitis. A lobar pulmonary infiltrate may be seen with a typical bacterial pneumonia. *(Fleisher and Ludwig, p. 745)*

51. (B)

52. (D)

Explanations 51 and 52

Short stature in an adolescent is a common reason for visiting the pediatrician or endocrinologist. Most short stature in adolescence is constitutional growth delay. These children will have normal growth velocity and delayed bone age. Growth is normal for the first 4–12 months, then decelerates to below the fifth percentile. These children will catch up to their peers in a slightly delayed fashion. Frequently, other family members have a history of short stature in childhood, delayed puberty, and eventual normal stature as adults. In contrast, children with familial short stature have a normal bone age and regular onset of puberty. These children will maintain their short stature as adults. Somatomedin-C (IGF-1) is commonly used as a surrogate measure for the end-organ effect of the pulsatile growth hormone release. In children with GH deficiency, the end-organ effect will be a low somatomedin-C level. An advanced bone age (advanced bone maturation) usually results in shorter final height. Chronic renal failure is a cause of growth delay, but not a common one *(Rudolph's Pediatrics, pp. 2014–2017; Behrman, p. 1851)*

53. (C)

54. (A)

Explanations 53 and 54

Pubarche in females is usually earlier than in males. Delayed puberty alone may be a pathologic condition; its presence in conjunction with short stature makes a pathologic state more likely. Males do, indeed, have adrenarche. Panhypopituitarism is a cause of puberty delay, but not a common one. Undiagnosed hypothyroidism can be a cause of pubertal delay, and thyroid function testing should be a part of the routine evaluation of this problem.

The onset of puberty in males is usually signaled by an increase in testicular volume. This is commonly seen in conjunction with lengthening of the phallus and thinning of the scrotal skin. As a result of puberty, the other findings (deepening of the voice, increased muscle mass, and increased facial hair) may be seen, but the first of the listed findings to appear is increased testicular volume. In females, puberty is usually signaled by the enlargement of breast buds. *(Rudolph's Pediatrics, pp. 2093–2105)*

55. (C)

56. (B)

Explanations 55 and 56

Polyuria in a prepubertal female may indicate the presence of a UTI. A UTI must be excluded as the first step. Polyuria may also indicate vulvovaginitis. Vulvovaginitis in a prepubertal female is usually irritation and hygiene related. The presence of dysuria with the polyuria would make the utility of checking a fingerstick glucose, as a screening test for diabetes, low yield.

The nightly use of bubble baths makes chemical urethritis the most likely cause of this girl's polyuria and dysuria. Diabetes mellitus would present typically with polyuria, polydipsia, weight loss, and decrease in energy. There would also be no dysuria unless there were a concomitant UTI. Diabetes insipidus is a very rare disease in childhood and would be unlikely in an otherwise healthy girl. The presence of a retained foreign body (typically toilet paper) is usually seen in conjunction with a vaginal odor and discharge as well. *(Rudolph's Pediatrics, pp. 607–611)*

57. (E) Pinworms (*Enterobius vermicularis*) are common nematodes (roundworms) found in children. It usually is a benign, incidental finding, but can present with perianal pruritus or small, white, thread-like worms on visual examination. Ascariasis is the most common roundworm infection in humans, but these worms are larger. *Toxocara canis* (dog roundworm) is another nematode and is the cause of visceral larval migrans. *D. latum* (fish tape worm) and *Taenia solium* (pork tape worm) are cestodes, which are long, flat worms. (*The Red Book, pp. 486–487*)

58. (D) Iron deficiency is a common finding. Most proprietary infant formulas have iron supplementation. Infants who are strictly breast fed may require oral iron supplementation. A total body iron deficiency can result in a microcytic, hypochromic anemia. Testing of total serum iron, ferritin, and total iron binding capacity can help clarify the body iron stores. (*Rudolph's Pediatrics, pp. 1525–1528*)

59. (B) The absence, or malabsorption, of zinc from the diet will result in zinc deficiency. The clinical entity is called acrodermatitis enteropathica. Symptoms may manifest during the transition from breast milk to cow's milk. The typical dermatologic manifestations of this are symmetrically distributed perianal and perioral (in a horseshoe pattern) dermatitis. The skin lesions are eczematous, dry, scaly, or psoriasiform. Children with vitamin C deficiency present with petechial hemorrhages of the skin and mucus membranes. Hypocalcemia does not include specific dermatologic changes. Tetany is a classic manifestation of hypocalcemia. Skin pallor is the most important sign of iron deficiency. Children with inadequate iodine in their diet may develop hypothyroidism. (*Rudolph's Pediatrics, pp. 1326; Behrman, p. 2249*)

60. (A) Parathormone (PTH), with vitamin D, is a major regulator of the serum levels of calcium. PTH is made in the chief cells of the four parathyroid glands and exerts effects mainly on the bone and kidneys to maintain adequate serum levels of calcium. (*Rudolph's Pediatrics, pp. 2142–2149*)

61. (C)

62. (D)

Explanations 61 and 62

Hypothyroidism results from inadequate thyroid hormone production or a defect in thyroid hormone receptor activity. Hypothyroidism can be congenital or acquired. Most infants with congenital hypothyroidism are asymptomatic at birth. Feeding difficulties, choking spells, and somnolence often present during the first month of life. Respiratory distress can also occur in part due to the large tongue and nasal obstruction. On physical examination, you may find a large abdomen, umbilical hernias, subnormal temperature, cold skin, murmurs, or bradycardia. Iodine is absorbed in the GI tract as iodide. Iodide is concentrated in the thyroid gland and four atoms are incorporated into each molecule of thyroxine. Profound dietary deficiency of iodine will result in hypothyroidism and is the most common cause of goiter in the world.

Rickets results from a deficiency of vitamin D. This condition predominately affects the long bones and skull. Vitamin C deficiency results in scurvy, a condition with impaired collagen formation. The clinical manifestations may include changes in the gums, loosening of teeth, brittle bones, and swollen joints. Pallor is the most important sign of iron deficiency anemia. Children may also have the desire to ingest unusual substances such as ice or dirt. Finally, hyponatremia and hypoglycemia are the prominent presenting signs of adrenal insufficiency in infants. (*Rudolph's Pediatrics, p. 2059; Behrman, pp. 184–186, 1872–1875*)

63. (D)

64. (B)

65. (A)

Explanations 63 through 65

Febrile seizures are the most common cause of seizures in childhood. These are classically seen early in an illness and when there is a rapid rise in the child's temperature. These seizures usually last less than 2–3 min (typical febrile seizures last no longer than 15 min) and have a very mild, short, postictal phase. Children who have seizures that are the result of bacterial meningitis will not subsequently be normal.

For typical febrile seizures, in an otherwise healthy and well-appearing child, no evaluation (outside of treating any underlying cause of the fever) is warranted. Blood and urine cultures would not be necessary in evaluation of the seizures, but they may be warranted in evaluation of the fever. An EEG and head CT will nearly universally be normal and are unwarranted.

A single typical febrile seizure routinely does not require any anticonvulsant therapy. If the child has had multiple febrile seizures, or the seizures are not typical, anticonvulsant therapy may be entertained. Prophylactic anticonvulsant therapy is usually initiated after the third febrile seizure. Occasionally children may have convulsions associated with fevers which do not fall into the typical features. Some criteria which would make a febrile seizure atypical would be prolonged duration (>15 min) and a prolonged postictal state (>30–60 min). *(Fenichel, pp. 18–19)*

66. **(B)** Relative immaturity of the lacrimal drainage system can result in the accumulation of debris in the nasolacrimal duct. This will manifest as a swelling inferior to the middle canthus. Dermoid cysts in children are commonly found as a subcutaneous nodule on the lateral portion of the eyebrow. Mucoceles are usually found as fleshy papules on the inner portion of the lower lip. Frontal encephaloceles are midline in location. *(Rudolph's Pediatrics, pp. 2366–2367)*

67. **(D)**

68. **(B)**

69. **(A)**

Explanations 67 through 69

The clinical scenario describes a classic presentation of RMSF (infection with *R. rickettsii*).

Typical symptoms include a summertime fever, headache, petechial rash, thrombocytopenia, and hyponatremia. This may be mistaken for a systemic enteroviral infection, or enteroviral encephalitis, but the presence of thrombocytopenia and hyponatremia would exclude this diagnosis. Still disease (systemic-onset juvenile rheumatoid arthritis (JRA)) would have an elevation of acute-phase reactants, including the WBC and platelet count. Fourteen years old is an unlikely age for Kawasaki disease, and the acute phase reactants would likewise also be elevated.

RMSF is a very serious infectious illness. Appropriate antimicrobial therapy, usually doxycycline, needs to be started as soon as the diagnosis is seriously considered, as this can prevent some of the more severe sequelae. The use of systemic corticosteroids has no place in the management of RMSF. Confirmation of RMSF is serologic. Rising IgG titers or the presence of IgM titers to *R. rickettsii* is a confirmation of RMSF. *(The Red Book, pp. 532–534)*

70. **(C)** The most common cause of otitis externa (OE) is *Pseudomonas aeruginosa*. Treatment for acute OE will involve topical antimicrobials which cover *P. aeruginosa*, often in combination with a topical steroid. For chronic OE, yeast becomes a more important pathogen, and therapy should be directed as such. *(Fleisher and Ludwig, p. 1571)*

71. **(C)**

72. **(A)**

73. **(D)**

Explanations 71 through 73

Repeating all serologies is important. The prior negative testing should be included in the medical record, but should not dissuade one from confirming the result. The collection of stool for ova and parasites (O+P) is an important evaluation but should not be the only testing performed. A CBC is not an adequate screen for infections. *(The Red Book, pp. 173–180)*

The diagnosis of FAS includes findings of characteristic facies, growth retardation, and CNS impairment. The characteristic facies of FAS includes flat philtrum, thin upper vermilion border, short palpebral fissures, micrognathia, microphthalmos, and microcephaly. (*Smith's Recognizable Pattern of Human Malformations, pp. 555–558*)

BCG is a common vaccine administered in countries outside of the United States. The presence of a positive reaction to a PPD in a child who has had a prior BCG is still concerning. The presence of a 15-mm reaction is considered positive and warrants a CXR and initiation of antituberculosis treatment. The negative CXR would indicate TB exposure, and INH alone is recommended. Sputum collection is usually unwarranted in asymptomatic children. (*The Red Book, pp. 642–660*)

74. (C)

75. (B)

Explanations 74 and 75

This represents an allergic contact dermatitis. The allergen is the oil on the leaf of certain plants (poison ivy). The reaction is a delayed-type hypersensitivity reaction (type 4) and may take up to 72–96 h after exposure to fully manifest.

Limited allergic contact dermatitis will usually warrant limited therapy. Oral antihistamines, taken on an as needed basis, can provide effective symptomatic relief. Topical antihistamines are usually not effective and, if added to oral antihistamines, can result in toxic effects. Steroids should be used sparingly on the face, and high-potency steroid should not be used at all on the face. Secondary infection is unlikely if good skin hygiene is used. (*Fleisher and Ludwig, pp. 1134–6*)

76. (B)

77. (A)

78. (C)

Explanations 76 through 78

This clinical vignette describes an adolescent female with PCOS. PCOS is commonly seen in obese adolescent females with anovulatory menstrual cycles, hirsutism, and generalized virilization (acne). Commonly PCOS patients will have glucose insensitivity and manifest features of type-II diabetes mellitus.

The diagnosis of PCOS may be difficult to ascertain. A pelvic ultrasound demonstrating "polycystic ovaries" (the string of pearls sign) may be quite helpful. Girls with PCOS will typically have elevated triglycerides, low HDL-cholesterol, and a suppressed prolactin. As indicated above, PCOS girls also often have glucose insensitivity and an abnormal glucose tolerance test.

The most effective therapy in PCOS involves lifestyle alterations (weight loss and exercise) and hormonal regulation of ovulation. The hypoglycemic agent metformin is now being used to assist in the management of PCOS. Occasionally subcutaneous insulin may be effective in controlling hyperglycemia, but this will not prevent diabetes mellitus. (*Rudolph's Pediatrics, pp. 249–252*)

79. (C) Vertically transmitted, or perinatally acquired, HIV is the most common mode of transmission in pediatric patients. Maternal health, maternal viral load, third trimester antiretroviral therapy, and mode of delivery all affect the rate of perinatal acquisition. (*The Red Book, pp. 360–382*)

80. (D) Gingival hyperplasia is a common side effect of chronic phenytoin administration. This will resolve with cessation of the medication. None of the other medications listed will result in this problem. (*Rudolph's Pediatrics, p. 1292*)

81. (B) Historically, Reye syndrome was a cause of hepatitis and encephalitis. It was seen in children with influenza or varicella who were given aspirin. Widespread knowledge of this issue, resulting in an almost complete cessation of the use of aspirin in children, has made Reye syndrome a very rare occurrence. (*Rudolph's Pediatrics, p. 1490*)

82. **(E)** Gray or brown teeth staining can be seen with the use of tetracycline in children who still have their primary teeth. Tetracyclines are usually safe as a single course in normal doses in younger children. The use of tetracyclines in children is typically safe after 8 years of age. Teeth staining can also be seen in the children of women who took tetracycline while pregnant. (*Rudolph's Pediatrics, p. 878*)

83. **(A)** Theophylline, a methylxanthine, has an excitatory effect on the CNS. This serious side effect, in conjunction with its very narrow therapeutic window, has made theophylline use very uncommon. The use of any of the other medications listed would be recommended before consideration of the use of theophylline. (*Fleisher and Ludwig, pp. 924–925*)

BIBLIOGRAPHY

American Academy of Pediatrics. *The Red Book, 2003 Report of the Committee on infectious Diseases*, 26th ed. Elk Grove Village, IL: American Academy of Pediatrics, 2003.

Behrman RE, Kliegman RM, Jensen HD. *Nelson Textbook of Pediatrics*, 17th ed. Philadelphia, PA: W.B. Saunders, 2004.

Fenichel, GM. *Clinical Pediatric Neurology*, 3rd ed. Philadelphia, PA: W.B. Saunders, 1997.

Fitzpatrick TB, Johnson RA, Wolff K, et al. *Color Atlas and Synopsis of Clinical Dermatology*, 4th ed. New York, NY: McGraw-Hill, 2001.

Fleisher GR, Ludwig S (eds.). *Textbook of Pediatric Emergency Medicine*, 4th ed. Baltimore, MD: Lippincott Williams & Wilkins, 2000.

Hoffman R, et al. *Hematology: Basic Principles and Practice*, 3rd ed. Philadelphia, PA: Churchill Livingstone, 2000.

Jones KL (ed.). *Smith's Recognizable Pattern of Human Malformations*, 5th ed. Philadelphia, PA: W.B. Saunders, 1997.

McMillin JA, et al. *Oski's Pediatrics: Principles and Practice*, 3rd ed. Philadelphia, PA: Lippincott Williams & Wilkins, 1999.

Rudolph CD, Rudolph AM, et al. (ed.). *Rudolph's Pediatrics*, 21st ed. New York, NY: McGraw-Hill, 2003.

CHAPTER 4

Obstetrics and Gynecology
Questions

1. A 23-year-old female presents to the emergency department with "abdominal cramping," nausea, and vaginal bleeding. A human chorionic gonadotropin level returns 5150 mIU/mL. A vaginal probe ultrasound is performed and notes no evidence of an intrauterine pregnancy, normal appearing ovaries, a mild amount of fluid in the cul-de-sac, and no evidence of ectopic gestation. The emergency department physician can exclude which diagnosis from the differential?

   (A) spontaneous abortion
   (B) ectopic pregnancy
   (C) singleton intrauterine pregnancy
   (D) ruptured ovarian cyst (corpus luteum)
   (E) molar pregnancy

2. Following tubal ligation what percentage of pregnancies are ectopic?

   (A) 1%
   (B) 5%
   (C) 30%
   (D) 50%
   (E) 75%

3. A 31-year-old female presents to her physician complaining of rapid onset of hirsutism, deepening of the voice, irregular menses, clitoral enlargement, and acne. Which of the following is the most likely cause of this clinical presentation?

   (A) polycystic ovary syndrome (PCOS)
   (B) Cushing's syndrome

   (C) type II diabetes mellitus
   (D) androgen secreting tumor
   (E) acromegaly

4. A 23-year-old female presents to her obstetrician/gynecologist complaining of inability to conceive. She has regular menstrual cycles, and her husband's semen analysis is normal. She undergoes a hysterosalpingogram that shows evidence of bilateral distal tubal obstruction. Which of the following is the most likely cause of acquired tubal damage?

   (A) appendicitis
   (B) pelvic inflammatory disease (PID)
   (C) salpingitis isthmica nodosa (SIN)
   (D) trauma
   (E) ruptured ovarian cyst

5. A 17-year-old female presents with delayed puberty. Her mother reports lack of menarche. On examination the patient is 59 in (4 ft 11 in) tall, has widely spaced nipples, a broad neck, and tanner stage I breasts. Which of the following tests is most likely to confirm the diagnosis?

   (A) karyotype
   (B) follicle stimulating hormone (FSH)
   (C) luteinizing hormone (LH)
   (D) cranial MRI
   (E) growth hormone (GH)

6. In order to prevent unintended pregnancy following an episode of unprotected intercourse, by when is it recommended that "emergency" oral contraception should be initiated?

   (A) 12 h
   (B) 24 h
   (C) 48 h
   (D) 72 h
   (E) 1 week

7. A 61-year-old female is diagnosed with osteoporosis by a screening dual-energy x-ray absorptiometry (DEXA) scan. Which of these is a risk factor for postmenopausal osteoporosis?

   (A) Black
   (B) does not exercise
   (C) obese
   (D) delivered three children
   (E) late menopause

8. A 5-year-old girl presents for evaluation of breast development, history of multiple bone fractures, and vaginal bleeding. Physical examination is notable for "café au lait" spots on her skin, tanner stage 2 breasts, and she appears tall for her age. What is the most likely cause of precocious puberty in this child?

   (A) acromegaly
   (B) McCune-Albright syndrome
   (C) ovarian cyst
   (D) ingestion of her mother's oral contraceptives
   (E) hyperparathyroidism

9. A 39-year-old obese female presents with irregular menstrual periods, mild acne and hirsutism, and acanthosis nigricans on the nuchal fold, axilla, and intertriginous areas (inner upper thighs). You suspect PCOS. Which of the following laboratory tests would be most important to perform to rule out a likely confounding diagnosis?

   (A) 2-h oral glucose tolerance test
   (B) testosterone
   (C) prolactin

   (D) dehydroepiandrosterone sulfate (DHEAS)
   (E) LH and FSH

10. A 17-year-old female presents with primary amenorrhea. On physical examination she has normal secondary sexual characteristics, scant pubic and axillary hair, and a blind ending vaginal pouch. A pelvic MRI indicates inguinal gonads and no uterus. Her karyotype is 46, XY. Which of the following is the most likely etiology of primary amenorrhea in this patient?

    (A) müllerian agenesis (Mayer-Rokitansky-Küster-Hauser syndrome)
    (B) Klinefelter syndrome
    (C) androgen insensitivity
    (D) Turner mosaic
    (E) Kallmann syndrome

11. A 15-year-old female presents to the emergency room (ER) with acute onset right lower quadrant pain and nausea. She recently became sexually active and is "in the middle" of her menstrual cycle. Physical examination is notable for generalized guarding, rebound, and 8/10 pain in both lower quadrants. A pelvic examination shows no vaginal discharge, a normal appearing cervix, and general pelvic tenderness, but the examination is limited by the patient's guarding. Her complete blood count is notable for a borderline elevated white blood cell (WBC) count, and a urinary β-human chorionic gonadotropin is negative. Pelvic ultrasound shows a 2-cm simple appearing cyst on the right ovary and a mild amount of fluid in the cul-de-sac. A computed tomographic (CT) scan cannot definitively visualize the appendix, confirms the presence of a 2-cm cystic structure in the right ovary, and otherwise notes normal anatomy. Which of the following is the most appropriate next step?

    (A) diagnostic laparoscopy
    (B) pelvic MRI
    (C) intravenous antibiotics
    (D) admission for serial physical examinations and pain control
    (E) discharge home on oral antibiotics

12. An amenorrheic 17-year-old female is diagnosed with Kallmann syndrome. Blood testing of this patient would indicate which of the following results?

    (A) FSH, LH, normal estradiol
    (B) high FSH, high LH, low estradiol
    (C) normal FSH, normal LH, normal estradiol
    (D) low FSH, low LH, normal estradiol
    (E) low FSH, low LH, low estradiol

13. A woman complains of amenorrhea following a dilation and curettage. Uterine synechiae (scarring) following a surgical procedure or infection is termed as:

    (A) Sheehan syndrome
    (B) Asherman syndrome
    (C) Fitz-Hugh-Curtis syndrome
    (D) Swyer syndrome
    (E) syndrome X

14. Implantation of the embryo into the endometrium occurs how many days after ovulation?

    (A) 1
    (B) 2
    (C) 4
    (D) 6
    (E) 10

15. The pregnancy risk factor category B for a drug indicates which of the following?

    (A) Controlled human studies demonstrate no risk to a fetus.
    (B) This drug should never be used by a pregnant female under any circumstances.
    (C) Evidence of human teratogenic risk exists but in some cases the known risks may be outweighed in some serious situations, such as life-threatening disease.
    (D) Animal-reproduction studies have not demonstrated fetal risk but there are no controlled human studies to assess the risk.
    (E) Animal-reproduction studies have demonstrated risk to a fetus and no controlled human studies are available.

16. A 26-year-old female with recurrent pregnancy loss undergoes a laparoscopy and hysteroscopy. She is found to have a müllerian anomaly with a heart-shaped uterus that has two uterine horns but one common cervix. The name of the uterine anomaly is:

    (A) didelphic
    (B) septate
    (C) unicornuate
    (D) bicornuate
    (E) müllerian agenesis (Mayer-Rokitansky-Küster-Hauser syndrome)

17. A 16-year-old female presents for secondary amenorrhea. She cannot remember the date of her last menstrual period. A pregnancy test returns positive. Which of the following is the most accurate way to determine an estimated gestational age?

    (A) measure a uterine fundal height
    (B) ultrasound measurement of fetus during the first trimester
    (C) ultrasound measurement of fetus during the second trimester
    (D) knowing the date of "quickening," or the date of first recognized fetal movement
    (E) pelvic (bimanual) examination

18. A patient with a persistent headache following a postpartum hemorrhage is diagnosed with Sheehan syndrome. If the patient were subsequently amenorrheic and infertile, what treatment would you recommend to assist this patient to conceive?

    (A) gonadotropin releasing hormone (GnRH) pump
    (B) clomiphene citrate
    (C) dopamine agonist
    (D) in vitro fertilization
    (E) gonadotropins (FSH and LH)

19. A 44-year-old female has a history of endometriosis resulting in chronic pelvic pain. She presents to you 6 months after her total abdominal hysterectomy and bilateral salpingo-oophorectomy. She reports continued pelvic pain. Which of the following would be your most appropriate recommendation for medical management?

    (A) GnRH
    (B) oral estrogens
    (C) oral progestins
    (D) tamoxifen
    (E) GnRH antagonist

20. The predicted length of the follicular phase of a patient with a consistent 34-day menstrual cycle is:

    (A) 14 days
    (B) depends on the length of the luteal phase
    (C) 16 days
    (D) 18 days
    (E) 20 days

21. Which of the following can induce menstrual bleeding in a 21-year-old anovulatory, amenorrheic woman with PCOS?

    (A) administration of progestins
    (B) administration of estrogens
    (C) withdrawal of progestin therapy
    (D) withdrawal of estrogen therapy
    (E) danazol

22. A 63-year-old woman with a grade 2 endometrioid adenocarcinoma of the uterus diagnosed by endometrial biopsy is taken to the operating room for surgical treatment with a total abdominal hysterectomy, bilateral salpingo-oophorectomy, and pelvic and paraaortic lymphadenectomy. No complications are noted intraoperatively. On postoperative day number one, the patient complains of numbness in her medial thigh. Your neurologic examination suggests absence of cutaneous sensation to the medial thigh and an inability to adduct her hip.

Which of the following is the most likely etiology for this clinical presentation?

    (A) femoral nerve injury
    (B) genitofemoral nerve injury
    (C) pudendal nerve injury
    (D) obturator nerve injury
    (E) peroneal nerve injury

23. A 41-year-old woman, recently diagnosed with a 2-cm, stage IB1 cervical cancer, undergoes a radical hysterectomy, bilateral salpingo-oophorectomy, and retroperitoneal pelvic lymph node dissection. Her surgery and postoperative course are uncomplicated. Four weeks postoperatively, she presents to the ER complaining of left leg swelling and left lower quadrant abdominal pain. On physical examination she is afebrile, has a normal WBC count, and you palpate a 5 × 4 cm mass in the left lower quadrant. You order a pelvic ultrasound that shows a 5 × 5 cm simple cyst in the left lower quadrant. Which of the following is the most likely diagnosis?

    (A) deep venous thrombosis (DVT)
    (B) pelvic abscess
    (C) lymphocyst
    (D) ovarian cyst
    (E) diverticular abscess

Questions 24 and 25

A 38-year-old woman presents to the ER with heavy vaginal bleeding. A pelvic examination using a speculum to visualize the cervix reveals a large, friable, fungating cervical mass. On bimanual examination, the mass extends to the right pelvic sidewall. A biopsy from a recent gynecologic visit reveals invasive squamous cell carcinoma of the cervix. An abdominal/pelvic CT scan shows enlarged pelvic lymph nodes and right hydronephrosis. Her hematocrit in the ER is 24%, but she is hemodynamically stable with a blood pressure (BP) of 124/70 and a pulse of 73. The cervical mass is actively bleeding.

24. Which of the following is the most appropriate immediate management of the vaginal bleeding in the ER?

  (A) vaginal packing soaked with Monsel's solution
  (B) vitamin K
  (C) transfusion of fresh frozen plasma (FFP)
  (D) uterine massage
  (E) supportive care with transfusion of packed red blood cells

25. Your initial treatment of the vaginal bleeding in the ER only partially controls the bleeding, and she is requiring frequent retreatment. The best definitive treatment to control the bleeding at this time is:

  (A) emergency bilateral hypogastric artery ligation
  (B) uterine artery embolization
  (C) emergency high-dose radiation therapy
  (D) emergency radical hysterectomy
  (E) loop excision electrocautery procedure (LEEP)

Questions 26 and 27

26. A 42-year-old woman who previously underwent a vaginal hysterectomy for persistent cervical dysplasia presents to your office for vaginal cytology. Her vaginal cytology is consistent with a high-grade squamous intraepithelial lesion (HGSIL). Which of the following is the most appropriate next step in management?

  (A) repeat vaginal cytology in 6 months
  (B) observation
  (C) random vaginal biopsies
  (D) intravaginal estrogen cream followed by repeat cytology
  (E) colposcopic examination of the vaginal canal

27. On speculum examination you visualize a 1 × 1 cm lesion at the left vaginal fornix. The lesion is acetowhite, slightly raised, with coarse punctation and bizarre branching vessels. You take a biopsy of the lesion and the pathology returns consistent with vaginal intraepithelial neopla-

sia (VAIN) 3, suspicious for invasion. Your next step in management is:

  (A) carbon dioxide (CO_2) laser
  (B) wide local excision of the lesion
  (C) intravaginal 5-flourouracil (5-FU)
  (D) intravaginal estrogen cream
  (E) total vaginectomy

28. A 61-year-old postmenopausal woman, who has been on continuous combined hormone replacement therapy for 5 years, presents to your office complaining of vaginal bleeding. Which of the following is the most appropriate next step in her management?

  (A) pap smear
  (B) endocervical curettage (ECC)
  (C) pelvic ultrasound
  (D) endometrial biopsy
  (E) dilation and curettage

29. You are consulted by a 55-year-old asymptomatic postmenopausal woman who has been on tamoxifen for 2 years following a diagnosis of breast cancer. She has no other risk factors for endometrial cancer but she was searching the Internet and found information about the risks of tamoxifen therapy. She inquires about endometrial cancer screening. You tell her that for asymptomatic women on tamoxifen, the screening recommendations for endometrial cancer are:

  (A) yearly pelvic ultrasounds
  (B) yearly endometrial biopsies
  (C) yearly gynecologic examinations
  (D) yearly pelvic CT scans
  (E) yearly hysteroscopy

30. In your internal medicine clinic you are caring for a 42-year-old woman with hereditary non-polyposis colon cancer (HNPCC), Lynch syndrome II, which is a hereditary, autosomal dominant, cancer syndrome that results from a mutation in a mismatch DNA repair gene. These patients have a lifetime risk of colon cancer nearly 60–80%, but are also at risk for several other malignancies. For which gynecologic malignancy is this woman most at risk?

(A) ovarian cancer
(B) breast cancer
(C) cervical cancer
(D) vulvar cancer
(E) endometrial cancer

31. A 37-year-old woman (gravida 3, para 3) presents with a 4-month history of postcoital spotting. On pelvic examination, you visualize a 2-cm friable lesion on the anterior lip of the cervix. The next most appropriate step is:

(A) colposcopy
(B) pap smear
(C) office biopsy of the cervical lesion
(D) cervical cone biopsy
(E) metronidazole vaginal cream followed by reexamination

Questions 32 through 34

32. A 22-year-old nulliparous woman who desires future fertility is found to have a pap smear consistent with HGSIL. Initial management should be:

(A) routine pap smear in 1 year
(B) random cervical biopsies
(C) colposcopy
(D) endometrial biopsy
(E) human papilloma virus (HPV) testing

33. The test you performed above was inadequate. What would be your next step in management?

(A) transvaginal ultrasound
(B) endometrial dilation and curettage
(C) ECC

(D) cold knife cervical conization
(E) repeat pap smear in 3 months

34. The final pathology report indicates a single focus of squamous carcinoma invasive into the cervical stroma to a depth of 2.0 mm. An ECC is negative. There is no lymphovascular space invasion, and the cone margins are negative. The most appropriate therapy for this patient is:

(A) radiation therapy
(B) simple hysterectomy with pelvic lymphadenectomy
(C) radical hysterectomy with pelvic lymphadenectomy
(D) radical trachelectomy
(E) observation with close follow-up

35. A 39-year-old woman with a long-standing history of normal pap smears undergoes a total abdominal hysterectomy for a large uterine fibroid and menorrhagia. Six months after her hysterectomy she had a negative vaginal pap smear from the vaginal apex. She presents to your clinic today for a routine physical examination. Based on the American College of Obstetricians and Gynecologists recommendations, this patient should have pap smears:

(A) yearly
(B) every 3 years
(C) every 5 years
(D) never again
(E) only if she develops risk factors

36. A 56-year-old thin, White woman, who has recently undergone a total abdominal hysterectomy, bilateral salpingo-oophorectomy, and pelvic lymphadenectomy for a stage IB, grade 1, endometrioid tumor of the uterus, presents to your office complaining of hot flashes and vaginal dryness. She wants advice about the use of estrogen replacement in women treated for endometrial cancer. The best treatment for this woman is:

(A) psychotherapy
(B) estrogen replacement therapy

(C) increased soy intake

(D) combination hormone replacement therapy

(E) referral to an endometrial cancer support group

Questions 37 and 38

A 43-year-old Black female (gravida 3, para 3) with a previous tubal ligation, presents to your office complaining of increasing menorrhagia, dysmenorrhea, and fatigue over the past 6 months. On examination, her vital signs are normal, and on abdominal examination you palpate a firm, mobile mass just below the umbilicus. On pelvic examination, there is a moderate amount of old blood coming from the cervical os. A urine pregnancy test is negative, her last pap smear was normal and her spun hematocrit today is 28%.

37. Which diagnostic test would be most cost-effective in confirming a diagnosis?

(A) pelvic MRI

(B) abdominal plain films

(C) pelvic ultrasound

(D) hysterosalpingogram

(E) office laparoscopy

38. Which pharmacologic agent would potentially result in an improvement in her hematocrit and help to decrease uterine size?

(A) oral contraceptive pills (OCPs)

(B) medroxyprogesterone

(C) nonsteroidal anti-inflammatory agents

(D) narcotics

(E) GnRH agonists

Questions 39 and 40

A 76-year-old White female (gravida 8, para 8) presents to her family practitioner complaining of vaginal pressure, dyspareunia, urinary incontinence, and difficulty emptying her bladder for the past 4 weeks. Seven years ago she had a vaginal hysterectomy for uterine prolapse. Her postvoid residual urine in the office measures 250 cm^3. On examination, her anterior vaginal wall prolapses 4 cm beyond the hymen.

39. The most likely etiology of her urinary retention is

(A) detrusor overactivity

(B) bladder outlet obstruction

(C) urinary tract infection (UTI)

(D) menopause

(E) spinal cord tumor

40. Which of the following would be the most appropriate action to take at this time?

(A) referral for immediate surgery

(B) abdominal and pelvic CT scan

(C) urinalysis with culture and sensitivity

(D) prescription for oxybutynin (Ditropan)

(E) urodynamic studies

Questions 41 and 42

A 14-year-old nulligravid female is brought to the ER by her parents with a 12-h history of severe, intermittent left lower quadrant pain. She has had nausea and vomiting for the past 2 h. On history, the patient experienced menarche at age 12 and denies past or current contact with a sexual partner. Her last normal menstrual period was 3 weeks ago. On examination, she is afebrile, pulse 100, BP 110/70, respiratory rate (RR) 20. She is visibly uncomfortable. She has no costovertebral tenderness, has diminished bowel sounds, her abdomen is nondistended, and exhibits rebound and guarding in both lower quadrants. She is unable to tolerate a pelvic examination due to pain. Laboratory values are as follows: WBC 13, hematocrit HCT 39, β-human chorionic gonadotropin (β-hCG) (–), urinalysis (UA) (–). A pelvic ultrasound shows a normal nonpregnant uterus, normal right adnexa, and an 8-cm left adnexal mass with a 3-cm solid component.

41. The next appropriate step in managing this patient would be:

(A) abdominal and pelvic CT scan

(B) social work referral for possible sexual abuse

(C) obtain liver enzymes, amylase, and lipase

(D) consultation for immediate surgical intervention

(E) discharge to home with pain medications

42. The most likely etiology of this patient's pain is:

(A) ectopic pregnancy
(B) acute appendicitis
(C) ovarian torsion
(D) pancreatitis
(E) somatization disorder

Questions 43 and 44

A 22-year-old White female (gravida 2, para 1, abortus 1) comes to your office with a 3-week history of lower abdominal pain and increased vaginal discharge. She has a prior history of an ectopic pregnancy at age 16. Her last menstrual period (LMP) was 7 days ago, and she has had unprotected vaginal intercourse with a new sexual partner several times over the past few weeks. Her temperature is 38.0°C; her vital signs are stable. She has bilateral lower quadrant tenderness but no peritoneal signs. On speculum examination she has foul smelling green discharge emanating from her cervix. She has cervical motion tenderness on bimanual examination and is tender in both adnexae. Her wet mount shows copious white cells. Her urine β-hCG is (−).

43. The most appropriate treatment regimen for this patient would be:

(A) metronidazole PO for 5 days
(B) gentamycin IV × one dose
(C) ceftriaxone intramuscular (IM) plus doxycycline PO for 14 days
(D) Diflucan PO × one dose
(E) ampicillin PO qid × 14 days

44. Most cases of PID are associated with:

(A) gonorrhea alone
(B) chlamydia alone
(C) *Candida albicans*
(D) herpes simplex virus
(E) polymicrobial aerobic and anaerobic bacteria from the lower genital tract

45. A 43-year-old morbidly obese woman presents to your office with a 3-week history of increasing vulvar burning. She has had no new sexual partners or practices. She has not noticed any change in her vaginal discharge. She has

attempted to medicate herself with over-the-counter antifungals, herbal creams, and old antibiotics, none of which have provided relief. On examination, her entire labia majora and minora are markedly erythematous and tender to the touch. Her vaginal mucosa appears to have normal rugae. Her vaginal pH is normal and whiff test is negative. The wet mount shows a few WBCs and normal squamous cells. The most likely diagnosis is:

(A) chemical dermatitis
(B) bacterial vaginosis
(C) PID disease
(D) atrophic vaginitis
(E) lichens sclerosis et atrophicus

46. A concerned mother brings her 5-year-old daughter to the ER because she noticed redness around her daughter's genital region while bathing her last night. The child has not complained of any discomfort, itching, bleeding, or inappropriate contact with other adults. On external inspection of her labia, you see the fusion of the labia minora and generalized erythema. The most appropriate treatment would be:

(A) surgical excision
(B) vaginoscopy and biopsies
(C) ice packs and sitz baths
(D) lidocaine ointment
(E) topical estrogen cream

Questions 47 through 49

A 70-year-old White woman has been faithful about taking 1200 mg of calcium, 400 IU of vitamin D supplements, and performing weight bearing exercise on a daily basis. Her hip T score from her current DEXA scan has changed from −2.0 SDs to −2.55 SDs compared with last year's test.

47. At this time you recommend:

(A) oral alendronate (a bisphosphonate)
(B) weekly GnRH injections
(C) discontinuation of her vitamin D
(D) glucocorticoid therapy
(E) IM testosterone

48. Which of the following statements is correct?

(A) With osteoporosis, serum calcium is low.
(B) With hyperparathyroidism, serum calcium is normal.
(C) With Paget disease, serum calcium is low.
(D) With renal failure, serum calcium is low.
(E) With osteomalacia, serum calcium is high.

49. Which of the following is associated with a reduced risk of osteoporotic fractures?

(A) family history of hip fractures
(B) estrogen deficiency
(C) body mass index of greater than 23
(D) tobacco use
(E) vision problems

50. A 25-year-old nulligravid female, whose last menstrual period was 4 weeks ago, is seen by her obstetrician-gynecologist (OB/GYN) for a left breast mass. The patient discovered it 2 weeks ago while in the shower. Her maternal aunt died of breast cancer at age 60, and the patient is very worried about this new finding. On examination, a mobile, nonerythematous, 3-cm nonsolid feeling mass is palpated in the left upper outer quadrant of her left breast. There is no nipple discharge, and the axillary lymph nodes are nonpalpable. Her right breast examination is normal. The patient wants you to schedule a mammogram that same day. You reply that:

(A) A surgical biopsy should be performed instead.
(B) A needle core biopsy can be done at the same time of her mammogram.
(C) Ultrasound would be a better imaging modality for her situation.
(D) In-office cyst aspiration is reassuring if the fluid is bloody.
(E) Antibiotics can treat her mastitis.

51. A 63-year-old Black female presents to your office complaining of leaking urine. She gets up at night five times to urinate and occasionally loses urine en route to the toilet. During the daytime she urinates every 45 min "to help prevent the leakage." She denies loss of urine with coughing or sneezing. She has not had dysuria or any other pelvic floor complaints. She has a family history of diabetes. She drinks several caffeinated beverages throughout the day. On examination, her postvoid residual urine is normal, and a urine dipstick shows 3+ glucose but is otherwise negative. Her abdominal and pelvic examinations are normal. You recommend:

(A) surgery for her incontinence
(B) antibiotics for a UTI
(C) diuretic therapy
(D) timed voids, decrease in caffeine intake, and screening for diabetes
(E) referral to a urologist for cystoscopy

52. A 31-year-old (gravida 1, para 1) female had a forceps-assisted vaginal delivery 3 months ago. Her infant weighed 4250 g. During the delivery she sustained a fourth degree perineal injury that was repaired. She now complains of fecal incontinence when her stools are loose, which happens several days a week. The most likely etiology for her fecal incontinence would be:

(A) Crohn disease
(B) a perianal abscess
(C) a vaginal hematoma
(D) a retained vaginal foreign body
(E) a rectovaginal fistula

Questions 53 through 55

You are asked to perform a high school physical examination for a 16-year-old female patient. She is on the track team. By history, she is healthy except for the fact that she has been amenorrheic for 4 months. She denies current or past sexual activity. On examination, she is 5 ft 9 in tall and weighs 115 lb. Her heart rate is 50 bpm. She has dry skin with lanugo. She has several sores in her mouth and obvious dental caries. She has several scratches on the backs of her hands. She is tanner stage III on breast examination. Her pelvic examination is remarkable for findings of urogenital atrophy. Her urine β-hCG is negative.

53. The most likely diagnosis for this patient would be:

(A) domestic abuse

(B) eating disorder

(C) hyperthyroidism

(D) herpes simplex virus serotype I

(E) congenital adrenal hyperplasia

54. At this point in time, appropriate management of this patient would include:

(A) laboratory assessment of electrolytes and an electrocardiogram

(B) intensive care unit (ICU) admission

(C) antipsychotic medication

(D) reassurance

(E) intramuscular Depo-Provera injection

55. This patient is at risk for developing:

(A) schizophrenia

(B) renal failure

(C) morbid obesity

(D) osteoporosis

(E) cholecystitis

Questions 56 and 57

A 22-year-old Black female (G_3P_{0020}) presents to your office for an initial obstetric visit in her third pregnancy. She reports a sure last menstrual period date approximately 6 weeks ago, with a history of regular cycles. Her two previous pregnancies ended in spontaneous abortions. She denies any significant medical or surgical history. She denies use of alcohol, tobacco, or illicit drugs, though she does report a history of IV drug use as a teenager. She is a full-time student. She reports that twins run in her family, but she does not have any family history of diabetes, hypertension, or congenital anomalies. On review of her prenatal labs that have already been drawn, you find that her human immunodeficiency virus (HIV) antibody test is positive. Her test results are otherwise normal.

56. You counsel the patient that:

(A) This result is a false positive due to pregnancy, and she does not need any further testing.

(B) She is infected with HIV and will need to begin treatment right away.

(C) She will require an additional, confirmatory test to determine whether or not she has HIV.

(D) She may have HIV, but she should wait until after she delivers her baby to have further testing.

(E) Because it has been years since she participated in high-risk behaviors, she is unlikely to have HIV.

57. Which of the following is recommended to reduce the risk of perinatal transmission of HIV from mother to infant?

(A) A scheduled cesarean delivery can reduce the risk of transmission if the maternal viral load is greater than 1000 copies/mL.

(B) All pregnant women with HIV should receive highly active antiretroviral therapy regardless of severity of HIV infection.

(C) No treatment is required; the risk of perinatal transmission of HIV is quite low.

(D) All patients with HIV should be required to have a cesarean delivery.

(E) Treatment of opportunistic infections such as *Pneumocystis carinii* pneumonia in the mother is most important in reducing the perinatal transmission of HIV.

58. A 34-year-old Black (G_1) presents to your clinic for an obstetric visit at 16 weeks estimated gestational age (EGA). She has a sure LMP and her estimated date of delivery (EDD) is in December. She is generally healthy and has not had any surgeries. She denies history of sexually transmitted diseases or abnormal pap smears. She has no significant family history. She does not smoke or use alcohol or illicit drugs. She works as an administrative assistant.

Her prenatal labs are as follows: blood type O+, antibody screen negative; hepatitis B surface antigen negative; HIV antibody negative; Rubella nonimmune; RPR (syphilis) nonreactive; pap smear within normal limits; urine culture negative.

Based on her lab results and history, you recommend that she receive which of the following injections during her pregnancy?

(A) measles, mumps, and rubella vaccine

(B) influenza vaccine

(C) hepatitis B vaccine series

(D) RhoGAM injection

(E) poliomyelitis vaccine

Questions 59 and 60

A 19-year-old Hispanic (G_2P_{1001}) at $35^4/_7$ weeks EGA presents for a routine prenatal visit. Her pregnancy has been uncomplicated. She reports good fetal movement and denies vaginal bleeding, loss of fluid, or contractions. She is excited about the arrival of her baby and is planning to breast-feed. Her past medical history is significant for chlamydia that was treated approximately 1 year ago. She is otherwise healthy. Her BP today is 110/60. Fundal height is appropriate. UA is negative.

59. The patient would like to discuss options for postpartum birth control. Which of the following would be an appropriate and effective option for postpartum birth control for this patient?

(A) combined OCP

(B) intrauterine device (IUD)

(C) progesterone-only pill

(D) no birth control is necessary as the patient will be breast-feeding

(E) rhythm method

60. The patient wants to know what complications she might experience from breast-feeding. You tell her that the most common complication of breast-feeding is mastitis. If she were to develop mastitis, which of the following treatments would be recommended?

(A) dicloxacillin by mouth plus discontinuation of breast-feeding

(B) discontinuation of breast-feeding only

(C) Flagyl by mouth plus discontinuation of breast-feeding

(D) dicloxacillin by mouth with continued breast-feeding

(E) no treatment is required for mastitis

Questions 61 through 63

A 30-year-old (G_2P_{0101}) presents to the clinic for a new obstetric visit. She has an unknown LMP. She reports that she discovered she was pregnant when she took a urine pregnancy test at home a month ago. She vaguely recalls having a period about 2 months ago, but is not sure exactly when that occurred. She reports that she is generally healthy. She had a previous delivery at 36 weeks estimated gestational age, though she reports her doctor was not really sure about her due date in that pregnancy. She reports that she had a normal spontaneous vaginal delivery in her previous pregnancy, and the child is healthy. Her postpartum course was complicated by depression, which has since resolved and not recurred. She denies history of sexually transmitted diseases or abnormal pap smears. She has no surgical history. She does not smoke, drink alcohol, or use illicit drugs. She does not have any family history of hypertension, diabetes, twins, or congenital anomalies. She does report that her mother has a history of depression.

61. Which of the following tests will provide the most useful information to determine this patient's EDD?

(A) pelvic examination

(B) serum FSH and LH

(C) serum quantitative β-human chorionic gonadotropin (β-hCG) level

(D) measurement of fundal height

(E) pelvic ultrasound

62. Given the patient's history of postpartum depression as well as her family history of depression, her risk of postpartum depression after this pregnancy is approximately:

(A) 50% or greater

(B) 5%

(C) 10%

(D) 20%

(E) less than 1%

63. Postpartum psychosis is a serious disorder that can occur in the early postpartum period. Patients with which of the following medical conditions are at increased risk of postpartum psychosis?

(A) multiparity

(B) anxiety disorder

(C) thyroid disease

(D) bipolar disorder

(E) advanced maternal age

Questions 64 and 65

A 24-year-old White G_1P_{1001} presents to your office 6 weeks after a normal spontaneous vaginal delivery at term. She reports that she has been unable to breast-feed her baby despite help from her pediatrician and a lactation consultant. On further questioning, you elicit that she has also experienced nausea, weakness, and weight loss. In addition, she reports dizziness when getting out of bed in the morning. On your examination, she has a waxy texture to her skin and periorbital edema. You also note decreased axillary and pubic hair, which she reports is a change for her.

64. She most likely has which of the following diagnoses?

(A) postpartum depression

(B) normal postpartum changes

(C) Sheehan syndrome

(D) PCOS

(E) medication reaction

65. This condition is most commonly associated with which of the following?

(A) obesity and increased facial hair

(B) postpartum hemorrhage

(C) acute thrombosis

(D) no specific association is known, this condition is idiopathic

(E) serotonin imbalance

Questions 66 through 68

A 28-year-old White G_1 presents to your office for an initial obstetric visit. She reports a certain last menstrual period that allows you to estimate that she is 9 weeks gestational age today. She denies bleeding, cramping, or other symptoms of concern. She is excited about being pregnant. She has already started taking her prenatal vitamins with folic acid. She reports no significant past medical history. In fact, she states that she has not been to a doctor in many years because she has not had any problems. She has had no surgeries. She does not smoke. She drank alcohol socially prior to pregnancy but has not consumed any alcohol since she became pregnant. She has family history of hypertension, but no other significant history is elicited.

On physical examination, her BP is 110/60. She is healthy appearing, and you have no significant findings on your examination. Your pelvic examination confirms uterine size consistent with stated dates. As part of a routine laboratory evaluation, you decide to check a thyroid stimulating hormone (TSH). The result comes back with a TSH of 0.4 (normal range 0.5–5.5) and a free T4 of 1.8 (normal range 0.7–2.0).

66. You counsel the patient that she most likely has:

(A) hypothyroidism

(B) hyperthyroidism

(C) normal thyroid function, with laboratory values altered by hormone interactions associated with pregnancy

(D) a drug reaction altering thyroid function

(E) a thyroid nodule

The patient returns to clinic for routine prenatal visits. At approximately 28 weeks' gestational age, you decide to recheck the patient's thyroid levels. At this visit, her TSH is 0.1, her total T4 is 15 (normal range 4.5–12.5), and her free T4 is 2.4.

67. What is the most likely cause of this patient's hyperthyroidism?

    (A) toxic adenoma
    (B) multinodular goiter
    (C) hyperemesis gravidarum
    (D) lymphocytic thyroiditis
    (E) Graves disease

68. What is the most appropriate management of this condition?

    (A) thyroid ablation with radioactive iodine
    (B) prescription for propylthiouracil (PTU)
    (C) prescription for propranolol
    (D) subtotal thyroidectomy
    (E) no intervention is necessary as the problem will go away after the pregnancy

Questions 69 and 70

A 25-year-old nulligravid woman presents as a new patient to your gynecology practice. She has recently moved to the area. She is a healthy woman with no medical problems and is currently using oral contraceptives without problems. She informs you that she and her husband are planning to start a family within the next year. On review, you find her family history is unremarkable, but she informs you that her husband's sister has cystic fibrosis.

69. What is the approximate prevalence of cystic fibrosis carrier state in White individuals?

    (A) 1 in 10
    (B) 1 in 25
    (C) 1 in 50
    (D) 1 in 100
    (E) 1 in 200

70. If she and her husband were both known to carry a cystic fibrosis gene mutation, what would be their likelihood of having a child with cystic fibrosis?

    (A) 100%
    (B) 75%
    (C) 50%
    (D) 33%
    (E) 25%

71. Preconception counseling is an important component of health care encounters with reproductive-age women. As a general recommendation, women of childbearing age should be advised to consume what dose of folic acid for prevention of neural tube defects?

    (A) 0.1 mg
    (B) 0.4 mg
    (C) 1 mg
    (D) 4 mg
    (E) Folic acid has only been shown to prevent the recurrence of neural tube defects in women who have previously had an affected child.

Questions 72 and 73

A 35-year-old woman with two prior term pregnancies presents for her first prenatal visit at 12 weeks' gestation. She recalls having had hypertension near the end of her first pregnancy. She believes her BP has been normal since, but admits that she rarely seeks preventive health care visits, and that her last examination by a physician was more than 2 years ago. Today, you find her BP to be 160/100.

72. Which of the following antihypertensive agents would be contraindicated for management of her hypertension during pregnancy?

    (A) labetalol
    (B) alpha-methyldopa
    (C) enalapril
    (D) nifedipine
    (E) hydralazine

73. Her BP comes under good control after initiating medication and remains well controlled until the 36th week, when her BP is noted to have risen again to 170/110. She is also noted to have 3+ proteinuria on urine dipstick testing. For which of the following complications is she at risk?

    (A) eclampsia
    (B) fetal macrosomia
    (C) abnormal progress of labor
    (D) postpartum hemorrhage
    (E) breech presentation

74. Which of the following agents is considered the first-line therapy for prevention of eclamptic seizures?

   (A) diazepam
   (B) phenytoin
   (C) magnesium sulfate
   (D) phenobarbital
   (E) carbamazepine

75. A woman with type 1 diabetes is at increased risk for having a fetus with which of the following congenital anomalies?

   (A) gastroschisis
   (B) duodenal atresia
   (C) cleft lip and palate
   (D) congenital heart defects
   (E) diaphragmatic hernia

76. Which of the following statements about diabetes in pregnancy is true?

   (A) The risk of spontaneous abortion is not increased when compared to women without diabetes.
   (B) The risk of congenital anomalies rises in relation to the maternal hemoglobin A1c.
   (C) The rate of stillbirth is unchanged when compared to nondiabetic women.
   (D) The risk of cesarean birth is unchanged when compared to nondiabetic women.
   (E) Glycemic control is not related to fetal macrosomia.

77. A pregnant woman presents to the emergency room at 20 weeks' gestation with an acute exacerbation of her chronic bronchial asthma. She complains of a cold of 1 week's duration and admits that she lost her inhaler 2 weeks ago. Her examination reveals a temperature of 38°C, respiratory rate of 40, pulse of 110, and fetal rate of 150. Her lung examination is notable for diffuse expiratory wheezes and a prolonged I:E ratio of 1:4. She is utilizing accessory muscles for breathing, which appears labored. Which of the following statements regarding asthma in pregnancy is true?

   (A) Asthma exacerbations are more common in pregnant women than in nonpregnant women of similar age.
   (B) Influenza vaccination is contraindicated in pregnancy.
   (C) Peak expiratory flow rate monitoring is unreliable for monitoring disease state during pregnancy.
   (D) In pregnant women, the arterial partial pressure of carbon dioxide ($PaCO_2$) is decreased on arterial blood gases compared to nonpregnant individuals.
   (E) Due to potential risks of fetal radiation exposure, chest radiography should not be performed to evaluate for underlying pneumonia in women with asthma exacerbation.

78. Which of the following maternal cardiac conditions is associated with the highest mortality rate during pregnancy?

   (A) mitral stenosis, New York Heart Association class 1-2
   (B) corrected tetralogy of Fallot
   (C) porcine prosthetic heart valve
   (D) mechanical prosthetic heart valve
   (E) pulmonary hypertension

79. Which of the following statements regarding seizures in pregnancy is true?

   (A) Women with a seizure disorder are at increased risk for eclampsia.
   (B) Carbamazepine would be a better anticonvulsant during pregnancy, as it is associated with lower risk of congenital anomalies.
   (C) Women who take valproate during pregnancy are at increased risk for both open neural defects and congenital heart disease.
   (D) Women who require multidrug therapy to control their seizures are at no greater risk for congenital anomalies than women on monotherapy.
   (E) It has been clearly demonstrated that women taking anticonvulsants benefit from higher doses of folic acid for prevention of neural tube defects.

80. The background rate of major congenital anomalies in a general obstetric population is closest to which of the following numbers:

(A) 0.1% (1 in 1000)

(B) 0.5% (5 in 1000)

(C) 1% (10 in 1000)

(D) 3% (30 in 1000)

(E) 7% (70 in 1000)

81. A patient presents to your office for an annual gynecologic examination. She is an obese, postmenopausal, White female who reports a 4-month history of vulvar pruritis. Otherwise, she is without complaint. On examination, she is noted to have a whitened plaque-like area involving the posterior fourchette. The area is nontender, raised, and approximately $2.0 \times 2.0 \times 0.5$ cm. What is the next step in the management of this patient?

(A) Prescribe a topical antimonilial cream.

(B) Obtain a viral culture for herpes simplex type II.

(C) Perform a vaginal wet mount.

(D) Obtain a punch biopsy from the center of the lesion.

(E) Prescribe a topical steroid cream.

82. A 27-year-old nulligravid single White female presents to your office for an annual examination. In taking her history, you learn that her mother died of ovarian cancer at the age of 63. There is no other family history of breast or ovarian cancer. The patient asks you to tell her what she can do to reduce her own ovarian cancer risk. What is the most effective strategy appropriate for this patient to reduce her risk?

(A) bilateral laparoscopic salpingo-oophorectomy

(B) daily aspirin use

(C) oral contraceptive therapy

(D) bilateral tubal ligation

(E) avoidance of breast-feeding following pregnancy

83. A 37-year-old multiparous White female, s/p bilateral tubal ligation, reports a family history remarkable for a mother diagnosed with

bilateral breast cancer at the age of 43, from which she ultimately died, and a sister diagnosed with epithelial ovarian cancer at the age of 47, for which she is currently undergoing chemotherapy. Secondary to this worrisome family history, the patient elected to undergo genetic testing and was found to be a BRCA1 carrier. In view of her carrier status, you inform her that:

(A) She has a 30–50% lifetime risk for the development of ovarian cancer.

(B) She has a 10% lifetime risk for the development of breast cancer.

(C) If she develops ovarian cancer, it will likely be 10–15 years later than the normal onset of ovarian cancer seen in the general population.

(D) She is at increased risk for the development of hereditary nonpolyposis colorectal cancer (Lynch family syndrome type II).

(E) She has a lower risk for the development of fallopian tube cancer than the general patient population.

84. A 62-year-old female with newly diagnosed International Federation of Gynecology and Obstetrics (FIGO) stage IIIC epithelial ovarian cancer is without evidence of visible remaining disease following a total abdominal hysterectomy, bilateral salpingo-oophorectomy, complete omentectomy, bilateral pelvic and paraaortic lymph node sampling, and rectosigmoid resection with reanastomosis. She is seen now for further treatment planning. The appropriate adjuvant chemotherapy indicated in this setting is:

(A) Cyclophosphamide and cisplatin.

(B) The patient has no visible remaining disease and thus requires no further therapy.

(C) Melphalan.

(D) Carboplatin and paclitaxel (Taxol).

(E) Tamoxifen.

85. A 64-year-old White female presents to your office with complaints of vulvar pruritis and pain. You examine her and find an ulcerated lesion in the medial aspect of the left labia majora, 3.0 × 1.5 cm, that is thickened and indurated. You biopsy this lesion and the findings confirm a squamous cell carcinoma of the vulva. The groin nodes are palpably normal bilaterally. The next step in the patient's management would be:

    (A) wide local excision of the lesion
    (B) chemotherapy
    (C) radiation therapy
    (D) radical vulvectomy with ipsilateral inguinofemoral lymphadenectomy
    (E) laser ablation

86. A 37-year-old female presented to your office with an ultrasound report suggestive of bilateral ovarian masses. You take her to the operating room for an exploratory laparotomy and note the left ovary to be replaced by an 8 × 9 cm neoplastic process. The right ovary appears to have a small 2 × 2 cm cystic process, similar in appearance to the left ovary, involving only a small portion of the right ovary. After obtaining pelvic and upper abdominal washings, you remove the left ovary and then perform a cystectomy on the right ovary, removing all visible disease without rupture. The frozen section on both resected specimens reveals a serous tumor of low malignant potential. The best procedure for the patient at this point is:

    (A) Termination of the procedure; await final pathology report on the resected specimens.
    (B) Total abdominal hysterectomy and right salpingo-oophorectomy.
    (C) Omentectomy and peritoneal biopsies.
    (D) Omentectomy, peritoneal biopsies, selected pelvic and peritoneal lymph node sampling.
    (E) Terminate procedure and prescribe postoperative chemotherapy.

87. A 65-year-old female presents with ascites, multiple peritoneal implants, and a large abdominopelvic mass. At laparotomy, she is found to have omental disease, splenic metastases, retroperitoneal lymphadenopathy, and bilateral pelvic masses with rectosigmoid involvement posteriorly and bladder involvement anteriorly. The appropriate surgical management for this patient would be:

    (A) bilateral salpingo-oophorectomy, followed by postoperative chemotherapy
    (B) total abdominal hysterectomy and bilateral salpingo-oophorectomy, followed by postoperative chemotherapy
    (C) complete omentectomy, retroperitoneal lymphadenectomy, total abdominal hysterectomy, and bilateral salpingo-oophorectomy, followed by postoperative chemotherapy
    (D) peritoneal stripping, splenectomy, complete omentectomy, retroperitoneal lymphadenectomy, total abdominal hysterectomy, and bilateral salpingo-oophorectomy, followed by postoperative chemotherapy
    (E) rectosigmoid resection with reanastomosis, peritoneal stripping, splenectomy, complete omentectomy, retroperitoneal lymphadenectomy, total abdominal hysterectomy, and bilateral salpingo-oophorectomy, followed by postoperative chemotherapy

88. A thin, 37-year-old patient undergoes a total abdominal hysterectomy and bilateral salpingo-oophorectomy for chronic menometrorrhagia. The procedure lasts 2 h. A Balfour retractor is utilized intraoperatively to assist with exposure. On the morning of postoperative day #2, the patient stands to get out of bed and collapses on the floor, her right lower extremity unable to support her weight. You are called to examine her. Your neurologic examination suggests an absence of deep tendon reflex in the right lower extremity, absence of cutaneous sensation to the anterior and medial thigh, and an inability to flex at the hip and extend at the

knee. The most likely etiology for this presentation postoperatively is:

(A) DVT
(B) intraoperative compression injury of the femoral nerve
(C) intraoperative stroke
(D) intraoperative transection of the sciatic nerve
(E) undiagnosed diabetes

Questions 89 through 91

You are called by the labor and delivery nurse to evaluate the fetal monitoring strip of a patient. She is a 24 year old G_1 female at 40 weeks gestation who went into spontaneous labor earlier today. She is currently on IV oxytocin (pitocin). You review the fetal monitoring strip shown in Fig. 4-1.

89. What fetal heart rate condition does this monitor strip reveal?

(A) late decelerations
(B) early decelerations
(C) variable decelerations

(D) hyperstimulation
(E) fetal tachycardia

90. What physiologic process causes this to occur?

(A) uteroplacental insufficiency
(B) umbilical cord compression
(C) compression of the fetal head
(D) maternal fever
(E) fetal acidosis caused by too frequent uterine contractions

91. What is the most appropriate management at this point?

(A) Reduction in the dose of oxytocin.
(B) Place the woman on oxygen 10 L via facemask.
(C) Reposition the patient from her back to her left side.
(D) Acetaminophen to reduce maternal temperature.
(E) Reassurance and continuation of current care.

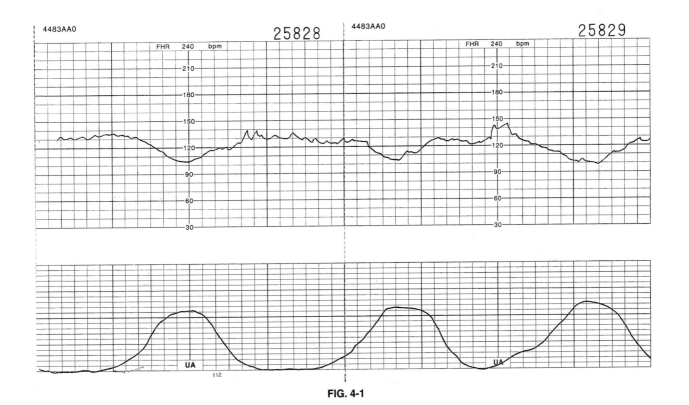

FIG. 4-1

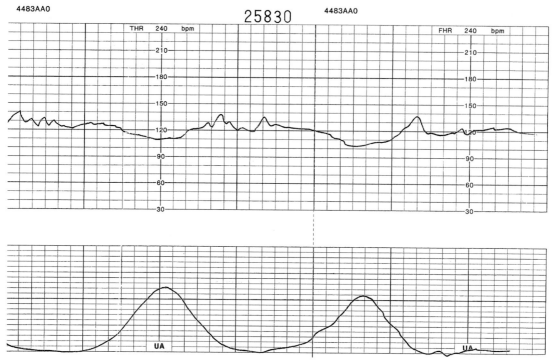

FIG. 4-1 (Continued)

Answers and Explanations

1. **(C)** Differentiating between an ectopic pregnancy, an early intrauterine pregnancy, or a miscarriage is a common dilemma for the emergency department physician. Transabdominal ultrasound can identify a normal intrauterine pregnancy when the β-human chorionic gonadotropin (β-hCG) level is greater than 1500 mIU/mL. Transabdominal ultrasound requires a β-hCG level of 5000–6000 mIU/mL before an intrauterine gestation can be confidently visualized. If the β-hCG is in excess of 1500 mIU/mL and a vaginal probe ultrasound shows no evidence of an intrauterine pregnancy then the patient does not have a normal singleton pregnancy. It is important to remember that a level of 3000 mIU/mL is required for vaginal probe ultrasound to rule out the less-likely possibility that the patient has a twin gestation. *(Beckmann et al., pp. 192–194)*

2. **(C)** Following tubal ligation pregnancy occurs about 1% of the time. This depends on the method used and the expertise of the surgeon. In general, 30% of pregnancies following tubal ligation are ectopic. A patient that presents with a positive pregnancy test following tubal ligation should be considered an "ectopic until proven otherwise." *(Beckmann, p. 353)*

3. **(D)** Androgen excess syndromes are common and usually characterized by one or more of the following problems: hirsutism, acne, weight gain, or irregular menses. PCOS is the most common disorder of androgen excess. Other syndromes that often result in signs and symptoms of androgen excess in adults include Cushing's syndrome and late-onset congenital adrenal hyperplasia. The classic presentation of a patient with an androgen-secreting tumor of the ovary or adrenal gland involves the rapid onset of symptoms. Late-onset congenital adrenal hyperplasia and an androgen-secreting tumor are the only disorders of androgen

excess usually resulting in clitoromegaly. *(Beckmann pp. 475–480)*

4. **(B)** PID is the most common cause of fallopian tube damage. The two most common pathogens are *Neisseria gonorrhea* and *Chlamydia trachomatis*. Other common causes of acquired tubal damage include endometriosis, previous pelvic surgery, and a ruptured appendix. *(Beckmann, pp. 500–501)*

5. **(A)** Numerous causes lead to delayed puberty. Common features of Turner syndrome include short stature, sexual infantilism, "shield" chest, "webbed" neck, high arched palate, increased carrying angle of the arms (cubitus valgus), short fourth metacarpal, and streak gonads. The diagnosis of Turner syndrome is established with a karyotype indicating 45, XO. Although the FSH would be elevated in Turner syndrome, it would not differentiate among the many causes of ovarian failure. *(Beckmann, p. 458)*

6. **(D)** The U.S. Food and Drug Administration (FDA) has approved the use of oral contraceptives as an effective method of postcoital contraception, often termed emergency contraception. The most common regimens involve two to four oral contraceptive tablets, depending on the dosage of the brand used, repeated 12 h later. Progestin-only regimens are also highly effective. Initiating treatment greater than 72 h after the event of unprotected intercourse is associated with a lower success rate. *(Beckmann, pp. 343–344)*

7. **(B)** Risk factors for postmenopausal osteoporosis include cigarette smoking, thinness, early menopause (natural or surgical), nulliparity, northern European heritage, some medications (e.g., glucocorticoids), high alcohol or caffeine intake, low dietary calcium consumption, and a family history of osteoporosis. Dietary calcium

and vitamin D supplementation and exercise (preferably weight bearing) are the classic lifestyle changes recommended to prevent or treat osteoporosis. (*Beckmann, pp. 487–488*)

8. **(B)** The McCune-Albright syndrome is due to a G-protein mutation in the α-subunit that causes constitutive stimulatory activity of the tissues. Affected tissues are autonomously active. Mutations have been found in many tissues including ovary, heart, liver, bone, intestine, adrenal glands, and pituitary adenomas. Sexual precocity, café-au-lait skin spots, and cystic bone lesions (polyostotic fibrous dysplasia) are the classic manifestations of McCune-Albright syndrome. (*Stenchever, p. 269; Speroff, p. 395*)

9. **(A)** PCOS is the most common endocrine disorder of reproductive age women. Common symptoms include oligo- or amenorrhea, acne, hirsutism, infertility, and weight gain. Common tests used to support the diagnosis of PCOS include LH to FSH ratio, testosterone, DHEAS, and pelvic ultrasound.

Acanthosis nigricans is a raised, velvety, tan skin lesion commonly seen on the back of the neck, in the axilla, and the intertriginous areas. Acanthosis nigricans is associated with hyperinsulinemia and is a sign that the patient is at significant risk for prediabetes and frank diabetes. Up to 30% of patients with suspected PCOS have prediabetes, and 8% are frank type II diabetics.

PCOS is a diagnosis of exclusion and requires ruling out other possible confounding diagnoses. Given the obesity and acanthosis nigricans in this patient, a 75-g, 2-h oral glucose tolerance test would be recommended. Other common confounding diagnoses in patients with PCOS include late-onset congenital adrenal hyperplasia (screened with a serum 17-hydroxyprogesterone), Cushing's syndrome (screened with a 24 h urinary free cortisol, or overnight dexamethasone suppression test), and thyroid disease. (*Beckmann, pp. 475–477*)

10. **(C)** Androgen insensitivity is an inherited disease resulting from the lack of functional androgen receptors. Gonadal function is that of normal testicles; however, there is no end-organ effect due to the lack of any functional receptors. Because the gonads produce müllerian inhibiting substance (MIS), the müllerian structures regress. Primary amenorrhea is therefore a common cause for presentation to a physician. Normal female secondary sexual characteristics and external genitalia result. This is due to the absence of any effect of endogenous androgens and the production of small, but adequate, amounts of estrogen, mostly from peripheral conversion of androstenedione. (*Stenchever, pp. 1106–1107*)

11. **(A)** Acute pelvic pain is a difficult diagnostic dilemma. An acute abdomen can result from appendicitis, ovarian torsion, ruptured ovarian cyst, ectopic pregnancy, PID, diverticular abscess, and other causes. Misdiagnosis of PID is common and the most likely diagnosis confused with PID is appendicitis. In the setting where the etiology of the acute abdomen is not certain, a laparoscopy is indicated both for diagnostic and, in many cases, therapeutic purposes. A pelvic MRI or serial examinations would further delay the diagnosis. In the case of ovarian torsion or appendicitis rapid diagnosis and treatment is critical to optimize outcomes. (*Beckmann, pp. 373–374*)

12. **(E)** Kallmann syndrome is a genetic problem due to failure of migration of olfactory and gonadotropin releasing hormone (GnRH) secreting neurons to make their appropriate connections in the brain. Classically, this leads to anosmia (inability to smell), delayed puberty, and amenorrhea. The GnRH is, therefore, not secreted, and pituitary FSH and LH release does not occur. In the absence of stimulation the ovaries do not produce significant estrogen. This is an example of hypogonadotropic hypogonadism, also termed hypothalamic amenorrhea. (*Stenchever, p. 1106*)

13. **(B)** Asherman syndrome describes intrauterine synechiae (scarring) of the uterine cavity following a surgery of infection of the uterine endometrium. Asherman syndrome is seen following uterine surgery (such as a uterine curettage or myomectomy), septic abortion, or other

endometrial cavity infection. The damaged endometrium scars together lead to impairment of the endometrial function. This may result in amenorrhea, dysmenorrhea, infertility, or miscarriage. If the scarring causes obstruction of outflow of menstrual tissue, then hematometra and dysmenorrhea can occur. Severe scarring leads to complete obliteration of the uterine cavity. (Stenchever, pp. 1109–1110)

14. **(D)** Following ovulation, fertilization of the egg by the sperm occurs in the fallopian tube. The embryo then divides and grows as it migrates down the fallopian tube and into the uterine cavity. As early as 6 days postovulation the embryo implants in the uterine endometrium. Trophoblast invasion then occurs allowing the embryo to burrow into the endometrium. A uteroplacental circulation is established by 11–12 days after ovulation allowing β-human chorionic gonadotropin to be detectable in maternal serum or urine. (Stenchever, pp. 7–9)

15. **(D)** The pregnancy risk factor category assists the physician and patient to understand the safety of the use of a medication during pregnancy. The summary of the categories is as follows: category A—controlled human studies demonstrate no risk to a fetus. Category B—animal-reproduction studies have not demonstrated fetal risk but there are no controlled human studies to assess the risk. Category C—animal-reproduction studies have demonstrated risk to a fetus and no controlled human studies are available. Category D—evidence of human teratogenic risk exists but in some cases the known risks may be outweighed in serious situations, such as life-threatening disease. Category X—this drug should never be used by a pregnant female under any circumstances. (Beckmann, p. 96)

16. **(D)** Müllerian anomalies result from either the lack of proper fusion or resorption of the paramesonephric (müllerian) ducts during organogenesis. Vertical abnormalities occur when the invaginating urogenital sinus—extending in a cranial direction from the introitus—and the müllerian structures—extending caudally—fail to canalize appropriately. Longitudinal defects occur when the two paramesonephric ducts either do not fuse appropriately or following fusion the intervening tissue is not reabsorbed completely. A didelphic uterus represents lack of fusion, and the patient has a duplicated cervix and each cervix is connected to a separate uterine horn. A unicornuate uterus results from aplasia of one of the paramesonephric ducts so that only one cervix connecting to a single uterine horn is found. A bicornuate uterus results from failure of the paramesonephric ducts to fuse cranially resulting in a single cervix but two separate uterine horns. A septate uterus occurs when fusion is completed but reabsorption of the intervening tissue is incomplete. (Stenchever, pp. 260–264)

17. **(B)** The most common way to establish a gestational age is a certain last menstrual period or, in some cases, a known date of conception (if infrequent intercourse or use of ovulation prediction method). During the first trimester, an experienced examiner, with a relatively thin and cooperative patient, can offer a reasonable estimate (±2 weeks) of gestational age by a pelvic examination if no other methods are available. The most accurate way to determine, or confirm, gestational age is by obstetric ultrasound. In the first trimester, transvaginal ultrasound is accurate to determine estimated gestational age within ±1–2 weeks. In the second trimester, transabdominal ultrasound is accurate to ±2 weeks. By the third trimester, because of normal variability within the population of fetal growth, transabdominal ultrasound is only accurate within ±2–3 weeks. For the same reason, fundal height becomes less accurate as the pregnancy progresses. Quickening, or the date of first fetal movement, is usually felt by 20 weeks but is quite variable. (Beckmann, pp. 82–84)

18. **(E)** Sheehan syndrome describes damage to the pituitary gland classically resulting from hypotension following a postpartum hemorrhage. The clinical picture is variable due to the fact that the damage may involve one or more of the various cellular subtypes in the pituitary gland that secrete either adrenocorticotropic hormone, GH, prolactin, TSH, or

LH/FSH. An amenorrheic patient with a history of Sheehan syndrome would not be expected to have functional pituitary gonadotropes so a GnRH pump or clomiphene citrate would not be useful because they both rely on a functional pituitary gland. Replacement of gonadotropins (LH and FSH) would be the best treatment option. *(Stenchever, p. 1116)*

19. **(C)** There are a number of effective medical therapies for pain due to endometriosis. These include GnRH agonists, danazol, progestins, and oral contraceptives. Surgical menopause obviates the use of GnRH agonists or antagonists because these medications cause suppression of ovarian function to be effective. Unopposed estrogen would be contraindicated in this patient because of its stimulatory effect on any remaining endometriosis. Tamoxifen has not demonstrated efficacy in the treatment of endometriosis. Progestins are effective at improving endometriosis symptoms due to their atrophic effect. *(Stenchever, pp. 542–552)*

20. **(E)** The luteal phase of the menstrual cycle, defined as beginning with the LH surge and ending with onset menses, is normally fixed at 14 ± 2 days. Therefore, the length of the follicular phase can fairly accurately be determined by subtracting 14 days from the total length of the cycle. In this case the length of the follicular phase is: $34 - 14 = 20$ days. *(Beckmann, pp. 444–454)*

21. **(C)** A patient who is anovulatory due to PCOS would be expected to have normal estrogen production. However, without corpus luteum formation following ovulation there is no significant progesterone production. The administration of progestins to this patient would not be expected to induce menstrual bleeding. Rather, the discontinuation of the progestin therapy would initiate the menstrual flow. *(Beckmann, p. 467)*

22. **(D)** In gynecology, the obturator nerve (L2-L4) is most commonly injured during retroperitoneal surgery for gynecologic malignancies. In this case, a pelvic lymph node dissection for endometrial cancer involves a retroperitoneal dissection into the obturator fossa to remove the obturator lymph nodes. The nodal tissue of the obturator fossa obscures the location of the obturator nerve and predisposes it to injury. Postoperatively, patients with an injury to the obturator nerve will present with sensory loss to the upper medial thigh and motor weakness in the hip adductors.

If an obturator nerve injury is recognized intraoperatively, immediate repair is the recommended treatment. However, with postoperative recognition, as in this case, treatment includes physiotherapy with neuromuscular electrical stimulation and electromyographic biofeedback, and exercise. Obturator nerve injury is a highly treatable condition, and complete recovery of motor strength is generally the result after physical therapy.

The femoral nerve is the most commonly injured nerve at the time of gynecologic surgical procedures, and it is usually injured at the time of laparotomy from inappropriate placement of lateral retractor blades. The retractor blades, when placed too deeply within the lateral pelvis, over the psoas muscle can compress the psoas muscle and the femoral nerve that runs within the muscle. Patients with injury to the femoral nerve will present with diminished or absent deep tendon reflexes, inability to straight leg raise, flex at the hips, or extend the knee. There may also be a loss of cutaneous sensation over the anterior thigh and the medial aspect of the thigh and calf.

The genitofemoral nerve (L1, L2) runs along the ventral surface of the psoas muscle, lateral to the external iliac artery. It is most likely injured during removal of a large pelvic mass, adherent to the pelvic sidewall, or during removal of the external iliac lymph nodes. When feasible, the nerve should be isolated and conserved. However, if removed or damaged, patients present with numbness of the ipsilateral mons pubis, labia majora, and skin overlying the femoral triangle. This nerve conducts sensory information only, thus there is no loss in motor function.

The pudendal nerve (S2-S4) also conducts sensory information only. Injury to the pudendal nerve results in a loss of sensation to the perineum. This is the nerve targeted by obstetricians for a pudendal block given during active labor to provide pain relief with vaginal delivery. Injury to the pudendal nerve at the time of vaginal surgery usually occurs in association with sacrospinous ligament fixation for vaginal vault prolapse. The surgeon can entrap the pudendal nerve within the suture used to secure the apex of the vagina to the sacrospinous ligament. Postoperatively, patients will complain of gluteal pain and perineal paresthesia or numbness.

The common peroneal nerve is the most frequently compressed nerve of the lower extremity. The peroneal nerve branches off the posterior tibial branch of the sciatic nerve just above the popliteal fossa and runs superficially across the lateral head of the fibula and down the lateral calf. This nerve can be compressed when patients are inappropriately placed in the lithotomy position with stirrups. Compression of the peroneal nerve occurs most commonly at the lateral fibular head and results in a foot drop and lateral lower extremity numbness or paresthesia. *(Irvin W, Andersen W, Taylor P, Rice L. Obstet Gynecol. 2004 Feb;103(2):374–382)*

23. **(C)** The incidence of lymphocyst formation following radical hysterectomy and pelvic lymphadenectomy ranges as high as 30%, but is less than 5% if only symptomatic cysts are counted. Risks for lymphocyst formation include lymphadenectomy, radiation therapy, lymph node metastases, and closure of the pelvic peritoneum. From a surgical standpoint, closure of the pelvic peritoneum traps the lymph fluid in the retroperitoneal space and prevents absorption by the peritoneal membrane. Most lymphocysts are small, asymptomatic, and clinically insignificant. Large lymphocysts can produce serious consequences including venous obstruction with DVT, ureteral obstruction, leg edema, and pain. Bilateral lymphocysts can cause obstructive renal failure. The diagnosis is made most easily and accurately by pelvic ultrasound. Large or symptomatic pelvic lymphocysts can almost always be managed by percutaneous drainage with a pigtail catheter placed under CT or ultrasound guidance.

A pelvic DVT following gynecologic surgery should be in the differential for this patient. Typically, DVT following pelvic surgery is asymptomatic, but the appearance of leg edema, pain, or tenderness in the calf, popliteal space, or inguinal triangle is highly suspicious. Erythema and fever are uncommon. A pelvic DVT is uncommon compared to a more distal DVT in the lower extremity venous system. Women with a pelvic DVT will not have the classic symptoms associated with a calf DVT. The diagnostic test to evaluate for a DVT would be a lower extremity venous duplex ultrasound.

In the absence of fever, an elevated WBC or diagnostic evidence of a bacterial infection in the cystic structure seen on pelvic ultrasound, the diagnosis of pelvic abscess cannot be confirmed. Typically a pelvic abscess arises within the first 7–14 days postoperatively. The cardinal clinical signs are fever, leukocytosis with a left shift, abdominal/pelvic pain, malaise, ileus, and perhaps a poorly defined mass. CT scan or ultrasound confirms the diagnosis.

An ovarian cyst is unlikely in this patient since she has had her ovaries surgically removed, and because the occurrence of the cyst occurred so rapidly following surgery. Occasionally, patients can have an ovarian remnant syndrome in which they have had their ovaries removed in the distant past, but a portion or remnant of the ovary was incidentally left at the time of surgery. Women who have this syndrome can then develop symptomatic benign or malignant ovarian masses in this remnant of ovarian tissue.

In the absence of fever, leukocytosis or gastrointestinal symptoms, the diagnosis of diverticular abscess cannot be confirmed. Diverticulitis is typically a disease of people over the age of 50. Diverticula of the colon are herniations of the mucosa, and diverticulitis is inflammation around the diverticular sac. Acute colonic diverticulitis is a characterized by fever, left lower quadrant pain, signs of peritoneal irritation, and leukocytosis. Rectal examination may reveal a mass. The inflammation often leads to constipation. The inflammation weakens the wall of the colon, and perforation of the sac may occur. If this perforation is walled off by the omentum or other neighboring structures, abscess formation occurs. Treatment of diverticulitis includes bowel rest, intravenous hydration, and broad-spectrum antibiotics. Treatment for a diverticular abscess includes intravenous antibiotics directed against gram-negative anaerobic bacteria, followed by surgical drainage or resection. *(Gynecologic Cancer Surgery by Morrow and Curtin. Churchill Livingstone Inc. 1996; Harrison's Principles of Internal Medicine, 14th ed., p. 1649)*

24.   (A)

25.   (C)

Explanations 24 and 25

A woman with advanced cervical cancer may present emergently with heavy vaginal bleeding. Often, the bleeding can be controlled for 24 h by packing the vagina with a packing soaked in Monsel's solution. The patient is kept on bedrest, and the packing is changed every 24 h. If packing the vagina does not control the bleeding, then emergent radiation therapy is warranted if the patient has not had previous radiation treatment. Hemorrhage is usually controlled within 24–48 h of initiating external beam therapy.

If radiation therapy fails, then the next best treatment is arterial embolization of either the uterine or hypogastric arteries. However, embolization may result in tumor hypoxia and decrease the sensitivity of the tumor to radiation. Arteriography with embolization may allow visualization of the bleeding vessel with direct embolization of the source. Arterial embolization has several risks including infarction of distal tissue, infection, and femoral artery thrombosis. If embolization is not available or not successful, bilateral hypogastric artery ligation is an option.

In this patient, surgical therapy with radical hysterectomy is not an appropriate treatment because this patient's disease has spread beyond the cervix. This procedure would

result in transection of the tumor and lead to further bleeding complications. This patient has at least a stage IIIB tumor, and the best treatment for her is chemoradiation. *(Prolog, Gynecologic Oncology and Surgery, 4th ed. American College of Obstetricians and Gynecologists, 2001)*

26.   (E)

27.   (B)

Explanations 26 and 27

VAIN is frequently found in women who have a history of cervical dysplasia. Although the etiology of VAIN has not been thoroughly elucidated, like CIN, it is thought that human papilloma virus (HPV) is the carcinogenic agent. Thus, when vaginal cytology is abnormal, the evaluation is very similar to that of an abnormal pap smear. It is important to assess the histologic severity and the extent of the lesion. To do this, the next step in management is a thorough colposcopic evaluation of the entire vaginal canal, especially because many patients will have multifocal disease. During colposcopy the application of acetic acid (4%) is useful. The speculum should be fully inserted to visualize the upper vagina and then slowly removed while rotating the speculum, being careful to view the entire vaginal mucosal surface. Most vaginal lesions are not grossly visible. However, a raised white epithelium may occasionally be seen. If a lesion is visible, then directed biopsy of the lesion is indicated to confirm the diagnosis.

In the presence of high-grade vaginal cytology, repeat cytology in 6 months, and observation are not viable management options given the concern for carcinoma in situ or for invasive carcinoma of the vagina. Random vaginal biopsies are also not likely to be helpful since they will most likely miss the involved area and lead to a false negative result. Intravaginal estrogen cream is reserved for use when there is no suspicion of invasion, the examination is consistent with vaginal atrophy, the woman is postmenopausal, and the cytology is consistent with low-grade VAIN. In this situation, vaginal atrophy can result in atypical cytology. Treatment with intravaginal estrogen cream followed by repeat vaginal cytology will often result in resolution of the atrophy and the abnormal cytology. Estrogen is not a treatment for VAIN 3, or high-grade VAIN.

Acceptable treatments for VAIN include wide local excision or partial vaginectomy, laser ablation, 5-flourouracil, estrogen cream, and total vaginectomy. Before deciding on a therapy, several factors should be considered including the patient's age and hormonal status, the grade of the lesion, the presence or suspicion of invasion, and the location, extent, and multifocality of the lesion. In this case, the patient is 42 years old and premenopausal, with a high-grade lesion suspicious for invasion that is relatively small and localized. Therefore, wide local excision is the best treatment option. Laser and 5-FU, which are obliterative procedures, should be avoided in the presence of invasion or a suspicion for invasion. If invasion can be ruled out, then these options are reasonable. Estrogen therapy is not an option for this patient since the lesion is high grade and she is premenopausal without evidence of atrophy. Estrogen is reserved for postmenopausal women with vaginal atrophy and low-grade VAIN without evidence of invasion. Finally, a total vaginectomy should be reserved for very large lesions, multifocal lesions that involve the entire vaginal mucosa, suspicion for invasion, or failure of other treatment modalities. In this young, premenopausal, sexually active woman with a localized lesion, a total vaginectomy is an over-aggressive treatment for her disease. (*Wright VC, Chapman W. Intraepithelial neoplasia of the lower female genital tract: etiology, investigation, and management. Semin Surg Oncol 1992;8:180; Wharton JT, Tortolero-Luna G, Linares AC, et al. Vaginal intraepithelial neoplasia and vaginal cancer. Obstet Gynecol Clin North Am 1996;23:325)*

28. **(D)** Vaginal bleeding in a postmenopausal woman may be caused by numerous etiologies including an endometrial polyp, endometrial hyperplasia, atrophic endometrium, a submucosal fibroid, or endometrial cancer to name a few. In this group of women, endometrial cancer must be ruled out. Although this woman may need a pap smear as part of her routine gynecologic screening, a pap smear is inadequate to rule out the diagnosis of endometrial cancer. ECC is a sampling of the endocervical canal, not of the endometrium. Thus, again, an ECC is not adequate to rule out endometrial cancer. The ECC is more commonly used in the workup for cervical dysplasia to assess extension into the cervical canal. A thickened endometrial stripe on pelvic ultrasound can aid in making the diagnosis of an endometrial abnormality, but the ultrasound itself is not diagnostic for endometrial cancer. A thickened endometrium on ultrasound may be the result of a submucosal fibroid, hyperplasia, a polyp, or endometrial cancer. A dilation and curettage is an outpatient surgical procedure that involves dilation of the cervix and a thorough sampling of the endometrium with a curette. This procedure will obtain adequate endometrial tissue to make a diagnosis of tissue. In general, this procedure is reserved for patients in which endometrial biopsy is unsuccessful or for patients who have continued symptoms with a negative endometrial biopsy. Endometrial biopsy is a simple office procedure for sampling the endometrium, and it is 95% accurate. Thus, it is the preferred method of sampling the endometrium to rule out endometrial cancer. (*Good AE. Diagnostic options for assessment of postmenopausal bleeding. Mayo Clin Proc 1997;72:345–349)*

29. **(C)** The current American College of Obstetricians and Gynecologists guidelines for screening women on tamoxifen for endometrial cancer state that no screening except for routine yearly gynecologic examinations should be performed in asymptomatic women. In symptomatic women with vaginal bleeding on tamoxifen therapy, endometrial biopsy is recommended. Tamoxifen directly affects the endometrium, and a pelvic ultrasound will reveal a thickened endometrium in 75% of asymptomatic women. The most common changes to the endometrium include benign cystic glandular dilation, stromal edema,

endometrial hyperplasia, and polyps. Approximately 20–30% of women will develop benign endometrial and endocervical polyps. Women on tamoxifen have a two- to threefold increased risk for endometrial cancer. Given the high rate of benign changes in the endometrium from tamoxifen, the usefulness of transvaginal ultrasound and endometrial biopsy is drastically diminished. In the setting of tamoxifen, ultrasound has only a 9% positive predictive value. However, the negative predictive value is 99%, meaning that if the ultrasound is normal, you may be 99% certain that there is no disease present. CT scans in general are less effective than ultrasound at evaluating the endometrial cavity, and they are not recommended for screening. Hysteroscopy will allow direct visualization with directed biopsy of the abnormal endometrium. However, again, the majority of lesions in women on tamoxifen will be benign, and a large number of hysteroscopies would be performed with the detection of very few cancers. Thus, this is not cost-effective and is a low yield diagnostic procedure in this group of women. Also, there is some debate as to whether hysteroscopy in the presence of endometrial cancer increases the risk for positive cytology and leads to a seeding of the peritoneal cavity with endometrial cancer cells by effluxing cancer cells from the endometrium out through the fallopian tubes into the abdominal cavity. *(Barakat RR. Tamoxifen and the endometrium. Cancer Treat Res 1998;94:195–207)*

30. **(E)** Women with HNPCC, Lynch syndrome II have a 20–40% lifetime risk of endometrial cancer. These women tend to get endometrial cancer at a much earlier age (median 46 years) compared to the general population (median 63 years). These women are also at risk for carcinomas of the ovary, breast, stomach, small bowel, pancreas, biliary tract, and transitional cell tumors of the urinary tract. Because of the inordinately high risk for endometrial and ovarian cancer in these patients, prophylactic hysterectomy and bilateral salpingo-oophorectomies are offered to women with this syndrome after the completion of childbearing. *(Vasen HFA, Wijnen JT, Menko FH, et al. Cancer risk in families with*

hereditary nonpolyposis colorectal cancer diagnosed by mutation analysis. Gastroenterology 1996;110:1020)

31. **(C)** An office biopsy of the cervical lesion should be taken immediately when a gross lesion is seen on physical examination. For smaller, less distinct lesions, colposcopy may be helpful in determining the best area to biopsy, but it is not always necessary for larger, distinct, gross lesions. A pap smear can be performed, but it cannot be relied on to detect invasive cervical cancer. Cervical cone biopsy is not indicated at this time, particularly because the diagnosis can be made by less invasive means with an office biopsy. Also, if a cone biopsy is performed and the cancer is invasive or more extensive than originally thought, a cone biopsy may affect the oncologist's ability to perform a radical hysterectomy or alter the effectiveness of vaginal brachytherapy. Finally, the use of metronidazole vaginal cream is not indicated in this patient since there is no evidence of a vaginal infection. *(Hillard PA. Benign diseases of the female reproductive tract: symptoms and signs. In: Berek, JS. (ed). Novak's Gynecology. 12th ed. Baltimore, MD: Lippincott Williams & Wilkins, 1996:331–397)*

32. **(C)**

33. **(D)**

34. **(E)**

Explanations 32 through 34

Current American Society for Colposcopy and Cervical Pathology (ASCCP) guidelines for treating a pap smear consistent with HGSIL is to perform colposcopy with directed biopsies if a lesion is seen. Routine pap smear in 1 year is an unacceptable option for this patient given her increased risk for developing cervical cancer. Random biopsies have a high false negative rate if there is no visible lesion to biopsy, thus, are not helpful. The pap smear is a screening test of the cervix, not the endometrium. There is no reason to suspect that this patient has endometrial pathology, therefore, an endometrial biopsy is not warranted. HPV testing is not recommended for high-grade pap smears. All high-grade pap smears require further investigation with colposcopy regardless of HPV status.

If colposcopy is unsatisfactory, meaning no lesion is identified, the full transformation zone is not visualized or the full extent of the lesion is not identified, then a diagnostic excisional procedure is warranted. A loop excisional electrocautery procedure (LEEP) would be appropriate. However, note that if your suspicion for cancer is high, the cauterized edges from a LEEP procedure can complicate the pathologic assessment of positive margins. A cold knife cervical conization can be performed in the operating room as an outpatient surgery and provides the best surgical specimen for pathologic evaluation. In this case, a transvaginal ultrasound, endometrial dilation and curettage, and ECC are all inappropriate options since they do not accurately evaluate the cervix, which is the primary site of concern. (*American Society for Colposcopy and Cervical Pathology [ASCCP], 2002*)

This patient has, by definition, microinvasive cervical cancer. Approximately 10–15% of patients in the United States with stage I cervical cancer will have a microinvasive cancer. Microinvasive cancer is defined as stage IA with invasion limited to a depth of 5 mm with lateral extent not to exceed 7 mm. Stage IA is further subdivided into stage IA1 with stromal invasion less than 3 mm and IA2 with invasion 3–5 mm in depth. Young patients with microinvasive squamous cell carcinoma of the cervix who desire future fertility can be treated with conization alone, provided that certain strict criteria are met. The cone specimen should be properly excised and then evaluated by an experienced pathologist. The tumor must meet the criteria for stage IA1 disease with invasion less than 3 mm and a lateral extent less than 7 mm. The cone margins must be negative, and there should be no lymphvascular space invasion.

Patients with stage IA1 disease who do not desire future childbearing should be treated with a simple hysterectomy. Thus, the other options including radiation, simple or radical

hysterectomy with pelvic lymphadenectomy, or radical trachelectomy would be overtreatment for this patient, and they would not preserve her fertility. (*Winter R. Conservative surgery for microinvasive carcinoma of the cervix. J Obstet Gynaecol Res 1998;24:433–436*)

35. **(E)** This patient, who had a hysterectomy for a benign condition, no longer needs pap smear screening as long as she is monogamous and does not develop risk factors for cervical dysplasia. The incidence for vaginal dysplasia after hysterectomy for benign disease is approximately 0.13%. Invasive carcinoma of the vagina is rare, and screening for this cancer is not cost-effective. However, women who had a hysterectomy for cervical dysplasia or cancer are at increased risk for vaginal dysplasia and should continue to have vaginal pap smears. It is also reasonable to reinitiate pap smear screening in women who had a hysterectomy for benign disease if they have new sexual partners or new risk factors. A pap test is also indicated if patients present with vaginal spotting or bleeding. (*McIntosh DG. Pap smear screening after hysterectomy. Compr Ther 1998;24:14–18*)

36. **(B)** The use of estrogen replacement in women previously treated for endometrial cancer represents a recent change in practice. For many women, the improvement in quality of life and the reduction in osteoporosis outweigh the possible risks of stimulating tumor growth. Most patients are diagnosed early with endometrial cancer and successfully treated with surgery. As a result, the risk-benefit ratio of estrogen replacement in these women has been reexamined. In a recent survey of the Society of Gynecologic Oncologists, 83% of the respondents approved estrogen replacement in stage I, grade 1 endometrial cancer. Data on the use of estrogen replacement therapy in women with endometrial cancer are limited primarily to retrospective studies. Three retrospective studies have concluded that estrogen replacement therapy is not detrimental to patients after treatment for endometrial cancer. There exists no data on which to base specific recommendations about estrogen replacement in these patients. The decision must involve a candid

discussion about risks and benefits to the patients and be individualized to each patient, taking into consideration the stage, grade, and histology of the tumor and their current hypoestrogenic symptoms and risk factors for osteoporosis. The delivery method of estrogen is also not clear. Some patients may want to use more natural products like soy, although the relief of symptoms with soy varies considerably. Others may complain more of vaginal dryness, and a vaginal estrogen cream may be more appropriate. The benefit of adding progesterone and giving patients combined hormone replacement therapy is also unclear. *(ACOG Committee Opinion. Estrogen replacement therapy and endometrial cancer. Washington, DC: American College of Obstetricians and Gynecologists, 1993)*

37. (C)

38. (E)

Explanations 37 and 38

Pelvic ultrasound is the least invasive and most cost-effective test to diagnose uterine fibroids. MRI is useful but not always readily available and much more expensive. Plain radiographs would not be helpful, and office laparoscopy impractical and potentially dangerous given the presumed size of her uterus. A hysterosalpingogram would only note filling defects within the uterine cavity and miss intramural or subserosal fibroids. *(Buttram VD and Reiter RC. Uterine leiomyomata: etiology, symptomatology, and management. Fertil Steril 1981;36:433–445)*

GnRH agonists have been used widely for preoperative treatment of uterine fibroids. They work by inducing amenorrhea, which improves hematologic parameters and decreases uterine volume. Although nonsteroidal antiinflammatory drugs (NSAIDs) may help decrease bleeding for some patients with fibroids, they have not been reliably shown to decrease fibroid size. The other agents (OCPs, progesterone, and narcotics) do not have these effects and generally are not effective in treating dysfunctional uterine bleeding caused by anatomic lesions such as fibroids. *(Stovall TG et al. GnRH agonist and iron versus placebo and iron in*

the anemic patient before surgery for leiomyomas: a randomized controlled trial. Obstet Gynecol 1995;86: 65–71)

39. (B)

40. (C)

Explanations 39 and 40

When pelvic organ prolapse occurs beyond the level of the hymen, anatomic obstruction of urine occurs in approximately 30% of patients. Over time, urinary stasis from obstruction can lead to UTIs(rather than the other way around). Detrusor hypocontractility, not overactivity, can be another long-term sequela of chronic urinary retention, enhanced by a stretch injury to the postsynaptic parasympathetics in the bladder wall. Menopause alone is not a risk factor for retention, and a spinal cord tumor is not likely in this patient without specific neurologic complaints or findings on physical examination.

Due to urinary stasis, she is at risk for a UTI. Left untreated, she could develop obstructive uropathy and/or pyelonephritis. Surgery is an option, but not without the prior consideration of nonsurgical options such as a pessary or intermittent clean, self-catheterization (if the problem were to persist). In the event of chronic retention, radiographic imaging would help to assess for upper tract obstruction (i.e., hydronephrosis). Oxybutynin is not appropriate, as it could compound urinary retention. Urodynamic studies could be helpful in the future to ascertain the exact cause of her retention (obstruction from the prolapse vs. chronic detrusor insufficiency vs. neurogenic bladder), but is not the first action to consider. *(Weinberger M. Differential diagnosis of urinary incontinence. In: Ostergard's urogynecology and pelvic floor dysfunction. 5th ed., Philadelphia, PA: Lippincott Williams & Wilkins, 2003, pp. 64–65; Coates KW et al., Uroflowmetry in women with urinary incontinence and pelvic organ prolapse. Br J Urolo 1997;80:217)*

41. (D)

42. (C)

Explanations 41 and 42

This patient is demonstrating acute peritoneal signs that require surgical intervention. Adding additional testing, either with radiology or more laboratory assessment would not alter the management at this point in time. Although some patients with chronic pelvic pain have a history of sexual or physical abuse, an assessment in the acute emergent setting does not take initial priority.

Although ovarian torsion can be enigmatic in its presentation, this patient demonstrates classic signs of intermittent pelvic pain and an ovarian cyst with a solid component. The 8-cm increase in ovarian size is likely due to vascular congestion from occlusion of the blood supply. Early intervention is more likely to result in salvaging viable tissue before the onset of irreversible tissue necrosis. The absence of fever and other GI symptoms, along with a left lower quadrant mass on ultrasound goes against the possibility of appendicitis or pancreatitis. Her pregnancy test is negative which generally excludes an ectopic pregnancy. (*Corfman RS, Davis J Bryant BJ. Ovarian surgery. In: Operative Gynecology, 2nd ed., Philadelphia, PA: W.B. Saunders, 2001, pp. 676–677*)

43. **(C)**

44. **(E)**

Explanations 43 and 44

PID is actually a spectrum of inflammatory disorders of the upper female genital tract. It includes endometritis, salpingitis, tubo-ovarian abscess, and pelvic peritonitis. While the sexually transmitted bacteria *N. gonorrhea* and *C. trachomatis* are often implicated, vaginal flora, including anaerobes, *Gardnerella vaginalis, Haemophilus influenza,* gram-negative rods, and others, are also associated with PID. The clinical diagnosis of acute PID can be difficult and imprecise. There is a wide range of variation in signs and symptoms, and many women have very mild or subtle symptoms only. Because of the difficulty with diagnosis and the potential for damage to reproductive health with even mild PID, one must keep a low threshold for the diagnosis. Empiric treatment for PID should be considered in sexually active young women, or other women at risk for STDs, if there is uterine, adnexal, or cervical motion tenderness, and no other cause of illness can be identified. Additional criteria that support a diagnosis of PID include temperature >101°F, mucopurulent cervical or vaginal discharge, presence of WBCs on wet prep of vaginal secretions, elevated ESR, elevated C-reactive protein, and documentation of infection with gonorrhea or chlamydia.

The treatment of PID should provide broad-spectrum coverage of gonorrhea, chlamydia, anaerobes, gram-negatives, and streptococci. Treatment should be initiated as soon as a presumptive diagnosis is made. Hospitalization should be considered when surgical emergencies (such as appendicitis) cannot be excluded, the patient is pregnant, the patient cannot tolerate or does not respond to outpatient treatment, the patient has severe illness (nausea, vomiting, and high fever), or the patient has a tubo-ovarian abscess. Sexual partners of women with PID should be evaluated and appropriately treated as well. (*www.cdc.gov/mmwr/preview/mmwrhtml/rr5106a1.htm*)

45. **(A)** History is critical in the evaluation and management of vulvar diseases. Given the fact that this patient has had exposures to numerous topical medications, it is likely that she has contact dermatitis of the vulva. Given the lack of hyphae on her wet mount and no apparent abnormal vaginal discharge, a candidal infection is less likely. She is obese and not in the average age range for menopause, thus atrophic findings are unlikely. The wet mount lacks clue cells that establish the diagnosis of bacterial vaginosis. (*Stenchever, pp. 487–488*)

46. **(E)** Labial agglutination is a clinical diagnosis, with a greater prevalence occurring in pediatric or elderly patients. Forced manipulations of the genital region are to be avoided, as the condition readily responds to topical estrogen therapy. (*Bacon JL. Prepubertal labial adhesions: Evaluation of a referral population. Am J Obstet Gynecol 2002;187(2):327–331*)

47. (A)

48. (D)

49. (C)

Explanations 47 through 49

This patient meets criteria for the diagnosis of osteoporosis, with a T-score falling below –2.5 standard SD. A T-score indicates the number of standard deviations below or above the average peak bone mass in young, healthy adults of the same gender. Bisphosphonate therapy has been shown to reduce vertebral and hip fracture risk in up to 50% of women with documented osteoporosis. GnRH therapy and discontinuation of her vitamin D therapy would worsen, not improve, this patient's bone density. Although testosterone may arrest further bone loss, the side effects of the medication are too great compared to any potential benefit. *(Schnitzer T et al. Therapeutic equivalence of alendronate 70 mg once weekly and alendronate 10 mg daily in the treatment of osteoporosis. Aging (Milano) 2000;12:1–12)*

For women who have osteoporosis the serum calcium level is generally normal. In premenopausal osteoporosis, or more severe cases of bone loss/fractures, the presence of metabolic bone disease should be considered. In hyperparathyroidism the serum calcium is elevated. With renal failure, as with osteomalacia, serum calcium is low. The serum calcium level is normal, and the alkaline phosphatase level is elevated in patients with Paget disease. *(Barbieri RL, Osteoporosis, ACOG Educational Bulletin No. 246, April 1998)*

The use of tobacco, a family history of mother or maternal grandmother with hip fractures, postmenopausal state without estrogen replacement, vision problems, and a body mass index of less than 23 are all increased risks for fractures. A body mass index of greater than 23 does not represent an increased risk for fracture. *(Ullom-Minnich P. Prevention of Osteoporosis and Fractures. Am Fam Physician 1999; 60:194–202)*

50. (C) By history and physical examination, this patient most likely has a breast cyst. Given her age, mammography is not helpful due to the density of her breast tissue. Ultrasound is more helpful in detecting fluid-filled breast masses. In-office aspiration would be both diagnostic and therapeutic if the fluid was not bloody. *(Agency for Healthcare Research and Quality. Diagnosis and management of specific breast abnormalities. Evidence Report/Technology Assessment 33. Rockville (MD): AHRQ; 2001. AHRQ publication no. 01-E-046; Lister D et al. The accuracy of breast ultrasound in the valuation of clinically benign discrete, symptomatic breast lumps. Clin Radiol 1998;53:490–492)*

51. (D) Clinically this patient is exhibiting signs and symptoms of overactive bladder syndrome, or urge incontinence. Her risk factors include her age, race, caffeine use, and potential abnormal glucose tolerance. Attention should first be directed toward treating any modifiable risk factors. She does not demonstrate findings or a history of stress urinary incontinence for which surgery might be appropriate. Diuretic therapy could worsen, rather than improve, her symptoms, and she does not have findings consistent with a UTI. *(Montella JM. Management of overactive bladder. In: Ostergard's Urogynecology and pelvic floor dysfunction. 5th ed., Philadelphia, PA: Lippincott Williams & Wilkins, 2003, pp. 293–306)*

52. (E) Maternal obstetric injury remains a major cause of rectovaginal fistula in women. For this patient, it is imperative to determine the presence or absence of a concomitant injury to the anal sphincter complex along with the possibility of a fistula. Crohn disease can be a cause of abdominal pain, diarrhea, anal abscess formation, and fecal incontinence. It would be very unlikely, and highly coincidental, for it to present in this manner. Perianal abscesses can lead to anal fistula formation and subsequent fecal incontinence, but most commonly present with exquisite pain. Fistulas and fecal incontinence would be later complications. Neither a vaginal hematoma nor a retained vaginal foreign body would result in fecal incontinence. *(Strohbehn K, Hackford A Aronson M. Surgical treatment of anal incontinence and rectovaginal fistulas. In: Operative Gynecology. 2d ed., Philadelphia: PA: W.B. Saunders, 2001, pp. 429–438)*

53. (B)

54. (A)

55. (D)

Explanations 53 through 55

Menstrual disorders, primarily oligo- and amenorrhea, are particularly common among women with eating disorders and are thought to be the result of hypothalamic hypoestrogenism. This patient demonstrates estrogen deficiency (decreased breast size, urogenital atrophy). Her dental caries, oral sores, and hand sores might be a result of self-induced vomiting. Hyperthyroidism would be considered in the differential diagnosis of a young woman with weight loss and menstrual irregularities. In contrast to persons with a medical condition that causes weight loss, those with an eating disorder express a disordered body image and, often, a desire to be underweight.

This patient requires additional investigation to assess for the possibility of inpatient admission. Patients with a prolonged, severe eating disorder are at risk for developing dehydration, electrolyte imbalance (especially hypokalemia), cardiac dysrhythmias, and hypothermia. Hospitalization would be considered for those who are severely dehydrated, who have marked electrolyte abnormalities, who are <75% of their ideal body weight, or who have a comorbid condition that would require hospitalization, such as a severe psychiatric disorder.

Although weight-bearing exercise favors bone formation, when excessive exercise and/or an eating disorder results in amenorrhea, estrogen levels fall. Subsequently, bone mineral density decreases. Persons with eating disorders are at increased risk for comorbid psychiatric conditions including depression, anxiety, obsessive-compulsive disorder, and personality disorders. *(Becker AE, et al. Eating disorders. N Engl J Med 1999;340:1092–1098)*

56. (C)

57. (A)

Explanations 56 and 57

Screening for HIV should be offered to all pregnant women as part of routine prenatal care. Screening for HIV infection is done using an enzyme immunoassay (EIA). If the screening test is positive, it may be repeated. Once the screening test is determined to be positive, a Western blot assay or immunofluorescent antibody assay (IFA) is done as a confirmatory test. If the confirmatory test is positive, the patient is then considered to be infected with HIV. Pregnant patients should be treated for HIV by the same standards as any other adult with HIV, though some consideration is given to selection of antiretroviral medications that are safest in pregnancy. Appropriate HIV-related care should not be deferred because of pregnancy.

For patients with significant HIV disease, the combination of elective scheduled cesarean and antiretroviral therapy has been shown to be more effective than antiretrovirals alone at reducing perinatal transmission of HIV. In the absence of any therapy, the risk of vertical transmission is estimated at 25%. With zidovudine therapy, the risk is decreased to approximately 5–8%. When zidovudine is given in combination with elective cesarean for appropriate patients, the risk is decreased to approximately 2%. *(Gabbe, Chap. 40; ACOG Compendium #234, May 2000; www.cdc.gov)*

58. (B) Influenza vaccination is recommended to all women who will be in the second or third trimester of pregnancy during the flu season. Poliomyelitis vaccination is not recommended for women in the United States unless they have some increased risk due to travel or exposure. Measles, mumps, rubella (MMR) vaccination is contraindicated in pregnancy secondary to a theoretic risk of teratogenicity from the rubella vaccine. MMR should be given to this patient postpartum. RhoGAM is recommended routinely during pregnancy in Rh negative women who are unsensitized to Rh factor.

In this case the patient is Rh positive. *(ACOG Committee Opinion #282, January 2003; www.cdc.gov)*

59. (C)

60. (D)

Explanations 59 and 60

The patient would be best served by a progesterone-only pill as it will be less likely to interfere with breast milk production. The rhythm method cannot be reliably used in the early postpartum period as normal menstrual cycles may not have resumed. An IUD would be contraindicated in this patient because of her recent history of chlamydia infection. Patients may not ovulate during breast-feeding but should not rely on breast-feeding alone as a form of contraception, as pregnancy can occur while breast-feeding. *(Koetsawang S. The effects of contraceptive methods on the quality and quantity of breast milk. Int J Gynaecol Obstet 25 (Suppl) 1987:115-127)*

Mastitis is a common complication of breast-feeding. It is characterized by fever, myalgias, and redness with pain in the affected breast. Antibiotic options include penicillin V, ampicillin, or dicloxacillin. Studies show that patients may continue to breast-feed while undergoing treatment for mastitis. *(Thomsen AC, Espersen T, Maigaard S. Course and treatment of milk stasis, noninfectious inflammation of the breast, and infectious mastitis in nursing women. Am J Obstet Gynecol 149:492, 1984; Gabbe, Chap. 21)*

61. (E)

62. (A)

63. (D)

Explanations 61 through 63

The pelvic ultrasound is the most reliable measurement of fetal gestational age in the absence of accurate dating by last menstrual period. A first trimester sonogram is thought to be reliable ±7 days. Given the patient's history, she is likely at least 2 months pregnant. hCG level at this gestation can be variable and is not a useful

method of pregnancy dating. A pelvic examination is useful to help confirm likely dating, but is not a reliable means of determining EDD. FSH and LH levels have no role in determining pregnancy dating. *(Savitz DA, Terry JW, Dole N, Thorp JM Jr. Comparison of pregnancy dating by last menstrual period, ultrasound scanning and their combination. Am J Obstetrics and Gynecology, Vol 187, No 6, Dec 2002; Gabbe, Chap. 10)*

The risk of postpartum major depression is estimated at 8–20% in all postpartum patients. In those with a previous history of postpartum depression, the risk is thought to be 50–100%. In patients who have had previous depression not associated with pregnancy, the risk of postpartum depression is 20–30%. Maternity blues is a milder psychologic reaction that can occur in the early postpartum period and is thought to occur in 70+ % of all postpartum patients. Patients with a history of bipolar disease have a higher risk of recurrence in the postpartum period, and these patients often present with postpartum psychosis symptoms. *(Nonacs R and Cohen LS. Assessment and treatment of depression during pregnancy: an update. Psychiatric Clinics of North America, Vol 26, No 3, Sept 2003; Gold LH. Postpartum disorders in primary care. Primary Care Clinics in Office Practice, Vol 29, No 2, March 2002; Gabbe, Chap. 21)*

64. (C)

65. (B)

Explanations 64 and 65

Sheehan syndrome is also known as postpartum pituitary necrosis. It is associated with severe blood loss during the early postpartum period. The patient with this syndrome may present acutely with hypotension and shock, though often it presents as in this case, with the more gradual onset of symptoms. *(Nader, S. Thyroid disease and other endocrine disorders in pregnancy. Obstetrics and Gynecology Clinics, Vol 31, No 2, June 2004; Gabbe, Chap. 33)*

66. (C)

67. (E)

68. (B)

Explanations 66 through 68

In question 66, this patient likely does not have thyroid disease. She is asymptomatic, has a normal physical examination, and her free T4 is normal. Human chorionic gonadotropin shares a chemical subunit with TSH. The circulating hCG can cause suppression of the thyroid. This is a transient change and does not represent true thyroid disease.

Graves disease is the most common cause of hyperthyroidism in pregnancy. It is the cause of 90–95% of such cases. Patients may complain of rapid heartbeat, weight loss, and GI symptoms such as nausea and vomiting. On examination, you may palpate diffuse thyromegaly and may note exophthalmos. The other listed causes of thyrotoxicosis are much less common in pregnancy, accounting for the remaining 5–10% of cases.

Treatment of this problem is necessary because thyrotoxic women are at increased risk of perinatal mortality, preterm delivery, and maternal heart failure. Treatment is typically with PTU or methimazole. Propranolol can be used initially to reduce symptoms but does not address the underlying problem. Surgery should be reserved for women who do not respond to medical therapy. Radioactive iodine is contraindicated during pregnancy as it can ablate fetal thyroid tissue, leading to the possibility of congenital hypothyroidism. *(Obstetrics and Gynecology Clinics, Vol 31, No 2, June 2004; Thyroid disease and other endocrine disorders in pregnancy. ACOG Practice Bulletin No. 32, Nov. 2001)*

69. (B)

70. (E)

Explanations 69 and 70

Cystic fibrosis is the most common hereditary condition in Whites with a carrier frequency of 1 in 25. The American College of Obstetricians and Gynecologists, the American College of Medical Genetics, and the National Institutes of Health have recommended that cystic fibrosis carrier screening be offered to all White couples either pregnant or considering a pregnancy, and that the availability of screening be discussed with members of other ethnic groups who have a lower frequency of cystic fibrosis carrier state.

Cystic fibrosis is inherited in an autosomal recessive fashion, so for a couple in which both mother and father are carriers the risk of having an affected child is 25% or 1 in 4. In the case presented, in which the husband's sister has cystic fibrosis, his likelihood of being a carrier is 2 in 3 (since he has an affected sibling, both of his parents are obligate carriers, and since he is not affected, he is either a noncarrier [1 in 3] or a carrier [2 in 3]). *(American College of Medical Genetics/American College of Obstetricians and Gynecologists/National Institutes of Health Standing Committee: Preconception and prenatal carrier screening for cystic fibrosis 2001)*

71. (B) In randomized control trials, the daily administration of 0.4 mg of folic acid in the periconception period was shown to prevent the first occurrence of open neural tube defects by approximately 70% as compared to placebo. For women who have previously had a fetus with an open neural defect, the recommended dose for prevention of recurrence is 4 mg and has been shown to have approximately 70% effectiveness in preventing recurrence. *(American College of Obstetricians and Gynecologists Practice Bulletin 44. Neural Tube Defects; Czeizel AE, Dudas I. New England Journal of Medicine 1992; 327: 1832–1835)*

72. (C)

73. (A)

Explanations 72 and 73

The angiotensin converting enzyme inhibitors (and angiotensin receptor blockers) are contraindicated in pregnancy due to their potential to cause decreased fetal renal perfusion, ultimately resulting in fetal oliguria, oligohydramnios, renal tubular dysplasia, and neonatal anuric renal failure, as well as defects in ossification of the fetal skull. These adverse effects occur during the second and third trimesters of pregnancy. If a pregnant woman conceives while taking an angiotensin converting enzyme inhibitor, she should be changed to another agent during the first trimester. *(Piper JM et al. Pregnancy outcome following exposure to angiotensin converting enzyme inhibitors. Obstetrics & Gynecology 1992;80:429)*

Preeclampsia, or pregnancy-related proteinuric hypertension, is associated with an increased risk for end-organ complications as a result of the increased vascular reactivity, third spacing of fluids (including peripheral and cerebral edema), and platelet activation. End-organ complications include oliguria, the syndrome of hemolysis, elevated liver function tests, and low platelets (HELLP) and eclamptic seizures. Fetal macrosomia occurs more commonly in pregnancies complicated by diabetes. Abnormal labor progress and postpartum hemorrhage as well as breech presentation are not more common in pregnancies complicated by preeclampsia. *(Gabbe SG, Niebyl JR, Simpson JL. Obstetrics: normal and problem pregnancies, 4th ed. 2002)*

74. **(C)** Magnesium sulfate has been demonstrated in randomized control trials to be superior to any other anticonvulsant agent in prevention of initial eclamptic seizures and prevention of recurrence of eclampsia *(Witlin AG, Sibai BM. Magnesium sulfate therapy in preeclampsia and eclampsia. Obstetrics & Gynecology 1998;92:883).* Phenytoin would be considered the best alternative in patients who had an absolute contraindication to magnesium sulfate therapy (such as women with myasthenia gravis).

75. **(D)** In general, women with diabetes mellitus are at increased risk for congenital abnormalities as well as spontaneous abortion, with the risk rising in direct relationship to the maternal hemoglobin A1c. The risk is particularly increased when the periconception hemoglobin A1c value exceeds 10 mg per cent. In addition to congenital heart defects, which are increased approximately fivefold over the general population (2.5% vs. 0.5%), open neural defects are thought to be 10 times more common (1% vs. 0.1%). *(Gabbe SG, Niebyl JR, Simpson JL. Obstetrics:*

normal and problem pregnancies, 4th ed. 2002; Reese EA, Hobbins JC. Diabetic embryopathy: pathogenesis prenatal diagnosis and prevention. Obstetrical and Gynecological Survey 1986;41:325)

76. **(B)** Women with preexisting diabetes, both type 1 and type 2, are at increased risk both for spontaneous abortion and congenital anomalies, and the risk for these rises in direct relation to the maternal hemoglobin A1c concentration. In general, women with diabetes are at increased risk for late pregnancy complications, including stillbirth and cesarean delivery. The likelihood of fetal macrosomia (birth weight greater than 4000 g) increases with worsening degrees of maternal glycemic control; the macrosomic fetus is at increased risk for birth trauma, including shoulder dystocia and resultant Erb's palsy. *(Albert TJ, Landon MB, Wheller JJ. Prenatal detection of fetal anomalies in pregnancies complicated by insulin-dependent diabetes mellitus. American Journal of Obstetrics and Gynecology 1996;174:1424)*

77. **(D)** Physiologic changes in respiration during pregnancy include reduced total lung capacity and functional residual capacity, increased inspiratory capacity and no change in the vital capacity. Increased progesterone causes a chronic hyperventilation, as reflected by a 30–40% increase in tidal volume and minute ventilation. This rise in minute ventilation results in a decrease in both alveolar and arterial carbon dioxide, with normal arterial partial pressure of carbon dioxide in pregnancy ranging between 27 and 32 mmHg. *(Lucius H, Gahlenbeck H, Kleine H et al. Respiratory functions, buffer system, electrolyte concentration of blood during human pregnancy. Respiratory Physiology 1970;9:311)* Overall the risk of asthma exacerbation is not thought to be higher in pregnancy. The peak expiratory flow rate correlates well with the forced expiratory volume in 1 s, which is an excellent way of monitoring disease state in both pregnant and nonpregnant individuals. *(Gabbe SG, Niebyl JR, Simpson JL. 2002)* The Centers for Disease Control recommends vaccination against influenza during the appropriate season for all pregnant women who will be in the second and third trimester

during the time of vaccine administration. This is a killed virus vaccine and has not been demonstrated to be associated with risk to the developing fetus. Similarly, the pelvic radiation dose of a single chest radiograph is approximately 50 mrad, which is well below the threshold of concern for fetal risk of 5 rad.

78. **(E)** Many women with underlying cardiac disease have increased risk for serious complications during the pregnancy, including maternal mortality. Clark et al. (*Critical Care Obstetrics, 2d ed.*) have classified maternal cardiac conditions into mortality groups. Group 1 conditions (including mild mitral stenosis, corrected tetralogy of Fallot, and porcine prosthetic valves) have a maternal mortality rate of less than 1%. Group 2 conditions, which include mechanical prosthetic heart valves, more severe degrees of mitral stenosis, uncorrected congenital heart disease, and mild Marfan syndrome, have a mortality rate of 5–15%. Group 3 conditions include those that have a mortality risk of 50% or higher and include pulmonary hypertension, complicated coarctation of the aorta, and Marfan syndrome with an abnormal aortic root.

79. **(C)** All anticonvulsant drugs are associated with at least some risk of congenital abnormalities. Most anticonvulsants are classified as FDA category D, indicating that there is some demonstrated fetal risk but that the maternal benefits of taking the medication may outweigh the risks to the fetus. Carbamazepine, which for a time was thought to have a lower risk for fetal anomalies than other agents such as phenytoin, is now known to have a risk as high or higher. It particularly contributes to an increased risk when it is part of multidrug therapy for women with epilepsy. While the risk of neural tube defects is known to be elevated in women with epilepsy, and particularly those taking anticonvulsant drugs, no data exist to show that higher doses of folic acid will prevent neural tube defects in this group of women. The risk of open neural tube defects in women taking valproate is thought to be 1% (or 10 times the risk in the general population),

and the risk of congenital heart disease is also increased. (*Nulman I, Scolnik D, Chitayat D et al. Findings in children exposed in utero to phenytoin and carbamazepine monotherapy: independent effects of epilepsy and medications. American Journal of Medical Genetics 1997; 68: 18; Lindhout D, Schmidt D. In utero exposure to valproate in neural tube effects. Lancet 1986; 2:1392*)

80. **(D)** A major congenital anomaly is defined as one that is not compatible with survival or one that requires major corrective surgery to restore normal function. The risk of such anomalies in a general obstetric population is usually reported to be between 2 and 3%. If minor congenital anomalies are included, 7–10% of pregnancies will be affected. (*Wilson JG, Fraser FC. (eds). Handbook of Teratology. New York, NY: Plenum, 1979*)

81. **(D)** The most common presenting symptom of vulvar cancer is vulvar pruritis. Women diagnosed with vulvar cancer typically experience a 6–12 month delay prior to diagnosis secondary to the hesitancy of physicians to biopsy the area in the office in order to establish a histologic diagnosis. Generally, women are prescribed antimonilial creams to address presumed intertriginous yeast infections, or topical steroid creams to relieve the inflammation and associated pruritis. Ultimately, in the absence of improvement, a biopsy will finally be performed and the diagnosis established.

Delay in diagnosis is the leading cause of preventable death in patients diagnosed with vulvar cancer, with the 5-year survival rate dropping off precipitously with advancing stage at diagnosis. (*stage I-90%, stage II-80%, stage III-50%, stage IV-15%*) Physicians should have a very low threshold to biopsy cutaneous abnormalities noted on the external genitalia in any patient presenting for a problem visit, or for routine gynecologic care. (*Vulvar squamous cell carcinoma: guidelines for early diagnosis and treatment. Am J Obstet Gynecol. 2003 Sep; 189(3 Suppl):S17–S23*)

82. **(C)** A meta-analysis of 20 studies published from 1970–1991 demonstrated a significant reduction in the risk of ovarian epithelial carcinoma with

the use of oral contraceptives. The risk of ovarian cancer decreased with increasing duration of oral contraceptive use: a 10–12% decrease in lifetime risk was noted with 1 year of use, a 50% decrease in lifetime risk noted with 5 years of use, and an 80% decrease in lifetime risk associated with 10 years of use. Oral contraceptive therapy has consistently demonstrated in epidemiologic studies the ability to decrease a woman's lifetime risk for the development of ovarian cancer. It is the most effective means of primary prevention in women at high risk for the development of ovarian cancer, short of physically removing the ovaries themselves.

Both hysterectomy and bilateral tubal ligation have been associated with a 30% decrease in the lifetime risk for the development of ovarian cancer. However, in women yet to complete their childbearing neither is a realistic option. Breast feeding and increasing parity have been shown to decrease a woman's lifetime risk for the development of ovarian cancer. There are some data to suggest that anti-inflammatory medications (aspirin, NSAID) may decrease the risk of ovarian cancer, but this has yet to be substantiated in epidemiologic studies. *(The estimated effect of oral contraceptive use on the cumulative risk of epithelial ovarian cancer. Obstet Gynecol 1994;83:419–425)*

83. **(A)** Though 85% of cancers develop spontaneously, approximately 10–12% will arise in patients with an inherited chromosomal defect that places them at increased risk for the development of certain types of cancers. Patients with an inherited defect in a tumor suppressor gene encoded on chromosome 2, for example, have an increased risk for the development of breast, ovarian, endometrial, and ovarian cancers and suffer from a syndrome known as hereditary nonpolyposis colorectal cancer, or Lynch family syndrome type II. Patients with an inherited defect in a tumor suppressor gene encoded on chromosome 17 (BRCA1), on the other hand, have an increased lifetime risk for the development of predominantly breast and ovarian cancer.

Patients with a BRCA1 chromosomal defect have a 30–50% lifetime risk for the development of ovarian cancer (compared to a 1.4% lifetime risk in the general patient population), a 60–80% lifetime risk for the development of breast cancer (compared to a 10% lifetime risk in the general patient), and an increased lifetime risk for the development of both fallopian tube cancer as well as peritoneal carcinoma. These cancers generally arise in affected women 10–15 years earlier than when seen in nonaffected women.

The risk for ovarian and breast cancer in carrier women is sufficiently high to warrant bilateral salpingo-oophorectomy once child bearing is complete, or by the age of 35, whichever comes first, as well as prophylactic bilateral mastectomy. An alternative to prophylactic surgery is a more vigilant screening program, with lifetime annual mammography beginning at the age of 25 and ovarian screening with annual or biannual ultrasound, CA-125 determination, and pelvic examination beginning at the age of 35. The efficacy of these screening programs is unproven. *(Understanding hereditary breast and ovarian cancer. Clin J Oncol Nurs. 2003 Sep–Oct;7(5):591–594)*

84. **(D)** All patients diagnosed with ovarian cancer require postoperative chemotherapy, with the exception of FIGO stage IA and IB disease. There is some debate as to whether patients with stage IC disease require postoperative chemotherapy. Two large studies (ICON I, GOG 157) would suggest an improvement in overall survival among this group of patients when given postoperative chemotherapy following surgical debulking.

For those patients requiring postoperative chemotherapy, the combination of carboplatin and paclitaxel represents the current standard. For several years the combination of cisplatin and cyclophosphamide had been considered the treatment of choice. However, in 1993 a large prospective randomized trial compared cisplatin and cyclophosphamide to cisplatin and paclitaxel in patients with advanced stage disease and found the combination of cisplatin and paclitaxel to be associated with a 50% improvement in median survival. Though this came to be accepted as the new chemotherapeutic standard for the management of ovarian cancer, the nephrotoxicity and neurotoxicity associated with the cisplatin prompted a second large prospective randomized trial, GOG 158. This study compared the efficacy of cisplatin and paclitaxel to carboplatin and paclitaxel in patients with advanced stage disease following optimal surgical debulking. The study found the two arms to be equivalent and actually suggested that the carboplatin/paclitaxel arm may even be superior to the cisplatin/paclitaxel arm in terms of overall survival. This has since become the standard chemotherapeutic management for advanced stage ovarian cancer.

Melphalan, an alkylating agent, was previously used in the treatment of patients with advanced stage ovarian cancer (response rate 35–60%) but has since been replaced by more effective chemotherapeutic agents. Tamoxifen is not used in the primary treatment of ovarian cancer, but rather as a third- or fourth-line agent (response rate 11–18%). *(Paclitaxel (Taxol)/ carboplatin combination chemotherapy in the treatment of advanced ovarian cancer. Semin Oncol. 2000 Jun; 27(3 Suppl 7):3–7)*

85. **(D)** The management of vulvar cancer is primarily a surgical one. In the setting of small volume disease, wide local excision with 2–3 cm margins is generally sufficient. For patients to be candidates for such conservative management, the lesion must be <2 cm in width, <1 mm in depth, with no lymphatic or vascular space invasion and nonpalpable groin nodes.

The majority of patients presenting with vulvar cancer, however, will require a radical vulvectomy and inguinofemoral lymphadenectomy to resect the primary lesion, as well as to evaluate for evidence of metastatic spread. If the lesion is midline, with a midline lesion defined as one less than 2 cm lateral to an imaginary vertical line drawn through the clitoris, urethra, and anal verge, the potential for metastatic spread to either groin is sufficiently high that both groins should undergo lymphadenectomy. If the lesion is lateralized, however, only the ipsilateral groin needs be dissected. If metastatic tumor is found in two or more groin nodes, postoperative radiation therapy to the involved groin(s) and ipsilateral pelvic nodes has been shown to improve survival.

(Contemporary management of primary carcinoma of the vulva. Surg Clin North Am. 2001 Aug; 81(4): 799–813)

86. **(D)** Borderline tumors of the ovary, or tumors of low malignant potential (LMP), represent approximately 15% of all epithelial ovarian tumors. The average age at diagnosis is 40 years of age, 15–20 years earlier than is the average age at diagnosis for the invasive ovarian counterpart.

Roughly 50% of all borderline tumors are serous. Because most borderline serous tumors occur in women of reproductive age and are classified as stage I at the time of diagnosis, treatment is usually conservative. Most patients can be managed with cystectomy or oophorectomy alone; in fact, cystectomy is the treatment of choice in the presence of bilateral borderline ovarian cystic tumors, or when only one ovary remains and fertility is desired. If the patient is perimenopausal, postmenopausal, or has no desire for fertility, hysterectomy with bilateral salpingo-oophorectomy is recommended.

When the diagnosis of borderline tumor is made on the basis of an intraoperative frozen section evaluation, a complete staging procedure is still recommended in the event the final pathology report reveals an invasive cancer. The staging information will be critical in that setting in order to determine the stage of disease present and the need for chemotherapy postoperatively. Surgical staging should include pelvic and abdominal cytology, random peritoneal biopsies (right hemidiaphragm, paracolic gutters, ovarian fossa bilaterally, cul de sac, and bladder flap), partial omentectomy, and lymph node sampling.

Unlike invasive ovarian neoplasms, chemotherapy has not been shown to be helpful in the management of ovarian tumors of low malignant potential. LMP tumors have such a low cellular turnover rate that any DNA damage that results following exposure to chemotherapy is easily repaired prior to S-phase associated DNA replication. *(Contemporary treatment of borderline ovarian tumors. Cancer Invest. 1999;17(3):206–210)*

87. (E) Despite decades of effort aimed at improving methods of early detection and diagnosis, the majority of cases of cancer of the ovary are not diagnosed until the disease has spread beyond the ovary. The surgical management of epithelial ovarian cancer consists of attempts at maximal surgical cytoreduction at the time of surgical exploration. The surgical goal is to remove all disease, such that at the completion of the debulking procedure no visible remaining disease is present. In order to accomplish this goal, extensive surgical procedures are often required in those patients presenting with advanced stage disease.

Griffiths et al. reviewed the theoretical basis for cytoreductive surgery. Complete removal of bulky ovarian tumor masses improves patient survival when compared to inadequate or incomplete surgical cytoreduction, in three specific ways:

1. Maximal surgical debulking enables the resection of hypoxic tumor sanctuaries in which viable tumor cells have the ability to escape exposure to adequate concentrations of chemotherapy postoperatively.
2. Maximal surgical debulking enables the resection of large tumor masses containing chemoresistant tumor clones that do not respond well to any form of postoperative chemotherapy.
3. Maximal surgical debulking enables the resection of large tumor masses, thereby reducing the tumor burden to such an extent that all remaining cells in the G0 resting state will now return to the actively dividing cell cycle, where they are more amenable to chemotherapeutic damage and ultimate cell kill.

Numerous investigators (Griffiths, Munnell, Delclos and Quinlan, Hoskins, Eisenkop) have consistently confirmed the biggest single prognosticator predicting how well a patient will respond, and how long they will live, following treatment for ovarian cancer is the volume of disease remaining following their initial surgical debulking. Patients left with residual deposits of disease >2 cm in diameter are considered suboptimally debulked and do no better than patients that have no surgical debulking proce-

dure performed. Optimal surgical cytoreduction, on the other hand, is defined as no residual deposit of disease remaining greater than 1 cm in maximal dimension. The smaller the residual disease remaining (no deposit >.5 cm, >no deposit >.25 cm, and so on), the longer the overall survival of the patient, with those left with no visible remaining disease having the longest overall survival of all as a rule. Given the immense amount of retrospective data supporting the importance of optimal surgical debulking in the patients overall outcome and survival, all attempts must be made at the time of initial surgical cytoreduction to obtain an optimal debulking, preferably one with no visible remaining disease at completion. (*Surgical management of ovarian cancer. Semin Oncol. 2002 Feb; 29(1 Suppl 1): 3–8*)

88. (B) The femoral nerve is the most commonly injured nerve at the time of gynecologic surgical procedures. The nerve can be injured at the time of laparotomy through the inappropriate placement of lateral retractor blades with fixed or self-retaining retractors. The retractor blades, when placed too deeply within the lateral pelvis, have the potential to directly compress the psoas muscle and thereby, the femoral nerve within the psoas muscle. The more prolonged the nerve compression, the more pronounced and long lasting the injury postoperatively. The femoral nerve can also be injured at the time of vaginal surgery as a result of inappropriate lithotomy positioning, with extreme hip flexion and maximal knee extension most commonly associated with injury.

The femoral nerve is a component of the lumbosacral nerve plexus and provides both motor as well as sensory function. Injury to the femoral nerve will present with diminished or absent deep tendon reflexes, inability to straight leg raise, hip flex, or knee extend. There may also be a loss of cutaneous sensation over the anterior thigh as well as the medial aspect of the thigh and calf.

Neurologic injuries following gynecologic surgical procedures are rare, complicating approximately 1–3% of all gynecologic surgical procedures. Once these injuries occur, postoperative physical therapy is generally required, often with braces, until neurologic function returns. Careful attention to retractor blade placement at the time of laparotomy and to appropriate lithotomy positioning at the time of vaginal surgical procedures can minimize the potential for neurologic injury at the time of surgery.

DVT will generally present with asymmetric lower extremity swelling postoperatively, but without associated motor or sensory neurologic deficits. An undetected cerebrovascular accident intraoperatively will generally present with more widespread central deficits than the focal lower extremity deficit seen in this example. Injury to the sciatic nerve will present with a different constellation of neurologic deficits, including inability to extend at the hip, flex at the knee, ankle dorsiflex, and evert. Undiagnosed diabetes can present with a variety of neurologic sequelae including peripheral neuropathy, nephropathy, and retinopathy. Rarely will undiagnosed diabetic neuropathy present with such a focal deficit as seen in this case scenario. *(Irvin W, Andersen W, Taylor P, Rice L. Minimizing the risk of neurologic injury in gynecologic surgery. Obstet Gynecol. 2004 Feb; 103(2):374-382)*

89. (B)

90. (C)

91. (E)

Explanations 89 through 91

The fetal monitoring strip in these questions shows the presence of early decelerations. Early decelerations are characterized by a gradual decrease in the fetal heart rate and gradual return to the baseline in association with a contraction. The onset and recovery of the heart rate are coincident with the onset and recovery of the contraction. These are thought to be due to vagal stimulation due to fetal head compression. They are not associated with fetal hypoxia or acidosis and no intervention, other than continued careful labor monitoring, is indicated.

Variable decelerations are caused by umbilical cord compression. They are characterized by the abrupt decrease in heart rate. The onset of the deceleration frequently varies in successive contractions, and they generally last less than 2 min. Late decelerations are gradual decreases in heart rate that begin at or after the peak of the contraction and return to baseline after the contraction has ended. It is often the first fetal heart rate abnormality seen in uteroplacental-induced hypoxia. Any process that causes maternal hypotension, excessive uterine activity, or placental dysfunction can induce late decelerations. Fetal tachycardia is defined as a baseline fetal heart rate of >160 bpm and is considered severe if the rate is >180 bpm. The most common cause of this is maternal fever, but it can also be due to fetal compromise, arrhythmias, or certain medications. Hyperstimulation is a nonreassuring heart rate pattern caused by the presence of frequent uterine contractions. This occurs most commonly in labors that are being augmented with oxytocin. The initial management includes reduction in the dose, or discontinuation, of the oxytocin. *(Cunningham et al., pp. 336–344)*

BIBLIOGRAPHY

Beckmann CRB, Ling FW, Laube DW, et al., *Obstetrics and Gynecology*, 4th ed. Baltimore, MD: Lippincot Williams & Wilkins, 2002.

Cunningham FG, et al. *Williams Obstetrics*, 21st ed. New York, NY: McGraw-Hill, 2001.

Gabbe SG, Niebyl JR, Simpson JL. *Obstetrics: Normal and Problem Pregnancies*, 4th ed., New York, NY: Churchill Livingstone, 2002.

Speroff L, Glass RH, Kase NG. *Clinical Gynecologic Endocrinology and Infertility*, 6th ed. Baltimore, MD: Lippincot Williams & Wilkins, 1999.

Stenchever M, et al. *Comprehensive Gynecology*, 4th ed. St. Louis, MO: Mosby, 2001.

CHAPTER 5

Psychiatry
Questions

Questions 1 and 2

A 29-year-old woman presents to the primary care clinic complaining of frequent headaches for several months. During the interview she appears tearful and withdrawn, with minimal eye contact and reluctance to answer questions. With further encouragement and support, she is able to describe intense feelings of sadness, along with significant insomnia, poor concentration, fatigue, anhedonia, and little appetite with a 20 lb weight loss.

1. Before she leaves the office, what is the most important question to ask her?

    (A) "Have you been drinking alcohol or using illicit drugs recently?"

    (B) "Have you been taking any over the counter medications?"

    (C) "Have you been treated for any medical conditions?"

    (D) "Have you ever felt like this before?"

    (E) "Have you had thoughts of hurting yourself?"

2. It is decided to begin treatment for her depressive symptoms with pharmacotherapy. Regarding the selection of the specific class of medication, a family history of what would be crucial?

    (A) allergies

    (B) depressive symptoms

    (C) manic symptoms

    (D) medical illnesses

    (E) substance abuse

Questions 3 and 4

A 40-year-old male is returning to the office for a follow-up visit. He is told about his blood work results, which are consistent with leukemia. He is informed that he should receive a bone marrow biopsy for further clarification. While being presented with this information, he remains silent, peering, and staring intensely. When finished, he comments "Doctors think they are so smart!" He then explains that he has been mistreated by physicians in the past and, in fact, has several malpractice suits pending. He feels that the biopsy was recommended only "because you want to use me in order to publish and further your career."

3. Based on the above, what is his most likely diagnosis?

    (A) antisocial personality disorder

    (B) narcissistic personality disorder

    (C) paranoid personality disorder

    (D) schizoid personality disorder

    (E) schizotypal personality disorder

4. When interacting with this patient, which of the following approaches would be most effective?

    (A) defend the recommendation by citing professional credentials

    (B) encourage him to speak with a psychiatrist to provide added support

    (C) interpret his anger as a defense against his fears of having leukemia

    (D) provide detailed information regarding his differential diagnosis

    (E) refer him to a colleague to avoid litigation

Questions 5 and 6

A 38-year-old married female is brought in to the primary care clinic by her husband. She is minimally responsive to questioning, head bowed, and staring at the floor. Most of the history is obtained from her spouse. He denies any known personal or family history of mental illness, but he claims for the past several months his wife has become increasingly depressed and withdrawn. Instead of taking part in her usual hobbies, she is lying around the house. "She tosses and turns" throughout the night. Her husband ensures that she eats a limited amount of food, but she has lost a significant amount of weight. She has been ruminating about guilty feelings regarding a number of issues and recently has been speaking about suicide, although she has no plan or intent. She has refused to come in to see a doctor. Her husband insisted that she come today, as she informed him that the devil has possessed her and told her she will "go to hell."

5. What is her most likely diagnosis?

    (A) bipolar disorder, depressed, with psychotic features
    (B) delusional disorder, somatic type
    (C) major depressive disorder, with psychotic features
    (D) schizoaffective disorder, depressed type
    (E) schizophrenia, paranoid type

6. What is the most effective pharmacologic treatment for this patient?

    (A) antidepressant alone
    (B) antidepressant and antipsychotic
    (C) antipsychotic alone
    (D) mood stabilizer alone
    (E) mood stabilizer and antipsychotic

Questions 7 and 8

A 16-year-old girl is brought into the family practice clinic for her yearly health maintenance examination. Her height is average and her weight is above average. When this is mentioned to her, she blushes and quickly states that she is trying to lose weight. When asked further about her dieting habits, she eventually admits to routinely eating large amounts of food at one sitting, such as two pizzas, a large sandwich, and a gallon of ice cream. She also confides that she frequently will self-induce vomiting in order to compensate but denies laxative use. She realizes that her behavior is unhealthy, but she feels "out of control."

7. Routine blood work would most likely demonstrate which of the following?

    (A) acidosis
    (B) hyperchloremia
    (C) hypernatremia
    (D) hypokalemia
    (E) leukopenia

8. After discussion of her condition with her parents, it is decided to begin her on psychotropic medication and refer her to an eating disorder program. What class of pharmacotherapy would be the most efficacious in this patient?

    (A) anticonvulsants
    (B) antipsychotics
    (C) benzodiazepines
    (D) mood stabilizers
    (E) serotonin-specific reuptake inhibitors (SSRIs)

Questions 9 and 10

A 4-year-old boy is brought into the emergency room by his mother for evaluation. When the child is asked regarding specific complaints, he looks anxiously away and states, "It hurts when I go peepee." His mother confidently adds that "He has another urinary tract infection (UTI)." She lists the antibiotics that he has been treated with in the past and then demands that he be admitted for a workup. On examination, his vitals signs are unremarkable except for a temperature of 102°F. His physical examination is notable for suprapubic tenderness and some evidence of recent urethral trauma. His urinalysis is consistent with a UTI. Further review of his medical chart reveals multiple emergency room visits for various physical complaints, including similar presentations for recurrent UTIs. Prior inpatient and outpatient assessments have not been able to adequately account for any underlying etiologies.

9. What is the most appropriate next step in the management of this patient?

   (A) admit to inpatient and notify child protective services

   (B) confront the mother regarding the suspicions

   (C) consult with a psychiatrist to speak with the mother

   (D) refer the patient to a urologist

   (E) treat the patient for a UTI and send home

10. What is the most likely explanation for the mother's behavior?

   (A) conscious production of symptoms to assume the sick role

   (B) conscious production of symptoms to obtain secondary gain

   (C) expectable reaction from a concerned parent

   (D) hysterical reaction from an overly concerned parent

   (E) unconscious production of symptoms due to unconscious conflict

Questions 11 and 12

A 19-year-old newly married female presents to the emergency room, accompanied by her spouse. She states that she awoke this morning to find that she could not move her legs. She denies any pain but claims that she is unable to feel anything below her abdomen. She denies any trauma or past medical history. She is 24 weeks' pregnant, has had an uneventful pregnancy, and only takes prenatal vitamins. She is concerned if her symptoms will get better and wonders whether the "baby is pulling on my spinal cord." Her neurologic examination is remarkable for 0/5 motor strength in her lower extremities bilaterally, with decreased sensation to light touch and pinprick below the level of her umbilicus. Her cranial nerves and reflexes are normal, and she does not display any upper motor neuron signs. A STAT MRI performed is read as normal.

11. Which of the following is the most likely explanation for her current symptoms?

   (A) conscious production of symptoms to assume the sick role

   (B) conscious production of symptoms to obtain secondary gain

   (C) pathology involving the central nervous system

   (D) pathology involving the peripheral nervous system

   (E) unconscious production of symptoms due to unconscious conflict

12. Which of the following is the most appropriate approach for this patient?

   (A) administer intravenous fluids, informing her it will cure her symptoms

   (B) admit her to the inpatient neurologic unit for further tests

   (C) confront the patient regarding the nature of her symptoms

   (D) obtain consultation with a psychiatrist in the emergency room

   (E) reassure her and suggest that her symptoms will improve

13. A 30-year-old woman with a prior history of depression is attending her postpartum follow-up appointment after the birth of her first child. She has no physical complaints and her examination demonstrates no significant problems. She appears anxious. When asked, she describes intrusive thoughts of wanting to harm her baby but quickly states, "I'm not like that. I would never do anything to hurt him."

Which of the following is the most appropriate next step in her management?

   (A) assess further for symptoms of psychosis and support system

   (B) begin immediate treatment with an antidepressant

   (C) call child protective services in order to have the child removed

   (D) hospitalize the woman immediately for further evaluation

   (E) reassure her that these thoughts are normal

Questions 14 and 15

An 80-year-old woman is admitted to the medical service for treatment of a UTI. While she is hospitalized, she is evaluated for confusion. On her mental status examination (MSE), she appears somnolent at times, fluctuating with an alert state. She is not cooperative, is hostile, and clearly is hallucinating at times. Her insight and memory are poor. The differential diagnosis includes both delirium and dementia.

14. Which of the following signs/symptoms is the most specific for delirium?

    (A) aggressiveness
    (B) fluctuating consciousness
    (C) poor memory
    (D) psychosis
    (E) uncooperativeness

15. Which of the following is the most appropriate pharmacotherapy for her behavioral management?

    (A) low dose diphenhydramine (Benadryl)
    (B) low dose donepezil (Aricept)
    (C) low dose haloperidol (Haldol)
    (D) low dose lorazepam (Ativan)
    (E) low dose risperidone (Risperdal)

Questions 16 and 17

A young White female, age unknown, is brought into the emergency room after being found unresponsive in the bus station. She is obtunded and her vitals signs are temperature 97.8°F, blood pressure 94/60, pulse 55, and respirations 8. Her physical examination is notable for a markedly underweight, poorly groomed woman. She appears pale with cold, dry skin, and mucous membranes. She is not cooperative with the examination. Her pupils are pinpoint and minimally reactive to light. Her cardiac examination demonstrates bradycardia without murmurs or rubs. Her lungs are clear with shallow breathing. Her abdomen appears to be slightly distended.

16. Intake of which of the following substances would most likely account for her presentation?

    (A) alcohol
    (B) anticholinergic
    (C) benzodiazepine
    (D) heroin
    (E) phencyclidine (PCP)

17. The next step in the management of this patient would be the administration of

    (A) disulfiram (Antabuse)
    (B) flumazenil (Romazicon)
    (C) naloxone (Narcan)
    (D) physostigmine
    (E) thiamine

Questions 18 and 19

A 30-year-old married male with a history of depression presents to the family practice clinic. He appears embarrassed and somewhat anxious during his appointment. He denies significant sadness or crying spells. He is sleeping adequately and eating well, without recent changes in his weight. His energy and concentration are normal, and he denies any suicidal or homicidal ideation. He claims to be compliant with his citalopram (Celexa), which he is taking for his depression, but he complains of "problems with sex."

18. Which of the following symptoms would this patient most likely exhibit?

    (A) decreased libido
    (B) painful intercourse
    (C) premature ejaculation
    (D) priapism
    (E) retrograde ejaculation

19. Consideration is given to switching the patient to another antidepressant in order to minimize his side effects. Which of the following would be the most appropriate medication to choose?

    (A) bupropion (Wellbutrin)
    (B) desipramine (Norpramin)
    (C) fluoxetine (Prozac)

(D) phenelzine (Nardil)

(E) venlafaxine (Effexor)

Questions 20 and 21

An 86-year-old woman is brought to the emergency room by her daughter. The patient is a poor historian with limited insight. Her daughter understands that she has a history of high blood pressure and is treated with an unknown medication. The patient has been living by herself in a retirement community. The daughter became concerned a year prior, when she noticed that her mother had seemed more confused. She had attributed this to "old age," but 2 weeks ago she noticed an abrupt worsening in her condition. Her mother now has difficulty recognizing close relatives and remembering information. For the past 2 weeks she has been getting lost, forgetting to turn off the stove, and has been unable to bathe herself. The daughter is concerned that she may inadvertently harm herself.

20. An MRI of the brain would most likely demonstrate which of the following findings?

(A) caudate nucleus atrophy

(B) dilated ventricles without atrophy

(C) frontotemporal atrophy

(D) generalized atrophy

(E) white matter infarcts

21. Which of the following will be the most likely course of her illness?

(A) gradual improvement

(B) rapid decline

(C) stable course

(D) steady worsening

(E) stepwise deterioration

Questions 22 and 23

A 67-year-old man is seen in the clinic for a scheduled visit. He complains of walking difficulties that have progressively worsened over many months. He also has noticed "shaking" of his hands, resulting in his dropping objects occasionally. He is greatly upset by these problems and admits to frequent crying spells. His only chronic medical illnesses are gastroesophageal reflux disease and hyperlipidemia. He is currently prescribed a proton-pump

inhibitor and cholesterol-lowering agent. His MSE is notable for little expression or range of affect. His vitals signs are within normal limits. On physical examination, there is a noticeable coarse tremor of his hands, left greater than right. His gait is slow moving and broad-based.

22. Which of the following brain structures is most likely affected in this man's condition?

(A) caudal raphe nuclei

(B) hippocampus

(C) locus ceruleus

(D) nucleus basalis of Meynert

(E) substantia nigra

23. Some time after initiation of treatment with the proper medication, he becomes agitated and is noted to be hallucinating. Which of the following medications would be the most appropriate to treat these new symptoms?

(A) clozapine (Clozaril)

(B) haloperidol (Haldol)

(C) risperidone (Risperdal)

(D) quetiapine (Seroquel)

(E) thioridazine (Mellaril)

Questions 24 and 25

The patient is a 24-year-old female medical student being seen in the student health center. She presents because she will be beginning her surgery clerkship next rotation and she gives a long history of becoming extremely anxious when faced with viewing blood or needles.

24. Which of the following hemodynamic responses will most likely occur when she participates in future operative procedures?

(A) initial bradycardia followed by hypotension

(B) initial bradycardia followed by tachycardia and hypertension

(C) initial bradycardia followed by tachycardia and hypotension

(D) initial tachycardia followed by bradycardia and hypotension

(E) initial tachycardia followed by hypertension

25. Which of the following treatment modalities would be the most effective for this individual?

(A) beta-blocker
(B) exposure therapy
(C) insight-oriented therapy
(D) SSRI
(E) supportive therapy

26. A 48-year-old man with no prior psychiatric history is seen in the acute care clinic because of concerns over having a sexually transmitted disease. He denies any dysuria, penile discharge, or lesions. His physical examination is unremarkable. When informed of this information, he insists on being tested. When inquires are made regarding his sexual history, he claims to be monogamous with his wife, who happens to be Senator Hilary Clinton. When confronted with the fact that she is already married to someone else and living in another state, he states that he married her 2 years ago in a "secret" ceremony. He adds that she flies in on weekends to have "conjugal visits," but he is afraid that she has been unfaithful to him and has given him a venereal disease. He has no medical problems and is not taking any medications currently. Further history reveals that he holds a steady job as a security guard. He lives alone in an apartment. He denies alcohol or illicit drug use. On MSE, he appears well-dressed and groomed. He is cooperative overall. His mood and affect are anxious. His thoughts are logical. He denies any suicidal or homicidal ideation, or any perceptual disturbances.

Which of the following is his most likely diagnosis?

(A) bipolar disorder, manic
(B) delusional disorder
(C) paranoid personality disorder
(D) schizoaffective disorder
(E) schizophrenia

Questions 27 and 28

The patient is a 7-year-old boy brought in for evaluation by his father. He has been concerned with his son's behavior. At school conferences, he has been told that his son will not stay in place and moves around the room despite being informed about the rules. He neither listens at home nor at school when given feedback. For example, he continues to have difficulty waiting in line, completing his homework, and cleaning up his toys, regardless of numerous consequences. In department stores, he will run around and grab at items, and this has resulted in his breaking merchandise on many occasions. The father states that his son has been this way "since he could walk" and is worried about his son's future.

27. Which of the following neurotransmitters is most likely implicated in the etiology and treatment of his condition?

(A) acetylcholine
(B) gamma-amino butyric acid (GABA)
(C) glutamate
(D) norepinephrine
(E) serotonin

28. Further history and school records are obtained, and a physical examination is performed. He is recommended to begin a first-line medication for his symptoms. His father has questions about the use of this particular agent. Which of the following statements is the most accurate regarding the pharmacotherapy for this disorder?

(A) Is absolutely contraindicated in patients with comorbid tics.
(B) The therapeutic effect involves paradoxical sedation.
(C) Would cause similar benefits if taken by a normal child.
(D) Will cause growth suppression if used during the school year.
(E) Will increase the future risk of substance abuse.

Questions 29 through 31

The patient is a 9-year-old girl brought into the urgent care clinic by both of her parents. Over the past 18 months they have noticed emerging "habits," including repetitive squinting and grimacing, along with associated clearing of her throat and grunting noises. These behaviors occur almost every day and frequently occur together. She has gotten increasingly teased because of her peculiarities and her anxiety has only worsened her symptoms. She has no major illnesses and is not taking any medications. Her physical examination is within normal limits with the exception of the above stereotypes.

29. Further history would most likely reveal which of the following comorbid diagnoses?

    (A) autistic disorder
    (B) major depressive disorder
    (C) obsessive-compulsive disorder (OCD)
    (D) panic disorder
    (E) conduct disorder

30. Which of the following would be the most effective pharmacotherapy for her presenting illness?

    (A) clonidine
    (B) haloperidol (Haldol)
    (C) lorazepam (Ativan)
    (D) methylphenidate (Ritalin)
    (E) paroxetine (Paxil)

31. A history of infection with which of the following organisms would be most likely in this patient?

    (A) herpes simplex virus
    (B) HIV
    (C) influenza virus
    (D) *Staphylococcus*
    (E) *Streptococcus*

Questions 32 and 33

The patient is a 26-year-old male graduate student presenting to his health maintenance organization. He is having ongoing difficulty completing his thesis. When he is working on the computer, he finds it necessary to print out and save every draft of his paper. Even though he realizes that it is unnecessary to do so, he feels compelled to read and reread all of his versions in case he made a mistake. As a result, he has been unable to move forward with his dissertation. He is consumed with doubts about his thesis, but at the same time he cannot throw away

discarded sections. In fact, his apartment contains stacks of paper spread throughout his rooms. He understands that these thoughts and behaviors are "not rational," and he is greatly distressed by them and the problems they have caused.

32. Which of the following would be the most appropriate pharmacotherapy for his condition?

    (A) alprazolam (Xanax)
    (B) bupropion (Wellbutrin)
    (C) citalopram (Celexa)
    (D) desipramine (Norpramin)
    (E) olanzapine (Zyprexa)

33. The patient does not wish to take medication but is interested in psychotherapy. Which of the following would be the most efficacious in reducing his symptoms?

    (A) behavioral therapy
    (B) eye movement desensitization and reprocessing (EMDR)
    (C) psychoanalysis
    (D) psychodynamic psychotherapy
    (E) supportive therapy

Questions 34 and 35

A 29-year-old married male is seen in the emergency room with the chief complaint of "I'm afraid I'm having a heart attack." He states for the past 2 months he has experienced recurrent episodes of chest pain and shortness of breath that last 10–20 min. He also describes associated tachypnea, lightheadedness, tingling in his extremities, nausea, diaphoresis, anxiety, and fears that he may die. These symptoms are now occurring almost daily but are not provoked by any situations or activities, such as exertion or exercise. He is significantly worried about having future episodes and is genuinely concerned that he will suffer a myocardial infarction. He denies having any medical illnesses or taking any medications. He drinks three beers on the weekends only and does not use illicit drugs. His physical examination reveals a slightly elevated blood pressure and pulse. An ECG demonstrates sinus tachycardia.

34. Which of the following medications would be most appropriate in the acute management of this patient's symptoms?

    (A) imipramine (Tofranil)
    (B) lorazepam (Ativan)
    (C) paroxetine (Paxil)
    (D) risperidone (Risperdal)
    (E) valproic acid (Depakene)

35. Which of the following medications would be most appropriate in the long-term management of this patient's symptoms?

    (A) imipramine
    (B) lorazepam
    (C) paroxetine
    (D) risperidone
    (E) valproic acid

36. A 55-year-old lawyer without past psychiatric history presents to her internist with complaints of insomnia. Since her husband suddenly passed away 5 weeks ago, she has had difficulty sleeping, frequently awakening throughout the evening. She subsequently finds herself tired during the day. When asked about her mood, she states that she is "sad" and she often will break down in tears when thinking about her husband. Although she feels that her job occupies her mind, she describes being distracted and making minor mistakes at work. Her appetite has diminished but her weight has not changed. While she feels "lost" and that her life is not enjoyable without him, she denies any suicidal ideation. She reluctantly admits to occasionally hearing her husband calling her name at nighttime. She understands that it is not real but still finds it comforting for her.

    Which of the following is the most appropriate next step in the management of this patient?

    (A) hospitalize her for further evaluation and treatment
    (B) initiate treatment with an antidepressant alone
    (C) initiate treatment with an antidepressant and antipsychotic

    (D) monitor her symptoms over the next several weeks
    (E) refer her to a psychiatrist for medication management

Questions 37 and 38

The patient is a 70-year-old man brought to the primary care clinic by his family over concerns that he has Alzheimer's disease. They have noticed a worsening of his memory over the past 6 months. He does not seem to want to get out of bed and he appears to have difficulty providing for his basic needs, such as cleaning, dressing, and cooking for himself. He is hesitant when talking, but it is unclear whether he is unable or unmotivated to speak. His family has also noticed that he appears depressed and is often seen crying. A MSE of the patient is performed to help determine whether he is suffering from a dementing illness or a depressive illness (pseudodementia).

37. Which of the following characteristics on MSE is most consistent with pseudodementia?

    (A) appears unconcerned during examination
    (B) attends poorly to questions on MSE
    (C) displays poor insight into symptoms
    (D) gives "don't know answers" to questions
    (E) performs consistently poorly to tasks

38. Further history, cognitive examinations, physical examination, and laboratory/radiographic studies are obtained. The results are consistent with Alzheimer's dementia. While the family had been able to take care of him initially, they have since returned to the clinic stating that they can no longer keep him at home. They feel that he is becoming much more agitated. He is staying up at night. Lately he has been rearranging the furniture, claiming to look for "the little people who are teasing me." They have noticed that he has difficulty walking, often moving slowly and dropping items. The family has pursued nursing home placement, but they wish to have something prescribed in order to help him sleep and keep him calm.

Which of the following medications should be avoided in this patient?

(A) buspirone (Buspar)

(B) donepezil (Aricept)

(C) lorazepam (Ativan)

(D) trazodone (Desyrel)

(E) risperidone (Risperdal)

Questions 39 and 40

A 12-year-old boy is brought into the office by his mother, who states "I can't deal with this anymore!" She appears exasperated, claiming that her son has been getting into more and more trouble over the past 15 months since the finalization of a particularly long and difficult divorce. He has been leaving the house at night without notifying his mother or telling his whereabouts. She suspects that he is responsible for the increased vandalism in the neighborhood. He has recently been caught shoplifting at a nearby store. His grades have always been poor, but he has just been suspended for missing classes and skipping school over the past year. He has often come home with evidence of having been in fights. She suspects that he may be hanging out with gang members. She is afraid of his ending up in jail and "becoming like his father."

39. A history of which of the following premorbid diagnoses would most likely be found in this patient?

(A) antisocial personality disorder

(B) attention-deficit/hyperactivity disorder (ADHD)

(C) autistic disorder

(D) childhood schizophrenia

(E) mental retardation

40. If untreated, which of the following diagnoses is most likely to transpire in this patient?

(A) alcohol dependence

(B) oppositional defiant disorder

(C) panic disorder

(D) schizoid personality disorder

(E) schizophrenia

Questions 41 and 42

A 19-year-old male United States Army veteran presents to the outpatient clinic. He recently returned from combat in Iraq where he was assigned to the infantry. While on patrol 1 month ago he witnessed several friends killed by a road-side bomb. Since that time he has had difficulty sleeping, with frequent awakenings after recurrent nightmares about the event. He finds himself "jumpy" at times, especially with loud noises. He stayed in his parents' house around the July 4th Holiday, as he became acutely anxious when hearing firecrackers. He has not spent time with friends or family. He refuses to watch any television or listen to the radio for fear of hearing news of more casualties. He complains of a sense of "numbness" and gets easily distracted. He denies suicidal ideation but sometimes feels that "my life ended over [in Iraq]."

41. Which of the following is the greatest risk factor for developing a chronic illness in this patient?

(A) history of childhood trauma

(B) lack of comorbid psychiatric disorders

(C) male gender

(D) no dissociation during the trauma

(E) premorbid schizoid traits

42. Which of the following medications as monotherapy is most likely effective to treat his symptoms?

(A) amobarbital (Amytal)

(B) haloperidol (Haldol)

(C) lorazepam (Ativan)

(D) sertraline (Zoloft)

(E) trazodone (Desyrel)

43. An 18-month-old boy is brought into the urgent care clinic by his mother who complains that he is "eating weird stuff." For the past few months since being able to walk, he has been found chewing and swallowing odd substances, such as hair, paper, paint, and string. She has been more concerned since she recently noticed him eating dirt and clay from around the foundation of their apartment in the projects. His appetite has been affected because of this and she is worried that he will become sick as a result.

Which of the following blood levels would most likely be decreased in this child?

(A) folic acid and lead
(B) folic acid and zinc
(C) iron and lead
(D) iron and zinc
(E) lead and zinc

44. A 14-month-old girl is brought into the primary care clinic by her parents. Her prior well-baby checks have been normal, but her parents have noticed that while she used to be "outgoing," she has now become shyer and less responsive. Whereas she had been beginning to walk, she has recently been falling more and unable to even stand up. Her mother noticed that she has been flapping her hands and that her sun hats have become too big for her.

Which of the following is the most likely diagnosis for this patient?

(A) Asperger disorder
(B) autistic disorder
(C) childhood disintegrative disorder
(D) fragile X syndrome
(E) Rett's disorder

Questions 45 and 46

A 60-year-old male with a history of chronic schizophrenia and multiple hospitalizations checks into the emergency room with complaints of "funny movements." He has been compliant with risperidone (Risperdal) 3 mg bid and he has been taking that dose for the last 6 years while living at a group home. He appears overweight but with adequate

hygiene. His thoughts are somewhat tangential but not grossly disorganized. He denies any paranoia, ideas of reference, or delusions. He denies perceptual disturbances or suicidal/homicidal ideation. His physical examination is unremarkable except for occasional involuntary blinking and grimacing, as well as rotation of his left ankle. He is greatly distressed about these "habits" and wishes something to be done about them.

45. Which of the following would be the most appropriate management for this patient?

(A) add benztropine to the risperidone
(B) continue the current dose of risperidone
(C) decrease the dose of risperidone
(D) discontinue the risperidone
(E) increase the dose of risperidone

46. The same patient is brought back to the emergency room via ambulance 1 month later due to "catatonia." According to his chart, he was maintained on his current dose of risperidone by his outpatient psychiatrist. On examination, he is unresponsive to questions. His vitals signs demonstrate a temperature of 103.5°F, blood pressure of 180/95, pulse of 105, and respirations of 20. His physical examination is notable for significant diaphoresis, muscular rigidity, and lack of cooperation with much of the examination.

Which of the following would be the most appropriate management for this patient?

(A) add benztropine (Cogentin) to the risperidone
(B) continue the current dose of risperidone
(C) decrease the dose of risperidone
(D) discontinue the risperidone
(E) increase the dose of risperidone

47. A 22-year-old male is brought into the emergency room by the police as he was found yelling in the middle of the street, naked. In the quiet room, he is unpredictable during the examination. He displays extreme lability, alternating between agitation with kicking the bed and listlessness. He is observed responding to internal stimuli and appears paranoid.

A limited physical examination demonstrates mildly elevated blood pressure and heart rate, nystagmus, ataxia, and muscle rigidity.

Intoxication with which of the following substances is most likely in this patient?

(A) alcohol
(B) cannabis
(C) heroin
(D) lysergic acid diethylamide (LSD)
(E) PCP

Questions 48 and 49

A 68-year-old widow presents to the primary care clinic for a routine appointment. Her current medical problems include hypertension, obesity, and chronic obstructive pulmonary disease. She has no significant psychiatric history, although she saw a psychologist for eight sessions after her husband died. She does not drink alcohol or use illicit drugs. She has smoked one and half to two packs of cigarettes per day for the past 45 years and she wishes to quit. She has heard about some of the options but is unsure which would be the most effective.

48. Which of the following strategies is most likely to succeed in helping her to quit smoking?

(A) abrupt cessation
(B) behavior therapy
(C) education
(D) medications such as nicotine replacement
(E) medications with group therapy

49. After being informed of the various choices, she decides to proceed with medication. Which of the following medications is most useful for tobacco cessation?

(A) bupropion (Wellbutrin)
(B) fluoxetine (Prozac)
(C) mirtazepine (Remeron)
(D) trazodone (Desyrel)
(E) venlafaxine (Effexor)

Questions 50 and 51

A 32-year-old female presents to the outpatient clinic with complaints of ongoing headaches. For the past 8 months she has had recurrent headaches, which she describes as bilateral, occipital, with a tight/squeezing pain, lasting for several hours and relieved with nonsteroidal anti-inflammatory medication. Further questioning reveals chronic feelings of fatigue and poor concentration. She admits to "constantly worrying" about her job performance as well as issues involving her relationship with a live-in boyfriend. In fact, her focusing on these concerns interferes with her sleep. As a result, she has on more than one occasion awakened with extreme panic, tremors, diaphoresis, nausea, and palpitations. Her medical problems include gastroesophageal reflux disease that is treated with famotidine. She drinks an occasional glass of wine and denies drug use.

50. Which of the following is her most likely diagnosis?

(A) generalized anxiety disorder
(B) major depressive disorder
(C) OCD
(D) panic disorder
(E) social phobia

51. After determining the diagnosis, consideration is given to initiating treatment with buspirone (Buspar) and/or a benzodiazepine. Which of the following statements is most accurate regarding the use of buspirone compared to a benzodiazepine?

(A) Patients on buspirone can develop tolerance and withdrawal with long-term use.
(B) Buspirone is more effective in reducing the cognitive symptoms of anxiety.
(C) Buspirone is often effective after a benzodiazepine has been tried.
(D) The time before the onset of action is approximately the same for buspirone and benzodiazepines.
(E) Buspirone should only be used as monotherapy.

Questions 52 and 53

The patient is an 18-year-old male brought into the emergency room in the early morning by his friends after attending a dance party. He is agitated, pacing the hallway but unsteady. Despite this, he claims to feel "wonderful," stating, "Everything will be alright." He also seems focused on seeing many colored flashes and hearing "all conversations at once." He has no known medical problems and is not taking any medication. He does admit to ingesting something early on, which he was told would help him "party all night." On physical examination, he has an elevated blood pressure and pulse, dilated pupils, and significant diaphoresis.

52. Which of the following is the most likely pharmacologic effect of the substance taken?

    (A) blockade of dopamine reuptake
    (B) blockade of glutamate receptors
    (C) increased activity of serotonin receptors
    (D) release of dopamine
    (E) release of dopamine and serotonin

53. This same patient is eventually admitted for detox and successfully completes a drug treatment program. He is attending college and performing well. He returns to the urgent care clinic with complaints of reoccurring experiences similar to those when he was "high," such as flashing lights, intensified sounds, and halos. He is greatly upset about these and he feels that they interfere with his studying. A complete physical examination and blood work (including toxicology screen) are negative.

    Which of the following medications should be most avoided in this patient?

    (A) carbamazepine (Tegretol)
    (B) clonazepam (Klonopin)
    (C) fluoxetine (Prozac)
    (D) haloperidol (Haldol)
    (E) valproic acid (Depakene)

Questions 54 and 55

The patient is a 48-year-old Vietnam veteran who has self-referred to the emergency room. He complains of feeling "depressed" and suicidal for the past several days. He admits to using "crack" cocaine daily for the past 3 weeks, although he is vague regarding how he obtains and affords his drugs. He also drinks several 40 oz beers three to four times per week and smokes marijuana "on occasion." He has been homeless, staying with "friends" and in shelters. He last used cocaine this morning and wishes to be admitted for detoxification.

54. Which of the following is most likely to be a comorbid diagnosis in this individual?

    (A) antisocial personality disorder
    (B) bipolar disorder
    (C) generalized anxiety disorder
    (D) major depressive disorder
    (E) schizophrenia

55. He is subsequently admitted to the mental health unit but the next day is evaluated for complaints of withdrawal symptoms. He complains of insomnia, listlessness, irritability, and worsening dysphoria. Which of the following would be the most appropriate treatment strategy for his current condition?

    (A) antidepressant treatment
    (B) benzodiazepine taper
    (C) education and reassurance
    (D) methadone detox
    (E) phenobarbital detox

Questions 56 and 57

A 6-year-old girl is brought in to the primary care clinic for evaluation by her foster parents, who are concerned that "something is wrong with her." They have noticed odd behavior, with repetitive words and phrases, and difficulty following directions. Her vitals signs are normal. Her physical examination is remarkable for a head circumference greater than the 90th percentile but a height less than the 30th percentile, large-appearing ears and significant flexibility in the joints.

56. Which of the following chromosomes is most likely abnormal in this patient?

    (A) 5
    (B) 15

(C) 18

(D) 21

(E) X

57. Which of the following is the most likely comorbid diagnosis in this patient?

(A) anorexia nervosa

(B) ADHD

(C) OCD

(D) oppositional defiant disorder

(E) Tourette's disorder

Questions 58 and 59

A 17-year-old boy is reluctantly taken to the family practice clinic by his mother, who is upset as "he is hanging out with the wrong crowd." She strongly believes that he has been smoking marijuana every day after school and on weekends with his friends. The patient appears irritated about the appointment but denies using any drugs or alcohol. His mother would like him to be counseled about the potential dangers of "smoking pot."

58. Which of the following physical effects are most consistent with cannabis intoxication?

(A) decreased respiration

(B) increased salivation

(C) lowered appetite

(D) normal motor function

(E) tachycardia

59. Which of the following would be the most serious potential long-term consequence of smoking cannabis in this individual?

(A) amotivational syndrome

(B) cerebral atrophy

(C) chromosomal damage

(D) lung cancer

(E) seizures

Questions 60 and 61

A 38-year-old married woman presents to her urgent care clinic complaining of "crying spells" for several weeks since the termination of her employment. She admits to feeling "down all the time," as well as difficulty falling asleep, poor energy, decreased appetite, "not being able to enjoy anything," and fears that her condition will never improve. She has begun to feel that "it wouldn't matter if I died," but she denies any suicidal plan or intent. She drinks one to two mixed drinks per week and denies any drug use. It is decided to begin antidepressant therapy with paroxetine (Paxil) 20 mg at bedtime.

60. If there is no significant improvement in her symptoms, but the medication is tolerated, after what length of time should a dosage increase be considered?

(A) 4 days

(B) 1 week

(C) 2 weeks

(D) 4 weeks

(E) 7 weeks

61. Which of the following side effects would be most likely to emerge after several months of treatment?

(A) headache

(B) inhibited orgasm

(C) loose stools

(D) nausea

(E) vivid dreams

Questions 62 and 63

An 8-year-old boy is brought in for evaluation by his parents who are worried about his behavior in school. Recently, he has become increasingly upset about attending school. Whereas he had always enjoyed being read to as a small child, he has appeared easily frustrated when reading or being asked to write. In fact, during those times he will often disrupt the class and this has led to his parents being asked to remove him from the school.

62. Which of the following tests would be the most useful in the evaluation of this child?

(A) Bender Visual Motor Gestalt Test

(B) Children's Apperception Test

(C) Reitan-Indiana Neuropsychological Test

(D) Rorschach Inkblots Test

(E) Wechsler Intelligence Scale for Children

63. Which of the following additional diagnoses most likely would be present in this patient?

    (A) ADHD
    (B) autistic disorder
    (C) major depressive disorder
    (D) mental retardation
    (E) tic disorder

Questions 64 and 65

The patient is a 52-year-old male presenting to the emergency room with complaints of severe leg pain. The patient states he has had ongoing left knee pain of 6 months duration, unrelieved by nonsteroidal anti-inflammatory medications (NSAIDs). He denies any trauma but claims to have arthritis. His vital signs are stable. Physical examination of his knee demonstrates no significant findings except for decreased range of motion but with little effort. There is no swelling, erythema, or signs of trauma. An x-ray is obtained which is read as "normal," without evidence of arthritis. When he is offered a trial of a NSAIDs and a referral to a specialty clinic, he becomes angry and walks out of the emergency room.

64. Which of the following is the most likely motivation for this patient's presentation?

    (A) conscious production of symptoms to assume the sick role
    (B) conscious production of symptoms to obtain secondary gain
    (C) false belief that he has arthritis
    (D) fear that he is suffering from a serious disease
    (E) unconscious production of symptoms due to unconscious conflict

65. Which of the following would be the most appropriate management should this patient return?

    (A) accusation regarding drug-seeking behavior
    (B) admission to a psychiatric facility
    (C) confrontation and further evaluation
    (D) notification of the police
    (E) referral to a psychiatrist

Questions 66 and 67

A 54-year-old woman is triaged to the emergency room for chest pain, rule-out myocardial infarction. She describes the sudden onset of left-sided, sharp chest pain with accompanying nausea, diaphoresis, palpitations, and tremulousness. On presentation, she appears somewhat disheveled and anxious, smelling of alcohol. On physical examination, her blood pressure and pulse are elevated. Her sclerae are injected and she looks flushed. She has a noticeable tremor of both of her hands. When asked about her last drink, she responds "late last night."

66. Which of the following laboratory tests would most likely be decreased in this patient?

    (A) alanine aminotransferase (ALT)
    (B) aspartate aminotransferase (AST)
    (C) gamma-glutamyl transpeptidase (GGT)
    (D) hemoglobin and hematocrit
    (E) serum triglycerides

67. Which of the following medications would be most helpful in decreasing her future cravings for alcohol?

    (A) disulfiram (Antabuse)
    (B) fluoxetine (Prozac)
    (C) lithium
    (D) naltrexone (ReVia)
    (E) risperidone (Risperdal)

68. A 26-year-old man is brought into the emergency room via ambulance, minimally responsive to questioning or examination. According to his girlfriend, he has a history of major depressive disorder (MDD) as well as alcohol dependence. He was found unconscious with a suicide note and many empty beer bottles. She also believes that he had taken "some other drug" that he purchased from a local drug dealer.

    Which of the following substances found in urine toxicology would be the most dangerous in this patient?

    (A) barbiturate
    (B) cannabis

(C) cocaine

(D) opiate

(E) PCP

Questions 69 and 70

A 26-year-old divorced woman is brought into the emergency room after being found wandering the streets aimlessly. She is a relatively good historian but gives few spontaneous answers to questions. She describes a 1-year history of the belief that she is being followed by "agents" of the Vatican, who watch her closely to "see if I'm a good Catholic." While they monitor her, they also use radio signals to tell her she is a "whore" and a "slut." Due to these experiences she has been unable to work. She is afraid to associate with others for fear of being "judged." She denies any medical problems and takes no medications. Her parents were divorced when she was an infant. She does not know anything about her father, but her mother has "manic-depression" and is taking lithium. Her MSE is notable for significant psychomotor slowing, paucity of speech, and a flat affect.

69. Which of the above features in this patient gives a better prognosis?

(A) age of onset

(B) family psychiatric history

(C) marital status

(D) mental status examination findings

(E) social history

70. With appropriate treatment, what is the likelihood for her leading a moderately well-functioning life?

(A) 0–20%

(B) 20–40%

(C) 40–60%

(D) 60–80%

(E) 80–100%

Questions 71 and 72

A 30-year-old man is seen in the primary care clinic. He complains of 3 months of "feeling down" that began soon after his job loss 6 months ago. His appetite has decreased and he has noticed his clothes are baggy on him. He has felt extremely distracted and fatigued. He attributes this to waking up at approximately 3:00 a.m. every day and then not falling back to sleep. While he has felt "lower than I've ever been," he denies any suicidal ideation. He does not have any past psychiatric history or current medical problems. He is subsequently begun on mirtazepine (Remeron) 15 mg at bedtime.

71. Which of the following symptoms will most likely be the last to improve?

(A) anergia

(B) hopelessness

(C) insomnia

(D) low concentration

(E) poor appetite

72. His illness is successfully treated and remits for 1 year. He returns to the clinic wishing to stop the medications. If he is tapered off the mirtazepine, which of the following are his approximate chances of developing a recurrence?

(A) 0–10%

(B) 10–30%

(C) 30–50%

(D) 50–80%

(E) 80–100%

Questions 73 and 74

The patient is a 25-year-old woman recently released from the hospital after her first manic episode. She is currently taking lithium 1200 mg per day, and her lithium level is 1.1 meq/L. She has a slight, but tolerable, tremor and has gained 5 lb, but she is otherwise tolerating the medication. She claims her mood is "pretty good." She is sleeping approximately 7 h per night. Her energy and concentration are adequate and she denies racing thoughts, talkativeness, or increased activity. She has no major medical problems and her only other medication is birth control pills. She does not consume alcohol or drugs. She is wondering "how long will I have to take medications for this problem?"

73. Which of the following should be the recommended time course for maintenance therapy in this patient?

    (A) 6 months
    (B) 1 year
    (C) 2 years
    (D) 5 years
    (E) life-long

74. This patient returns to the clinic 6 months later. She has continued to take the lithium and her level remains at 1.2 meq/L. She states that for the past several weeks she has become increasingly sad. She is now sleeping over 10 h per night but still feels tired. She is having difficulty focusing on her schoolwork and she doesn't eat more than one meal a day. She has not enjoyed pursuing her usual hobbies and feels that "life is not worth living," although she denies any suicidal plan or intent.

    Which of the following would be the most appropriate next step in the management of this patient?

    (A) add lamotrigine (Lamictal)
    (B) add sertraline (Zoloft)
    (C) add valproate (Depacon)
    (D) decrease lithium
    (E) increase lithium

Questions 75 through 77

A 68-year-old retired male is accompanied by his son and daughter to a family practice clinic. They are concerned about their father's health, as they have noticed him becoming gradually more "confused" over the past year. While he had always been capable of managing to live alone, he has not been keeping up with his bills. The patient explains that he needs his bifocals but both of his children quickly interrupt, stating that he has glasses but continues to misplace them. In fact, he also frequently loses his keys and forgets to shut his door. The management of the condominium has complained because they recently found him wandering around the lobby and pool in the middle of the night while dressed in his underwear. He has no medical problems and takes only an aspirin daily. His MSE is significant for defensiveness to questioning with some irritability. His mini-mental state examination is 19/30, with notable memory deficits and word-finding difficulties. His children are upset about his condition and would like something prescribed to help him to calm down and sleep at night.

75. Which of the following medications should be most avoided in this patient?

    (A) diphenhydramine (Benadryl)
    (B) donepezil (Aricept)
    (C) haloperidol (Haldol)
    (D) lorazepam (Ativan)
    (E) trazodone (Desyrel)

76. An MRI performed would most likely demonstrate which of the following findings?

    (A) atrophy of frontal and temporal lobes
    (B) caudate nucleus atrophy with cortical atrophy
    (C) diffuse cortical atrophy with dilatation of ventricles
    (D) dilatation of cerebral ventricles without cortical atrophy
    (E) subcortical white matter infarcts

77. Which of the following will be the most likely course of his illness?

    (A) gradual progression
    (B) no worsening
    (C) rapid progression
    (D) steady improvement
    (E) stepwise progression

Questions 78 through 80

An 82-year-old woman is admitted to the surgical ward after suffering a fracture of her right hip due to a fall down her stairs. Her surgery and recovery are uneventful, but 3 days later, the nurses are frustrated, as she does not let them take her vitals or draw blood. On interview, she appears drowsy, but this alternates with occasional agitation. She is unable to answer questions well and is only oriented to person. She also picks at the empty air, then begins yelling and swinging at the nurse who is present.

78. An electroencephalogram (EEG) performed on this patient would most likely show which of the following?

    (A) diffuse slowing
    (B) localized spikes
    (C) low-voltage fast activity
    (D) random activity
    (E) triphasic delta waves

79. Which of the following is the most important in managing this patient?

    (A) haloperidol (Haldol) to decrease agitation
    (B) lorazepam (Ativan) to regulate sleep

    (C) soft restraints to prevent injury
    (D) techniques to promote orientation
    (E) treatment of underlying condition

80. Which of the following most likely represents her mortality rate in 6 months after discharge?

    (A) 0–20%
    (B) 20–40%
    (C) 40–60%
    (D) 60–80%
    (E) 80–100%

Answers and Explanations

1. (E)

2. (C)

Explanations 1 and 2

This woman likely suffers from a major depressive episode. While asking about substance abuse, current medications, medical problems, and a past history of depression are very important in a complete psychiatric evaluation, assessment of suicidality is essential. The risk of suicide in patients with MDD is about 20 times higher than those without the illness. The estimated lifetime risk of suicide is approximately 15% in those individuals with MDD.

The choice of a specific antidepressant may be influenced by many factors, including prior response in the patient or a family member and comorbid medical problems or substance abuse in the family (and therefore potentially the patient). If a patient or family member has a history of manic symptoms or bipolar disorder, consideration should be given to beginning a mood stabilizer prior to initiating antidepressant therapy, as antidepressants can cause a switch into mania in those individuals. (*Practice Guideline for the Assessment and Treatment of Patients with Suicidal Behaviors, 2003, APA; Practice Guideline for the Treatment of Patients with Major Depressive Disorder, 2000, APA*)

3. (C)

4. (D)

Explanations 3 and 4

This patient clearly presents with a paranoid stance, although he is not overtly psychotic. Individuals with antisocial personality disorder are usually more dishonest, aggressive, and exploitative in their attitudes. Narcissistic patients may become easily offended by interactions when not feeling as though they are being treated as "special," but they do not display as much overt mistrust. Patients with schizoid and schizotypal personality disorders appear indifferent or odd, usually with a detached attitude. Patients with paranoid personality disorder display a pervasive suspiciousness toward others, continuously feeling slighted and bearing grudges, not unusually in the form of litigiousness (DSM IV).

Becoming defensive will likely only serve to "confirm" the patient's suspicions. A referral to a psychiatrist, while theoretically helpful, is usually not beneficial given the primitive and inflexible defenses (projection, denial, and so on) seen in these individuals. While the patient may have worsening paranoia as a consequence of his fears of having cancer, presenting him with this while he is upset may make matters worse. In fact, the patient may then feel even more accused and become angrier. Referral to a colleague would be indicated for a second opinion to further cultivate trust, but doing so in order to solely avoid a lawsuit may also be seen as defensive and "having something to hide." Individuals with paranoid personality disorder respond best to an empathic, not overly friendly and very professional attitude. Answering all questions with full disclosure of information pertaining to diagnosis, treatment, and prognosis can serve to strengthen the therapeutic alliance in these patients.

5. (C)

6. (B)

Explanations 5 and 6

While patients with bipolar depression do present with psychotic features, this individual does not give any history of manic episodes, making the diagnosis difficult at this time. Bizarre delusions (those that cannot possibly exist in life) and auditory hallucinations are not consistent with delusional disorder. Schizoaffective disorder, depressed type, includes both psychotic as well as depressive symptoms. However, the psychotic symptoms must last at least 1 month and occur in the absence of a depressed mood. The diagnosis of schizophrenia also requires at least 1 month of active psychosis but a total of 6 months of attenuated or residual symptoms. Although a depressed mood is very commonly seen in schizophrenia, the total duration of depression is brief overall compared to the psychotic symptoms. This patient presents with major depression with psychotic features, consisting of a depressed mood with neurovegetative symptoms for at least 2 weeks, as well as psychotic symptoms, which are only present along with the mood symptoms (DSM IV).

Mood stabilizers alone or with antipsychotic medications are not the first-line treatments for major depression with psychotic features, but rather for mania with or without psychotic features. Studies have demonstrated that the combination of antidepressants and antipsychotics is more effective in treating major depression with psychotic features than pharmacotherapy alone (*Practice Guideline for the Treatment of Patients with Major Depressive Disorder, 2000, APA*).

7. (D)

8. (E)

Explanations 7 and 8

This patient is suffering from bulimia nervosa, categorized by recurrent episodes of binge eating associated with compensatory behaviors including self-induced emesis, diuretic or laxative abuse. Because of the repeated vomiting of gastric fluids, patients are prone to develop various electrolyte abnormalities, such as hypochloremic alkalosis or hypokalemia.

Hypernatremia and leukopenia are not commonly seen.

Anticonvulsants, such as valproic acid and carbamazepine, as well as mood stabilizers such as lithium, may be helpful for treating comorbid bipolar disorder but are not in and of themselves efficacious in the treatment of bulimia nervosa. Similarly, antipsychotics and benzodiazepines may be used in cooccurring psychotic or anxiety disorders, but do not help with binging or purging. Antidepressants, especially the SSRIs, have been shown to be successful in decreasing both the binging and purging behaviors (*Synopsis, pp. 748, 750*).

9. (A)

10. (A)

Explanations 9 and 10

The child's mother demonstrates factitious disorder by proxy, categorized by a parent or caretaker intentionally inducing an illness in someone under their care. Confronting the mother in the emergency room setting would likely lead to defensiveness, denial, and anger. The mother could possibly leave abruptly with the child. Having a psychiatrist present in this situation may also create a similar result. While a referral to urology and treatment of the infection may be indicated and appropriate, it does not address the immediate concern, which is the mother's abuse of her son. As factitious disorder by proxy is considered a form of child abuse, the physician has the legal obligation to notify child protective services. Admitting the boy to the hospital will both enable treatment of his medical illness and provide time for the proper authorities to intervene if necessary.

The conscious production of symptoms for secondary gain (e.g., avoidance of work, school, jail, military service) is the rationale behind malingering. Although the mother's apparent concern for her child may appear expectable, her elaborate methods of abusing her son demonstrate significant pathology. The unconscious production of symptoms or signs due to unconscious conflict is the classic drive in conversion disorder. The motivation for factitious disorder is believed to be the purposeful production of an illness in order to assume the sick role.

11. (E)

12. (E)

Explanations 11 and 12

This young woman would be diagnosed with conversion disorder. The conscious production of symptoms to assume the sick role is the motivation underlying factitious disorder. Malingering is not a diagnosable mental illness but is the conscious inventing or exaggerating of physical or psychiatric symptoms in order to obtain secondary gain, such as disability benefits, or avoidance of work or a prison sentence. Given her unremarkable MRI, normal reflexes, absence of pathologic reflexes, coupled with the hemianesthesia along her umbilicus, her presentation is not consistent with either central or peripheral nervous system pathology. The apparent stressors relating to a new marriage and pregnancy are likely related to the genesis of her symptoms. Conversion symptoms are created through the unconscious production of neurologic symptoms due to unconscious conflict.

While administering a "placebo," such as intravenous saline, may resolve her symptoms, it is both dishonest and unethical. Admission to neurology is unnecessary unless there is a concern regarding an actual underlying or comorbid disease. It may also serve to reinforce the somatization of her conflict. Confronting a patient with conversion disorder often results in a subsequent worsening of symptomatology. Consultation with a psychiatrist may be useful in helping the patient cope with the stress of her dysfunction but, in the emergency room, may also lead to feelings of not being believed and an increase in symptoms. Many cases of conversion disorder spontaneously remit, but recovery may be significantly facilitated through support, reassurance, and actual suggestion that improvement will occur (*Synopsis, p. 650*).

13. (A) Although antidepressant treatment may be appropriate if the patient is suffering from a depressive illness, further questioning would have to be made prior to that determination. Postpartum depressive symptoms are not uncommon and they may not require treatment. If there is felt to be immediate danger to the child, calling child protective services would certainly be indicated. Having intrusive thoughts does not equate with acting on the thoughts, and thoughts similar to those in this case are not unusual given the stress of a newborn. Again, more information would need to be obtained. On the other hand, premature reassurance regarding the thoughts of harm without knowing additional facts might be dangerous if the patient is harboring a plan or intent to harm her child. Hospitalization may be necessary if the patient is suffering from postpartum psychosis or is suicidal. Only by gathering further history and symptoms, especially focusing on a support system and possible psychotic symptoms, can the clinician determine if there is significant cause for concern. Postpartum psychosis is considered a psychiatric emergency because of the risk of harm to the infant and usually requires immediate hospitalization.

14. (B)

15. (E)

Explanations 14 and 15

This case demonstrates a classic presentation for delirium. Delirium can present with many symptoms, including aggressiveness, hostility, memory impairment, psychotic symptoms (especially visual hallucinations) and overall uncooperativeness, such as pulling out IVs and getting out of bed. While these symptoms are common in delirious patients, they are not specific for delirium and can be seen in many psychiatric illnesses, including dementias, psychotic disorders, substance-use disorders, personality disorders, and others. The hallmark of delirium is a fluctuating level of consciousness over time, ranging from sedation to agitation.

Diphenhydramine can be sedating but, due to its anticholinergic side effects, it can also worsen delirium and cause urinary retention and constipation, especially in the elderly. Donepezil, or other anticholinesterase inhibitors, may be indicated for mild-to-moderate dementias, especially Alzheimer's dementia. It is not indicated for the treatment of delirium and it would be difficult to diagnose a dementing illness in the context of a delirious state. Giving benzodiazepines such as lorazepam may be useful for agitation caused by a delirium, but they can also disinhibit a patient and cause further agitation, especially in older individuals. A benzodiazepine would be the preferred treatment of alcohol withdrawal delirium (delirium tremens), however. A low dose of antipsychotic would be the best choice to decrease the agitation in a delirious patient. While a high-potency medication, such as haloperidol, can be used, it is more likely to cause extrapyramidal side effects than a second generation (or atypical) antipsychotic, such as risperidone.

16. (D)

17. (C)

Explanations 16 and 17

Alcohol and benzodiazepine intoxication commonly present with disinhibited behavior, slurred speech, poor coordination, and nystagmus, but not typically with dry mucous membranes or constricted pupils. Patients with anticholinergic overdose classically demonstrate psychotic symptoms and dry skin, similar to the above case. However, on physical examination, they usually show dilated pupils, warm skin, and tachycardia. PCP intoxication also manifests itself with vertical or horizontal nystagmus, dysarthria, and even coma, but it will usually cause hypertension or tachycardia (DSM IV). This case is a typical presentation of opiate (such as heroin) overdose. The clinical triad is coma/unresponsiveness, pinpoint pupils, and respiratory depression. Other signs may include hypothermia, hypotension, and bradycardia.

Disulfiram is an oral, nonemergent medication that blocks aldehyde dehydrogenase to cause a noxious reaction in those who consume alcohol while taking it. It is useful as a deterrent to drinking alcohol but not indicated for alcohol or opiate overdose. Flumazenil is a benzodiazepine receptor antagonist used to reverse the symptoms of overdose with benzodiazepines, especially the sedation and respiratory depression. It would have no effect on overdose on opiates unless concurrent benzodiazepines have been ingested. Intravenous thiamine is indicated for the treatment of Wernicke's encephalopathy, due to thiamine deficiency in alcoholics. The classic triad consists of oculomotor disturbances, ataxia, and delirium. Although individuals with chronic opiate dependence are often malnourished, thiamine would not prevent complications with overdose. Physostigmine is an anticholinesterase inhibitor used in the emergency treatment of anticholinergic toxicity, but it could be dangerous in opiate overdose, as it can cause further hypotension. Naloxone, an opiate antagonist given intravenously, is the treatment of choice for the urgent management of heroin overdose, as it rapidly reverses the sedation, respiratory depression, hypotension, and bradycardia seen in cases similar to the patient above (*Synopsis, pp. 454, 908, 1014, 1046*).

18. (A)

19. (A)

Explanations 18 and 19

Many psychotropic medications, including most of the antidepressants, cause a variety of sexual dysfunction symptoms. Both painful intercourse and retrograde ejaculation are not seen with antidepressant therapy. These are usually caused by other classes of medications, medical conditions, or surgical procedures. Premature ejaculation is not caused by antidepressants and, in fact, may actually be helped by antidepressants, especially SSRIs. Priapism is an uncommon side effect seen in patients treated with trazodone and even more rarely with the other antidepressants. Decreased libido is a frequent sexual side effect seen in individuals taking antidepressants, especially

SSRIs. Other sexual problems caused by these medications include decreased erection and delayed ejaculation.

Almost all of the antidepressants, including the tricyclic antidepressants like desipramine and the monoamine oxidase inhibitors such as phenelzine, can cause sexual dysfunction. Fluoxetine is a SSRI that commonly causes sexual dysfunction. Venlafaxine is a serotonin and norepinephrine reuptake inhibitor that has also been shown to cause similar problems with sexual performance. Bupropion, an effective antidepressant with questionable dopaminergic properties, not only causes little to no sexual dysfunction but also helps to treat antidepressant-induced sexual dysfunction (*Synopsis, pp. 707, 709, 711, 1029*).

20. (E)

21. (E)

Explanations 20 and 21

This is a case of dementia, vascular type (multiinfarct dementia), caused by poorly controlled hypertension. Atrophy of the caudate nucleus is seen in Huntington's chorea, which accounts for the movement disorder and dementia that are seen in that illness. Dilated ventricles without atrophy are characteristic of normal pressure hydrocephalus (NPH), one of the potentially reversible causes of dementia. The triad consists of a dementia, gait disturbance, and urinary incontinence. Pick's disease is a gradually progressing dementia, displaying marked but preferential atrophy of the frontal and temporal lobes of the brain. Generalized atrophy can often be seen with neuroimaging in Alzheimer's dementia. Vascular dementia classically will show lacunar infarcts of the white matter on MRI.

With the exception of reversible causes (e.g., NPH, metabolic causes, or heavy metal toxicity), improvement is unusual in dementing illnesses. A rapid decline is common in dementias due to prion infection, such as Creutzfeldt-Jakob disease. Stable dementias are also unusual, most notably seen in dementia due to a head injury. Both Alzheimer's and Pick's dementias demonstrate a steady wors-

ening of the illness over many years. The multiple small infarcts causing vascular dementia correspond to a stepwise deterioration in functioning of the patient.

22. (E)

23. (D)

Explanations 22 and 23

This patient suffers from Parkinson's disease, a disorder involving decreased dopaminergic transmission. The caudal raphe nuclei are the origin of the serotonergic system in the brain. The hippocampus is responsible for emotional and memory processing. The locus ceruleus is the location of the norepinephrine cell bodies. The nucleus basalis of Meynert is where the neurotransmitter acetylcholine originates. The nigrostriatal system originates in the substantia nigra. It is the primary dopaminergic tract in the central nervous system and is significantly affected in Parkinson's disease.

The concern with treating agitation and psychosis in patients with Parkinson's disease is that antipsychotics block certain dopamine receptors, which can subsequently worsen the Parkinson's symptoms. While clozapine has minimal extrapyramidal symptoms (EPS), its risk of agranulocytosis and need for regular blood monitoring make it not as practical as a first-line agent. Haloperidol is a high potency neuroleptic. It is efficacious in treating psychotic symptoms and reducing agitation, but its potency also presents a significant risk of worsening the Parkinson's disease. Risperidone is an atypical, or second generation, antipsychotic. Although the risk of EPS at low doses is less than with haloperidol, risperidone tends to still be more of a problem when compared with other atypical medications. Thioridazine is another older antipsychotic. While its lower potency creates less EPS and, therefore, less likelihood of worsening Parkinson's symptoms, it has significant anticholinergic side effects that may worsen the confusion. A more concerning risk is prolongation of the QTc interval on ECG, potentially causing a ventricular arrhythmia. Quetiapine is a second generation antipsychotic medication with essentially no EPS. This gives it a unique advantage in treating the psychosis and/or agitation in Parkinson's patients without also worsening the movement disorder.

24. (D)

25. (B)

Explanations 24 and 25

This woman experiences symptoms consistent with a specific phobia, blood-injection-injury type. While all other phobias are characterized by a sympathetic discharge causing tachycardia and hypertension, blood-injury type classically displays a vaso-vagal response. This would be represented by an initial tachycardia, followed by bradycardia and hypotension.

Due to the sympathetic discharge, individuals with certain phobias, most notably social phobia, can sometimes be managed with the use of beta-blockers, especially when a known exposure will occur. Beta-blockers could worsen the symptoms of blood-injury phobia, however, given the vaso-vagal nature of the response. Insight-oriented and supportive therapies are not particularly helpful with treating phobias, as phobias usually require specific behavioral techniques. SSRIs can be efficacious in certain anxiety disorders, such as social phobia, panic disorder, and generalized anxiety disorder, but they are not useful for phobias such as blood-injury type. Exposure therapy is considered to be the optimal treatment for phobias in general, especially specific phobias. In this therapy, the patient is exposed to particular phobic stimuli of an increasingly anxiety-provoking nature, along with certain relaxation techniques.

26. (B) Bipolar disorder usually has its onset in late adolescence or early adulthood. A manic episode consists of symptoms such as decreased need for sleep, increased energy, talkativeness, and an elevated or irritable mood. Individuals with paranoid personality disorder are chronically mistrustful and suspicious. Although they can distort reality, they are not overtly delusional as in the above case. Both schizoaffective disorder and schizophrenia display overt psychotic symptoms, including delusions, hallucinations, and disorganization. Patients with schizoaffective disorder additionally have either a major depressive or manic episode, while patients with schizophrenia require significant social or occupational impairment. Neither of these criteria is present in the above case. The patient demonstrates delusional disorder, which consists of a nonbizarre delusion (i.e., one that could actually exist), without significantly impaired function, odd behavior, or the presence of a major mood disorder. The age of onset for delusional disorder is commonly during middle age, whereas evidence of the other disorders is generally present at a much earlier age.

27. (D)

28. (C)

Explanations 27 and 28

This boy suffers from ADHD. Acetylcholine is involved in some cases of delirium as well as Alzheimer's disease. GABA more than likely plays a role in anxiety disorders, as it is the most prevalent inhibitory neurotransmitter in the brain. Conversely, glutamate is the most common excitatory neurotransmitter. It has been studied in relation to schizophrenia, because PCP (which affects glutamate receptors) causes a schizophrenic-like psychosis. Serotonin is associated with numerous mental illnesses, including anxiety disorders, depressive disorders, impulsivity, and schizophrenia. Norepinephrine (and possibly dopamine) is the neurotransmitter thought to be involved in the pathophysiology and treatment of ADHD. Norepinephrine plays a role in attention, and stimulant medications, which are very effective in treating ADHD, increase the release of both norepinephrine and dopamine.

Stimulants, such as methylphenidate, are considered to be the first-line treatment for ADHD. Although they can increase the frequency of tics in patients with an underlying tic disorder, they are not absolutely contraindicated in those particular patients. The risk-benefit ratio of using these medications must be discussed with the patient's caregivers. Stimulants may inhibit some growth in children, but the use of drug holidays has been shown to provide adequate time to make up that growth. The use of stimulants has not been shown to increase the risk of future substance abuse. Indeed, stimulant pharmacotherapy may actually lower the risk when compared to untreated ADHD. It was previously believed that stimulants exert their therapeutic effect through a paradoxical sedation. This is not considered to be the case. In fact, similar improvements in attention and behavior can be seen if persons without ADHD take stimulants. The positive effect is therefore one of degree, rather than a qualitative difference (*Synopsis, pp. 106, 107, 1224, 1228*).

29. (C)

30. (B)

31. (E)

Explanations 29 through 31

This patient has Tourette's disorder, characterized by the existence of both motor and vocal tics, present for 1 year. There is not a significantly increased comorbidity for autistic disorder, MDD, panic disorder, or conduct disorder. There is a very high comorbidity, however, for both ADHD and OCD in individuals with Tourette's disorder.

Lorazepam, a benzodiazepine, may be useful in the short-term management of the anxiety associated with Tourette's, but it is not indicated for the treatment of the tics themselves. Methylphenidate, a stimulant, may be used if there is associated ADHD along with the tic disorder, but it may increase the frequency of tics. Paroxetine, a SSRI, is used in treating both depressive disorders and OCD, but it is not indicated for treatment of Tourette's disorder. Clonidine, an alpha-2 adrenergic agonist, can be somewhat helpful in reducing some symptoms of Tourette's. The most efficacious, and first-line, treatment for Tourette's disorder is the use of dopamine antagonists, such as antipsychotics like haloperidol.

The etiology of several disorders, among them Tourette's and OCD, may be related to an autoimmune process. It is believed that infection with certain microorganisms, specifically streptococcal infections, may act synergistically with a genetic vulnerability to cause those mental illnesses. The full significance of this in terms of diagnosis, prevention, or treatment of these conditions has yet to be determined (*Synopsis, p. 1247*).

32. (C)

33. (A)

Explanations 32 and 33

This patient has OCD. Benzodiazepines such as alprazolam may be helpful for the acute anxiety associated with OCD, but are not a first-line medication to reduce the obsessions or compulsions. Although antipsychotics like olanzapine are sometimes used in conjunction with other psychotropics in patients with severe, intractable OCD, they are not recommended as monotherapy given their significant side effects. Antidepressants that mostly affect norepinephrine, such as bupropion and desipramine, are not particularly effective in treating OCD. Serotonergic drugs, such as citalopram and the tricyclic clomipramine, have been proven to improve both obsessions and compulsions. Because of this fact, OCD is therefore thought to involve the serotonergic system.

EMDR is a treatment used specifically for posttraumatic stress disorder. Although psychoanalysis and psychodynamic (or insight-oriented) psychotherapies may be beneficial for some individuals with OCD, there have not been enough studies to document their effectiveness. Supportive psychotherapy can be useful in helping the patients to cope with their severe anxiety and limitations, but it does not particularly address the obsessions and compulsions, themselves. Behavioral therapy has consistently demonstrated its success in treating OCD and studies have shown it to be as efficacious as pharmacotherapy (*Synopsis, p. 623*).

34. (B)

35. (C)

Explanations 34 and 35

This patient is most likely experiencing panic attacks as part of panic disorder. While tricyclic antidepressants, such as imipramine, and SSRIs, such as paroxetine, are both effective in the treatment of panic disorder, therapeutic benefit for both may require several weeks. Antipsychotic medications such as risperidone have not been shown to be effective in panic disorder. Their side effects and potential long-term toxicity deem them inappropriate. Valproic acid and other anticonvulsants/mood stabilizers have not been studied as extensively in this patient population, and any positive effect would also likely be delayed for several weeks. Benzodiazepines, such as lorazepam and alprazolam, have been shown to be effective in the treatment of panic disorder. Their more rapid onset of action (hours to days) make them ideally suited for the immediate and acute management of panic attacks.

Imipramine and other tricyclic antidepressants have demonstrated their efficacy in panic disorder. The disadvantages are several: the need to increase up to a therapeutic dose over time, a significant side effect profile, and their lethality in overdose. While benzodiazepines like lorazepam are also effective in the long-term treatment of panic disorder, their potential for abuse and withdrawal if/when tapered make them less than ideal overall. It is not unusual to initiate a benzodiazepine for more immediate relief of anxiety along with another agent that will require a longer time period until its benefits become apparent. Neither risperidone nor valproic acid is an appropriate first-line psychotropic in the management of panic disorder. Given their proven efficacy, reduced side effects, lack of abuse potential and safety in overdose, paroxetine, as well as the other SSRIs, are the most suitable choice for the long-term pharmacotherapy of panic disorder (*Practice Guideline for the Treatment of Patients with Panic Disorder, 1998, APA*).

36. (D) This is a woman who is suffering from bereavement, which is not a diagnosable mental illness. Bereavement is considered to be a normal grief reaction to the death of a loved one. Hospitalization would only be indicated if the patient were imminently dangerous to herself (or others) or if she were unable to take care of herself. As she is not suicidal and functioning adequately at work, hospitalization would be neither necessary nor helpful. Beginning an antidepressant would be appropriate if treating MDD. While she exhibits some symptoms consistent with MDD, it has been less than 2 months since the sudden death of her spouse and her complaints are not as pervasive as those seen in MDD (DSM IV). Another factor favoring bereavement over MDD in this patient is the lack of a prior history of depression or current suicidality. Pharmacotherapy with both an antidepressant plus antipsychotic would be the treatment of choice if she were suffering from MDD with psychotic features. Although she does have occasional perceptual disturbances, this phenomenon is not unusual in uncomplicated bereavement. Her insight and lack of other psychotic symptoms, such as delusions or disorganization, are not consistent with a major psychotic illness. Individuals with bereavement do not usually require referral to a psychiatrist unless there is another existing mental disorder or complicating problem. Given the time-limited nature of bereavement, monitoring her symptoms over time is the most appropriate approach for this patient. Referral to grief therapy, either individual or group, may also be helpful. If the patient's symptoms worsen, continue for more than 8 weeks, or there is major impairment in functioning or dangerousness, then referral to a psychiatrist or hospitalization may be warranted.

37. (D)

38. (E)

Explanations 37 and 38

Older patients with cognitive decline due to depression, sometimes called pseudodementia, display characteristic findings on MSE.

They usually are greatly concerned about their problems, even emphasizing their difficulties when compared with demented patients, who attempt to hide or minimize their deficits and appear unconcerned. Patients with pseudodementia are able to attend well to the tasks despite their cognitive complaints. Individuals with dementias, however, have significant difficulty with attention and concentration. Patients with depression are more likely to demonstrate good insight into their presumed memory loss than those with dementia, who will commonly deny that there is anything wrong with them. On tests of cognition, those individuals with pseudodementia will present inconsistent results, sometimes performing better than others. Patients with dementia, however, will consistently perform poorly on various tests that address the same function.

This patient displays characteristics of Lewy body disease, a dementia that may be related to Alzheimer's dementia. The classic triad of Lewy body dementia is a fluctuating course, peduncular hallucinations (visual hallucinations of small people, animals, or objects), and parkinsonian features. These patients tend to be very sensitive to extrapyramidal side effects and, therefore, antipsychotics such as risperidone should be avoided or sparingly used (*Synopsis, pp. 333, 340*).

39. (B)

40. (A)

Explanations 39 and 40

This patient exhibits the criteria for conduct disorder. Antisocial personality disorder can only be diagnosed in a person who is over age 18. In fact, the diagnosis of antisocial personality disorder requires evidence of conduct disorder prior to age 15 (DSM IV). Children with autism, schizophrenia, and mental retardation may display aggressive or disruptive behavior, but these illnesses do not necessarily predict future conduct disorder. Patients with ADHD and learning disorders are at an increased risk of developing conduct disorder as they get older.

It is not uncommon for patients with conduct disorder to have a history of oppositional defiant disorder (ODD) as a younger child. Indeed, the disorders are often thought of as on a spectrum, with ODD early on, followed by conduct disorder and eventually antisocial personality disorder. Having conduct disorder does not by itself predict panic disorder, schizoid personality disorder, or the development of schizophrenia. If left untreated, there is a significantly increased risk of developing a substance use disorder, which also predicts a worse prognosis (*Synopsis, p. 1237*).

41. (A)

42. (D)

Explanations 41 and 42

This patient is experiencing symptoms of post-traumatic stress disorder (PTSD). The greatest predictor of future symptoms is the proximity, severity, and duration of the trauma. There are other risk factors, however, including any premorbid or comorbid psychiatric illnesses. Females are more likely to develop PTSD than males. Dissociation during the trauma is believed to interfere with the laying down of memories, which may increase the likelihood of future anxiety symptoms. The presence of certain personality characteristics, including borderline, paranoid, and antisocial personalities, may also make someone more vulnerable to developing PTSD. A history of childhood trauma, whether physical, sexual, or emotional, is a strong predictor of future PTSD.

Administering amobarbital, or an amytal interview, has been sometimes used in conjunction with psychotherapy to help individuals work through their traumatic event. It has not been used as a treatment alone, however, given its addicting potential and lethality in overdose. Antipsychotics such as haloperidol have little evidence to support their use in PTSD symptoms, but they may be used acutely to manage agitation or violence. Lorazepam can also be used in a similar manner, but given the high comorbidity of substance abuse in patients with PTSD, this is not a recommended solo treatment. Trazodone, in lower doses, can be used to help treat insomnia in these individuals. Treatment of the PTSD symptoms, however, would likely require a full antidepressant dose, which carries significant side effects, such as daytime sedation and orthostasis. Sertraline, and the other SSRIs, are very effective and well-tolerated treatments for PTSD. SSRIs have been shown to improve all of the symptom clusters of PTSD (i.e., reexperiencing symptoms, avoidance of stimuli, and increased arousal). Based on their efficacy, tolerability, lack of abuse potential, and safety in overdose, they are considered to be first-line agents for treating PTSD (*Synopsis, pp. 624, 630*).

43. **(D)** This toddler has developed pica, the eating of nonnutritive substances. Decreased levels of folate may be associated with depression and dementia in adults but is not seen in cases of pica. The eating of lead-based paint can be present in children with pica, but this would lead to lead toxicity, with elevated levels of lead. Iron and zinc deficiency are considered to be potential causes of pica, especially when toddlers or children are noticed eating dirt and clay. Because of this, blood levels of both should be determined (*Synopsis, p. 1242*).

44. **(E)** Asperger disorder is a pervasive developmental disorder (PDD) manifested with impairments in social interaction and stereotyped behaviors, without the additional language abnormalities seen in autism. Childhood disintegrative disorder is also a PDD characterized by normal development until age 2, followed by a rapid decline in the use of language, motor skills, and social interaction. Fragile X syndrome is a genetic syndrome displaying mental retardation, characteristic physical features, and a high rate of PDD. The above patient displays a history consistent with Rett's disorder, a progressively worsening PDD seen only in females. Rett's patients routinely demonstrate normal development until at least 5 months of age, with subsequent head deceleration, stereotyped hand movements, loss of social engagement, gait difficulties, and impaired language (DSM IV).

45. **(C)**

46. **(D)**

Explanations 45 and 46

The patient has likely developed tardive dyskinesia (TD), a late-occurring movement disorder associated with chronic antipsychotic use. Adding an anticholinergic agent like benztropine would be indicated for treating an acute dystonia but is not effective for TD. Continuing the current dose of his antipsychotic will not lessen his movements, and increasing it will more than likely worsen them over time. Discontinuing his psychotropic will not reduce his dyskinesia and it will provide a high risk for relapse of his psychosis. Once an individual has TD, reducing the dose (if clinically indicated) may minimize the progression or even improve the abnormal movements.

The patient displays features consistent with neuroleptic malignant syndrome (NMS), a life-threatening condition associated with antipsychotic therapy. Adding benztropine will not treat NMS. Immediate discontinuation of the antipsychotic is recommended. Initiation of dantrolene, a muscle relaxant, as well as bromocriptine, a dopamine receptor agonist, may also be used to manage the patient (*Synopsis, pp. 1059–1060*).

47. **(E)** This patient presents with agitation and psychosis, likely caused by intoxication with a substance of abuse. While intoxication with alcohol can cause unsteadiness and belligerence, it does not present with hypertension and tachycardia. Cannabis can cause tachycardia and feelings of paranoia but, by itself, does not usually spur violence or grossly disorganized behavior. Intoxication with heroin or other opiates more often presents with drowsiness or apathy rather than the overt psychotic symptoms and sympathetic discharge seen in the above case. While LSD and other hallucinogens obviously cause psychotic symptoms, the nystagmus and muscular rigidity are not as common. Patients are not characteristically as hostile as in the case example. PCP use classically presents with the unpredictability, paranoia, and

aggressiveness similar to the above case. It is not uncommonly mistaken for schizophrenia. Physical findings may include nystagmus, hypertension, tachycardia, ataxia, and muscular rigidity (DSM IV).

48. (E)

49. (A)

Explanations 48 and 49

The quit rates for abrupt cessation and education/advice are quite low when used alone. The rates increase significantly with behavioral interventions or the use of medications, such as nicotine replacement. The highest quit rates are likely seen with the combination of medications plus behavioral therapy, such as group therapy (Synopsis, p. 446).

The reinforcing aspects of nicotine addiction are thought to involve the dopaminergic system in the central nervous system. This may be one reason why bupropion, which likely increases dopamine activity, is very effective in helping patients to quit smoking. The other antidepressants listed have not demonstrated efficacy for nicotine dependence.

50. (A)

51. (B)

Explanations 50 and 51

The patient does not complain of significant depression, anhedonia, problems with appetite, or guilt consistent with MDD. She also does not complain of specific obsessions or compulsions necessary for OCD, such as fears of dirt, hurting individuals, need for symmetry. While she does have panic attacks, they are not unexpected, relating to her worries about aspects of her life. She also does not have the ongoing fear of having more attacks characteristic of panic disorder. Social phobia consists of fears of acting in an embarrassing or humiliating way in public, which are not apparent in the above case. She complains of symptoms of excessive anxiety and worry about a number of activities,

associated with other cognitive and physical symptoms. This case fits the criteria for generalized anxiety disorder (GAD) (DSM IV).

Both buspirone and benzodiazepines are very effective in treating GAD. Buspirone has a large advantage in not being an addicting medication like benzodiazepines. Buspirone has been shown to be less effective in treating GAD after a benzodiazepine has been tried. Another disadvantage to buspirone is that, while the onset of action for benzodiazepines is within hours, buspirone requires several weeks to improve the anxiety symptoms. Because of this, a helpful strategy for managing GAD is to initiate treatment with both buspirone and a benzodiazepine, with the plan to taper the benzodiazepine as the buspirone starts to help. Buspirone has been shown to help reduce the cognitive symptoms of GAD more than the somatic symptoms (Synopsis, p. 635).

52. (E)

53. (D)

Explanations 52 and 53

This patient most likely ingested MDMA (ecstasy) at a rave. Cocaine likely causes its effects through blockade of dopamine reuptake, which is responsible for its reinforcing, and therefore, highly addicting nature. PCP intoxicated individuals can often be agitated, but they typically will also display nystagmus and, not infrequently, violent behavior. PCP works through blockade of glutamate receptors. Hallucinogens are thought to increase the activity of the serotonin system and they do not necessarily present with the feelings of euphoria seen in the above case. Amphetamine intoxication, by causing the release of dopamine, can appear similar to the above case but florid perceptual disturbances are not as frequent. Ecstasy, classically taken at raves, acts as an amphetamine and a hallucinogen, thereby creating feelings of well-being or euphoria, as well as causing hallucinations. Its dual nature is likely due to its neurophysiologic effects of releasing both dopamine and serotonin in the brain.

This patient gives a history consistent with hallucinogen persisting perception disorder (flashbacks), characterized by the reexperiencing of perceptual disturbances after cessation of use. Although there is no medication that definitively treats the flashbacks, various drugs may be helpful. These include anticonvulsants, like carbamazepine and valproic acid, or benzodiazepines like clonazepam. Antidepressants such as fluoxetine would be indicated if the patient displayed a depressive disorder in addition. Antipsychotics, including haloperidol, are to be avoided as they have been shown to actually worsen the symptoms of flashbacks (*Synopsis, pp. 414, 440*).

54. (A)

55. (C)

Explanations 54 and 55

There frequently are comorbid diagnoses in individuals with cocaine dependence. Affective disorders (including bipolar and major depression) as well as anxiety disorders are not uncommonly seen in cocaine addicted patients. Schizophrenia is not appreciably increased in this patient population. Antisocial personality disorder is the most likely associated diagnosis in patients with cocaine dependence.

Antidepressant treatment may be indicated if there is a comorbid depressive illness, but it will not specifically alleviate any withdrawal symptoms. A benzodiazepine taper would be necessary if this patient were displaying significant alcohol withdrawal symptoms. A methadone detox is often used for patients who are having severe opiate withdrawal but is not appropriate for cocaine withdrawal. A phenobarbital detox can be used to prevent withdrawal from benzodiazepines and can also be used (less frequently) for alcohol withdrawal. Unlike alcohol, benzodiazepine or barbiturate withdrawal, withdrawal from cocaine is not life-threatening and does not require pharmacologic intervention. Education about cocaine addiction and withdrawal, as well as reassurance regarding the likely short duration of symptoms, are all that are needed (*Synopsis, p. 429*).

56. (E)

57. (B)

Explanations 56 and 57

This patient displays the classic phenotype for fragile X syndrome: a large, long head, long ears, short stature, hyperextensible joints, and macroorchidism (in males). Lacking part of chromosome 5 is the cause of cri-du-chat syndrome, characterized by microcephaly, low-set ears, and severe retardation. Chromosomes 15 and 21 are involved in Down syndrome, the most common single cause of mental retardation. It displays slanted eyes, epicanthal folds, and a flat nose. Fragile X syndrome results from a mutation on the X chromosome.

Fragile X syndrome is the second most common single cause of mental retardation, with individuals affected having mild-to-severe mental retardation. It is also associated with various comorbid diagnoses, including learning disorders, autism, and approximately a 75% rate of ADHD (*Synopsis, pp. 1163, 1165*).

58. (E)

59. (D)

Explanations 58 and 59

Cannabis is one of the few substances of abuse that does not affect the respiratory rate. Consuming marijuana classically produces symptoms of a dry mouth and increased appetite (the munchies). Contrary to what is sometimes claimed, intoxication with cannabis does significantly impair motor function and, therefore, interferes with driving ability. It also can cause tachycardia (DSM IV).

Amotivational syndrome is a potential, but controversial, long-term effect of heavy cannabis use. It is characterized by apathy and boredom. Cerebral atrophy, chromosomal damage, and seizures have also been reported but not confirmed in individuals with chronic cannabis use. The most concerning medical consequences of smoking cannabis over the long-term are similar to those from smoking tobacco, such as lung cancer and respiratory disease *(Synopsis, p. 425).*

60. (D)

61. (B)

Explanations 60 and 61

This woman likely suffers from MDD. Treatment with a SSRI is considered to be first-line therapy. Although the neurovegetative symptoms of depression (e.g., insomnia, change in appetite, anergia, poor concentration) can sometimes improve after several days of initiating pharmacotherapy, the feelings of depression and hopelessness may take up to 4–6 weeks to significantly improve. As long as she is tolerating the SSRI, the urge to quickly increase the dose should be avoided so as to minimize side effects. On beginning the SSRI, education and reassurance should be provided to the patient regarding the expected time until remission.

Most patients tolerate treatment with SSRIs, although there are characteristic side effects. Many of these, such as headaches, gastrointestinal disturbances, and vivid dreams transpire at the start of treatment and may resolve over days to weeks. Sexual dysfunction, such as impotence or inhibited orgasm, not uncommonly occurs after several weeks to months of treatment with SSRIs and can continue with ongoing treatment.

62. (E)

63. (A)

Explanations 62 and 63

This child may have reading disorder, a type of learning disorder characterized by reading achievement below expected given measured intelligence and age (DSM IV). The Bender Visual Motor Gestalt Test is not a diagnostic test, but it may be used to identify perceptual performance difficulties. Projective psychologic tests, such as the Children's Apperception Test and the Rorschach, are not useful for intelligence testing and not as validated as instruments. The Reitan-Indiana Neuropsychological

Test is helpful for children with suspected brain damage. In diagnosing learning disorders, it is essential to measure intelligence in order to compare the results with any discrepancies in achievement. The Wechsler Intelligence Scale for Children is one of the most widely used for this purpose.

Many patients with learning disorders, such as reading disorder, have comorbid axis I disorders. It is not uncommon to find other learning disorders, such as mathematics disorder, present as well. Conditions such as autistic disorder and mental retardation make it difficult to diagnose a learning disorder. If another deficit in functioning is present, the learning difficulties must be in excess of those associated with it (DSM IV). Depressive symptoms are not unusual in individuals with learning disorders, given the problems with school performance and peer relationships. Tic disorders are not significantly increased in those with reading disorder. ADHD is highly correlated with reading disorder, in up to 25%, and there may be a relationship between their two etiologies *(Synopsis, pp. 1158–1159, 1181).*

64. (B)

65. (C)

Explanations 64 and 65

This case is a characteristic presentation for malingering. Consciously producing symptoms in order to assume the sick role is the motivation behind factitious disorder. There is no evidence of psychotic symptoms as would be seen in delusional disorder. Hypochondriasis involves the preoccupation with fears of having a serious illness rather than the focus on complaints of pain. The unconscious production of symptoms due to unconscious conflict is the hallmark of conversion disorder, which presents with a neurologic deficit. Malingering, which is not considered a mental illness, is defined as the intentional production of symptoms motivated by external incentives, such as avoidance of work, military duty, jail, or obtaining drugs (as in the above case) (DSM IV).

In cases of suspected malingering, accusations or law enforcement involvement will likely result in further hostility and harm to any therapeutic alliance. Referral for admission to a mental health facility or to a psychiatrist may also have the same effect and are not warranted unless another mental illness or safety concerns are present. While limit setting is absolutely necessary in these individuals, a professional demeanor must be maintained. Gentle confrontation coupled with a focus on understanding their underlying problems (leading to their feigning illness) are the most helpful approaches. A fuller evaluation may be necessary to determine whether or not there is an additional mental illness or substance dependence that will need to be treated.

66. **(D)**

67. **(D)**

Explanations 66 and 67

As alcohol is metabolized by the liver, heavy use causes inflammation of the liver. Enzymes such as ALT and AST are not uncommonly elevated with alcohol abuse, although they are not specific to either liver damage or alcohol. GGT is more specific for recent, heavy alcohol use. Triglycerides are also elevated in alcoholics. A low hemoglobin and hematocrit, either from blood loss due to gastritis or from a macrocytic anemia, are a result of chronic alcohol consumption.

Disulfiram is used in individuals with alcohol dependence. As it inhibits acetaldehyde dehydrogenase, causing a deleterious reaction when combined with alcohol, it is used as a deterrent and not for cravings. Antidepressants, lithium, and antipsychotics have not been shown to reduce cravings. Naltrexone, an opiate antagonist, has shown some positive results in decreasing cravings. The presumed mechanism is blockade of opiate receptors, thereby interfering with the reward cycle.

68. **(A)** Even large amounts of cannabis do not cause death. Cocaine, PCP, and opiates can certainly be lethal in overdose, particularly when combined with alcohol. However, because of their similar effects on the GABA receptors in the brain, barbiturates (and benzodiazepines) are especially deadly when added to alcohol in an overdose.

69. **(B)**

70. **(B)**

Explanations 69 and 70

This patient meets criteria for schizophrenia. Factors leaning toward a poorer prognosis include an earlier onset of symptoms, nonmarried status, negative symptoms (e.g., flat affect, poverty of speech, thought blocking, poor attention), and poor psychosocial/occupational functioning. Factors weighing toward a more positive prognosis include a later onset, good premorbid functioning, mood symptoms, married status, and a family history of mood disorders (such as bipolar disorder in the above case).

Even with appropriate antipsychotic treatment, the likelihood of maintaining a high level of functioning is low. Studies indicate that with treatment, approximately 50% of patients will still exhibit significant symptomatology and display poor functioning. Only 20–40% of patients with schizophrenia will be able to lead somewhat unimpaired lives (*Synopsis, pp. 485, 497*).

71. **(B)**

72. **(D)**

Explanations 71 and 72

This patient presents with a major depressive episode. He is appropriately begun on an antidepressant, namely mirtazepine. With all antidepressants, the first symptoms to improve over days to weeks will be the neurovegetative symptoms, such as insomnia, anergia, appetite, and concentration. Unfortunately, the depressed mood and hopelessness are often the last symptoms of depression to remit.

Like many other psychiatric as well as medical illnesses, MDD tends to be a recurrent illness. While individual episodes are very treatable, there is a high risk of recurrence without continued treatment. After having a single episode of depression, studies indicate approximately 50–85% of individuals will develop subsequent episodes of major depression *(Practice Guideline for the Treatment of Patients with Major Depressive Disorder, 2000, APA).*

73. (E)

74. (A)

Explanations 73 and 74

This woman has bipolar disorder, most recent episode manic, and she has been stabilized on lithium. Bipolar disorder is a chronic mental illness, with a high number of future episodes (mania and depression) likely. Because of this, after one episode of mania, it is generally recommended to continue on maintenance treatment indefinitely in order to minimize the risk of future recurrences.

This woman has now developed an episode of bipolar disorder, depressed. While adding an antidepressant such as sertraline may help the depression, there is always a risk of provoking a manic episode. Adding another mood stabilizer in order to treat the depression has little data to support it. Decreasing the lithium will not help her depression and it may enable her to become more vulnerable to a switch into mania. As her lithium level is therapeutic, increasing the dose will likely only add to her side effects and may lead to toxicity. Lamotrigine has been found to be beneficial in treating bipolar depression and does not appear to increase the likelihood of causing a manic episode, as other antidepressants do. It is recommended as a first-line treatment for depressive episodes in bipolar patients *(Practice Guideline for the Treatment of Patients with Bipolar Disorder, APA).*

75. (A)

76. (C)

77. (A)

Explanations 75 through 77

This patient presents with dementia, most likely Alzheimer's type. Alzheimer's dementia is caused, in part, by a deficiency in acetylcholine. Medications with significant anticholinergic effects are expected to worsen the cognitive deficits and confusion. Donepezil may help with mild-to-moderate dementia, improving the cognition and possibly agitation. Low dose haloperidol, lorazepam, and trazodone may help with sleep and/or behavioral problems, but diphenhydramine should be avoided given its anticholinergic side effects.

Preferential atrophy of the frontotemporal regions is consistent with Pick's disease, which may present similarly to Alzheimer's disease. Huntington's disease, another cause of dementia, is characterized by a severe movement disorder. It demonstrates striking atrophy of the caudate nucleus, along with possible cerebral atrophy. Dilatation of the ventricles without atrophy is the hallmark of NPH, one of the few potentially reversible causes of dementia. The classic triad of NPH is dementia, gait disturbance, and urinary incontinence. The second most common cause of dementia is vascular dementia, often caused by uncontrolled hypertension, which results in multiple small infarcts of the white matter surrounding the ventricles. Alzheimer's dementia, the most common cause of dementia, is characterized by diffuse cerebral atrophy and dilatation of the ventricles.

Stable dementias without progression are unusual. They are seen sometimes in patients after head trauma. Rapid deterioration of functioning is seen commonly in prion diseases, such as Creutzfeldt-Jakob disease. A steady improvement is only possible in reversible causes, such as metabolic etiologies. Stepwise progression is classically observed in vascular dementia, thought to be caused by lacunar infarcts. Most dementias, including Alzheimer's, display a gradual but steady deterioration in cognition and overall functioning.

78. **(A)**

79. **(E)**

80. **(B)**

Explanations 78 and 80

This patient exhibits signs and symptoms of delirium. An EEG is very sensitive for delirium. Localized spikes would be seen in a patient with seizure activity. Random activity is characteristic of the normal, awake state. Low-voltage fast activity is very specific to delirium secondary to alcohol or sedative/hypnotic withdrawal. Triphasic delta waves are characteristic for delirious states caused by hepatic failure. All other causes of delirium, however, demonstrate diffuse slowing on EEG.

Medications, such as antipsychotics and benzodiazepines, may be helpful in reducing the agitation often seen in delirium. Soft restraints may also be necessary to permit the treatment team to perform appropriate examinations, tests, or procedures and to prevent pulling out intravenous access, feeding tubes, and so on. Behavioral interventions, including pictures, lights, clocks, calendars, and so on, may be employed to reinforce orientation to person, place, and time. The primary and essential approach in the management of patients with delirium, however, is to determine and treat the underlying cause.

The presence of a delirium is a poor prognostic sign. The mortality rate for 1 year after a delirium is approximately 50%. The mortality rate for 6 months after an episode of delirium is approximately 25% *(Synopsis, p. 324)*.

BIBLIOGRAPHY

American Psychiatric Association. *Diagnostic and Statistical Manual of Mental Disorders*, 4th ed., Text Revision. Washington, DC: American Psychiatric Association, 2000.

American Psychiatric Association. *Practice Guideline for the Assessment and Treatment of Patients with Suicidal Behaviors*. Washington, DC: American Psychiatric Association, 2003.

American Psychiatric Association. *Practice Guideline for the Treatment of Patients with Bipolar Disorder*, 2nd ed. Washington, DC: American Psychiatric Association, 2002.

American Psychiatric Association. *Practice Guideline for the Treatment of Patients with Borderline Personality Disorder*. Washington, DC: American Psychiatric Association, 2001.

American Psychiatric Association. *Practice Guideline for the Treatment of Patients with Major Depressive Disorder*, 2nd ed. Washington, DC: American Psychiatric Association, 2000.

American Psychiatric Association. *Practice Guideline for the Treatment of Patients with Panic Disorder*. Washington, DC: American Psychiatric Association, 1998.

Sadock BJ, Sadock VA. *Kaplan and Sadock's Synopsis of Psychiatry*, 9th ed. Philadelphia, PA: Lippincott Williams & Wilkins, 2003.

CHAPTER 6

Preventive Medicine
Questions

Questions 1 through 3

A 50-year-old male presents to your office for a routine annual physical examination. He has no specific complaints for this visit other than wanting to be checked for all the usual stuff. His last visit with you was a year ago for a physical examination. At that time his examination was normal. You performed blood work that was within normal limits and included a total cholesterol of 172 with a high-density lipoprotein (HDL) of 45 and low-density lipoprotein (LDL) of 100. He reports that he had a tetanus shot 5 years ago.

Past medical history:	Unremarkable
Past surgical history:	1. Appendectomy at age 17 2. Vasectomy at age 43
Medications:	Daily multivitamin
Allergies:	NKDA (No known Drug Allergies)
Family history:	Father died at age 78 of a heart attack Mother is alive at age 76. She has hypertension and osteoarthritis Brother aged 48 without known chronic medical condition Children aged 16, 14, and 8—no known chronic medical illness
Social history:	Married, employed as an accountant; college graduate Denies tobacco or recreational drug use Drinks one alcoholic drink (either beer or wine) a day Does not exercise on a regular basis

1. Which of the following office examinations would be recommended for this patient?

   (A) measurement of his blood pressure
   (B) abdominal palpation to screen for abdominal aortic aneurysm
   (C) testicular examination to screen for testicular cancer
   (D) whole body skin examination to screen for skin cancer
   (E) palpation of the thyroid gland to screen for thyroid cancer

2. Which of the following tests would be recommended for this patient?

   (A) fasting lipid panel
   (B) chest x-ray
   (C) electrocardiogram (ECG)
   (D) glaucoma screening by measurement of intraocular pressure
   (E) fecal occult blood test

3. Which of the following interventions would be recommended for this patient?

   (A) pneumococcal vaccine
   (B) tetanus toxoid vaccine
   (C) complete cessation of all alcohol intake
   (D) beta-carotene supplementation to prevent cancer and heart disease
   (E) screening for depression with a patient-completed questionnaire

Questions 4 through 6

A 65-year-old White female presents to the office for her annual gynecologic examination. She has been a patient of yours for many years. She also sees you on a routine basis for treatment of hypertension and hypothyroidism. Her last pap smear was 5 years ago and she has never had an abnormal pap smear. She had a mammogram 1 year ago that was normal. She does not perform self-breast examination. She is without complaint today.

Past medical history:	1. Hypertension for 15 years 2. Graves disease, treated with radioactive iodine thyroid ablation at age 50
Ob/GYN history:	1. Menarche at age 14 2. Four term pregnancies with vaginal deliveries (at age 22, 25, 27, and 32) 3. Total abdominal hysterectomy and bilateral salpingoopherectomy (TAH/BSO) age 47 for fibroids 4. On estrogen replacement therapy from age 47 to 55
Past surgical history:	1. Appendectomy at age 16 2. Total abdominal hysterectomy/bilateral salpingo-oophorectomy (TAH/BSO) as noted above
Medications:	1. Hydrochlorothiazide 25 mg daily 2. Levothyroxine 0.1 mg daily 3. Potassium chloride 20 meq daily
Allergies:	None
Family history:	Parents, siblings unknown as patient was adopted Children are alive and well without known chronic medical conditions
Social history:	Widowed for 5 years, has not been involved in a sexual relationship since the death of her husband; retired school teacher; college educated; does not smoke cigarettes, drink alcohol or use drugs; walks 30–45 min a day for exercise

4. At this visit you should

   (A) perform a pap smear
   (B) recommend that she restart estrogen replacement therapy
   (C) tell her that she can reduce her risk of dying of breast cancer by performing self-breast examinations monthly
   (D) order a bone density test to screen for osteoporosis
   (E) send a urine culture as a screening test for asymptomatic bacteruria

5. Which of the following conditions results in the most deaths of American women over the age of 65?

   (A) breast cancer
   (B) ovarian cancer
   (C) lung cancer
   (D) cardiovascular disease
   (E) pneumonia

6. Which of the following vaccinations would be routinely recommended for this patient?

   (A) hepatitis B vaccine
   (B) measles, mumps, rubella (MMR) if patient does not recall having the measles
   (C) pneumococcal conjugate vaccine (PCV-7)
   (D) pneumococcal polysaccharide vaccine (PPV-23)
   (E) hepatitis A vaccine

Questions 7 through 9

A 40-year-old male comes to your office as a new patient to get established for care, as he recently moved into your city from another state. He has been on medical therapy for type 2 diabetes mellitus for 3 years and has had good glycemic control. He takes metformin 500 mg bid and reports having fasting glucose levels of less than 100 on home monitoring. He has records from his previous physician that show that he had a dilated eye examination 6 months ago that was normal and a hemoglobin A1c (HgbA1c) level of 6.2 that was taken 3 months ago. He has no known history of coronary artery disease. His last fasting lipid measurement was 14 months ago. You order a fasting lipid panel today and get the following results:

Total cholesterol: 235 mg/dL
Triglycerides: 210 mg/dL
HDL cholesterol: 45mg/dL
LDL cholesterol: 162 mg/dL

7. Your management today should include

   (A) institution of a low-carbohydrate diet
   (B) increasing his dosage of metformin
   (C) starting the patient on insulin therapy
   (D) continuing his current care without change
   (E) starting the patient on a hydroxymethylglutaryl-coenzyme A (HMG-CoA) reductase inhibitor (statin)

8. The patient follows up in 2 months and has been compliant with your recommendations. Results of a repeat fasting lipid panel are as follows:

   Total cholesterol: 160 mg/dL
   Triglycerides: 140 mg/dL
   HDL cholesterol: 48 mg/dL
   LDL cholesterol: 98 mg/dL

   Your recommendations for today are

   (A) continue his current regimen without change
   (B) add nicotinic acid
   (C) add a fibric acid
   (D) refer the patient to a dietician for counseling
   (E) increase the dosage of his HMG-CoA reductase inhibitor

9. Recommended goal levels of LDL cholesterol in an adult patient with type 2 diabetes mellitus are

   (A) 160 mg/dL
   (B) 130 mg/dL
   (C) 100 mg/dL
   (D) 70 mg/dL
   (E) 50 mg/dL

Questions 10 through 13

A 42-year-old male presents to the office for a refill of the nasal steroid medication that he uses every spring to control his allergies. You notice on the vital signs taken by the nurse that his blood pressure is 150/95. Except for some sneezing and nasal congestion, the patient has no symptoms. He has no other medical history and his only medication is a nasal steroid. He does not smoke cigarettes, does not drink alcohol, and does not exercise. His body mass index is 24 kg/m².

10. Initial management at this time should include

   (A) institution of therapy with a beta-blocker or thiazide diuretic
   (B) repeat blood pressure in each arm after he sits quietly for 5 min
   (C) recommendation to start taking a baby aspirin a day
   (D) a treadmill exercise stress test to stratify his risk for coronary artery disease
   (E) discontinuation of his nasal steroid

11. The patient returns for a follow-up visit and his blood pressure is 146/94. You diagnose him with

   (A) elevated blood pressure without hypertension
   (B) prehypertension
   (C) stage 1 hypertension
   (D) stage 2 hypertension
   (E) stage 3 hypertension

12. Further evaluation at this point should include

   (A) 24-h urine collection for protein and creatinine clearance
   (B) renal artery Doppler studies to evaluate for renal artery stenosis
   (C) an ECG
   (D) an echocardiogram to evaluate for ventricular hypertrophy
   (E) a serum measurement of thyroid-stimulating hormone (TSH)

13. Of the options listed, the most appropriate management at this point would be

  (A) recommendation of a low salt diet and follow up in 9–12 months
  (B) increasing the dosage of the previously started antihypertensive medication
  (C) initiating therapy with a calcium channel blocker
  (D) initiating therapy with a thiazide diuretic
  (E) no intervention is warranted at this time

Questions 14 through 17

A recent study compared two drugs—exemestane and tamoxifen—for the treatment of estrogen-receptor positive breast cancer in postmenopausal women. At the end of the study, 91.5% of the women treated with the drug exemestane and 86.8% of the women treated with tamoxifen were disease free ($P < 0.001$).

14. What is the relative risk of developing recurrent breast cancer in a woman treated with exemestane compared to a woman treated with tamoxifen?

  (A) 90%
  (B) 72%
  (C) 64%
  (D) 36%
  (E) 4.7%

15. What is the relative risk reduction for the development of recurrent breast cancer for women taking exemestane compared to women taking tamoxifen?

  (A) 95.3%
  (B) 72%
  (C) 64%
  (D) 36%
  (E) 4.7%

16. What is the absolute risk reduction (ARR) for the development of recurrent breast cancer for women taking exemestane compared to women taking tamoxifen?

  (A) 95.3%
  (B) 72%
  (C) 64%

  (D) 36%
  (E) 4.7%

17. What is the number needed to treat (NNT) with exemestane compared to tamoxifen to prevent one breast cancer recurrence?

  (A) 79
  (B) 50
  (C) 36
  (D) 21
  (E) 14

Questions 18 through 21

You are evaluating a journal article describing a new test for the diagnosis of congestive heart failure (CHF). In the study described, 250 consecutive patients were given the test. Of the 250 subjects, 106 tested positive for CHF and 144 tested negative. All 250 subjects were then evaluated by expert cardiologists who were blinded to the results of the experimental test. These cardiologists determined that of the 106 persons who tested positive, 95 actually had CHF. Further, the cardiologists found that of the 144 who tested negative, 2 truly had CHF.

18. What is the sensitivity of this test for the diagnosis of CHF?

  (A) 98%
  (B) 93%
  (C) 75%
  (D) 61%
  (E) 39%

19. What is the specificity of this test for the diagnosis of CHF?

  (A) 39%
  (B) 61%
  (C) 75%
  (D) 93%
  (E) 98%

20. What is the positive predictive value (PPV) of this test for the diagnosis of CHF?

  (A) 99%
  (B) 93%

(C) 90%

(D) 85%

(E) 77%

21. What is the negative predictive value (NPV) of this test for the diagnosis of CHF?

(A) 99%

(B) 93%

(C) 90%

(D) 85%

(E) 77%

Questions 22 through 25

In your role as a physician in a community health center, you agree to perform sports preparticipation examinations on students from the local high school. You have several scheduled for today.

Your first appointment is with a 16-year-old male who is planning to run on the cross-country team in the Fall and play baseball in the Spring. He reports that one time he "blacked out" while running, but he has never had chest pain while exercising and he is one of the top runners on the team. He has no known medical history, denies alcohol, tobacco, recreational drug, or performance-enhancing drug use. He had a cousin who died at the age of 21 of "some kind of heart disease," although your patient is not sure of any details. On examination, he is healthy appearing and has normal vital signs, with a pulse rate of 72 and a blood pressure of 100/65. Auscultation of his heart reveals no cardiac murmur while he is lying down, a soft systolic murmur when he stands, which increases on having the patient perform a Valsalva maneuver. The remainder of his examination is normal.

22. At this point, your most appropriate management option is

(A) allow unrestricted participation in sports

(B) allow participation in noncontact sports

(C) allow him to play baseball but not run cross-country

(D) restrict him from all athletic participation until he is evaluated by a cardiologist

(E) restrict him from competitive athletics but allow him to participate in gym class

23. Your next appointment is with a 15-year-old female who plans to play basketball and volleyball. She has no significant medical history, denies a family history of premature cardiac deaths, and denies tobacco, alcohol, recreational drug, or performance-enhancing drug use. She reports having regular menstrual cycles. On examination, she is 72 in. tall, weighs 150 lbs, and has an arm-span of 77 in. Her vital signs are normal. She has a high-arched palate, pectus excavatum, and long, slender fingers. Her cardiac, pulmonary, abdominal, and dermatologic examinations are normal.

Your management at this point should include further evaluation for the possible diagnosis of

(A) Turner syndrome

(B) Marfan syndrome

(C) the female athlete's triad

(D) type 1 diabetes mellitus

(E) atlanto-axial instability

24. Appropriate diagnostic testing would include

(A) chromosomal analysis

(B) echocardiography

(C) serum calcium measurement

(D) fasting plasma glucose

(E) cervical spine x-rays with flexion and extension views

25. Your last patient of the day is a 16-year-old male who plans to play on the football team. He has no complaints today, no significant medical history, and no concerning family history. He denies the use of tobacco, alcohol, or any kinds of drugs. His physical examination is entirely normal.

Appropriate management at this time would include

(A) urine drug screen

(B) diphtheria-tetanus vaccine (dT) if he has not had one since age 5

(C) serum hepatitis C antibody test if he is sexually active

(D) screening ECG

(E) urinalysis

26. Which of the following conditions results in the most deaths each year in the United States?

   (A) acquired immuno deficiency syndrome (AIDS)
   (B) breast cancer
   (C) motor vehicle accidents
   (D) occupational injuries
   (E) medical errors

Questions 27 and 28

A metaanalysis of randomized-controlled trials was published comparing two methods of managing postterm pregnancies. The question studied was whether the routine induction of labor at 41 weeks' gestation would result in improved maternal or fetal outcomes compared with expectant management. The authors reported that the odds ratio for caesarian delivery rate in the induction group compared to the expectant management group was 0.88 with a 95% confidence interval (CI) of 0.78–0.99. A second outcome studied was perinatal mortality. For this outcome the odds ratio for the induction group compared to the expectant management group was 0.41 with a 95% CI of 0.14–1.18.

27. Which of the following statements is true?

   (A) There was a statistically significant reduction in the number of caesarian deliveries in the induction group compared to the expectant management group.
   (B) There was a statistically significant reduction in perinatal mortality in the induction group.
   (C) There was no statistically significant difference for either outcome.
   (D) There was a statistically significant increase in the number of caesarian deliveries in the induction group compared to the expectant management group.
   (E) There was a statistically significant decrease in both the number of caesarian deliveries and perinatal mortality in the induction group.

28. The authors assessed the study as being underpowered for the outcome of perinatal mortality. Possible ways to increase the statistical power of a study include

   (A) using P-value to determine statistical significance in place of 95% CI
   (B) performing a "case-control" study in place of a metaanalysis of randomized-controlled trials
   (C) reporting the results as a relative risk in place of an odds ratio
   (D) performing a subgroup analysis
   (E) increasing the number of subjects enrolled in a study

Questions 29 through 31

While you are working in the community health center, a 40-year-old male presents to you as a referral from the dental clinic. The patient reported on the intake history form that he has been told that he has a heart murmur. The dentist refused to allow him to have a dental examination and cleaning until he was cleared by a medical doctor. Other than being told by a physician in the past that he had a heart murmur, the patient has no medical history and does not take any medications. He has never had any cardiac testing done and has never had cardiac surgery. He denies chest pain, palpitations, dyspnea, or any other symptoms. On examination, he has normal vital signs and a normal general examination. On auscultation of his heart you hear a 2/6 systolic ejection murmur at the left upper sternal border without radiation.

29. For which of the following conditions would bacterial endocarditis prophylaxis be recommended?

   (A) cardiac pacemaker
   (B) isolated secundum atrial septal defect
   (C) previous coronary artery bypass graft
   (D) bicuspid aortic valve
   (E) history of rheumatic fever without valvular dysfunction

30. An echocardiogram reveals that this patient has a lesion for which bacterial endocarditis prophylaxis would be indicated. For which one of the following dental procedures is bacterial endocarditis prophylaxis recommended?

   (A) fluoride treatments
   (B) taking of oral impressions
   (C) taking of dental x-rays
   (D) dental implant placement
   (E) postoperative suture removal

31. For which of the following nondental procedures would bacterial endocarditis prophylaxis be indicated?

   (A) balloon angioplasty
   (B) bronchoscopy with a flexible bronchoscope
   (C) urethral dilation
   (D) laparoscopic bilateral tubal ligation
   (E) circumcision

Questions 32 and 33

An 8-year-old boy is brought into the emergency room with a laceration of his right arm. According to his parents, he received the injury when he fell on the ground while playing at the family farm about 1 h ago. He has no known history of any medical problems. His parents say that they have not brought him to the doctor in years. On questioning, they report that he only received one of his "baby shots" and they are not sure which one that was. On examination, he is healthy appearing. He is appropriately apprehensive but calm and consolable. His right arm has a 5 cm linear laceration with visible soil particles in and about the wound. The remainder of his examination is unremarkable. You carefully clean and irrigate the wound and then primarily repair the laceration with sutures.

32. What immediate tetanus prophylaxis would be recommended in this case?

   (A) IM injection of adult diphtheria-tetanus toxoid (Td) vaccine only
   (B) IM injection of both adult Td vaccine and tetanus immune globulin

   (C) IM injection of single antigen tetanus toxoid only
   (D) IM injection of tetanus immune globulin only
   (E) IM injection of both adult Td vaccine and tetanus immune globulin and antibiotic prophylaxis with oral metronidazole

33. For this child, what would be the recommended "catch-up" immunization schedule to protect against tetanus?

   (A) Td vaccine today and booster every 5 years
   (B) Td vaccine today, repeat Td in 6 months then booster every 10 years
   (C) Td vaccine today, repeat Td in 4 weeks and 6–12 months then booster every 10 years
   (D) Td vaccine today, repeat in 2 months, 4 months, 15–18 months, and 5 years and then booster every 10 years
   (E) tetanus immune globulin IM every 5–10 years

34. Which of the following statements regarding vaccinations of pregnant women is true?

   (A) Women who will be beyond the first trimester of pregnancy during flu season should routinely receive the inactivated influenza vaccine.
   (B) Pregnancy is an absolute contraindication to the hepatitis B vaccine.
   (C) Women who test negative for rubella at their initial prenatal visit should routinely receive a rubella vaccine during their second trimester of pregnancy.
   (D) Pregnant women who have not completed a tetanus-diphtheria (Td) primary series should start this series in the immediate postpartum period.
   (E) Women who receive a rubella vaccination within 4 weeks of becoming pregnant should be advised of the high risk having a baby with congenital rubella syndrome.

Questions 35 and 36

A 50-year-old male presents to your office after reading an article on the Internet stating that a recent study showed that the drug finasteride can prevent prostate cancer. He asks you to prescribe this medication for him. You review the article and find the following information: a randomized-controlled trial of men over the age of 55 with normal prostate-specific antigen (PSA) readings was performed comparing finasteride and a placebo. At the end of the study, 18% of the men in the finasteride group and 24% of the men in the placebo group had developed prostate cancer.

35. How many men need to be treated with finasteride to prevent one case of prostate cancer (NNT)?

   (A) 6
   (B) 10
   (C) 17
   (D) 24
   (E) 32

36. Further review of the article reveals that 6.4% of the men in the finasteride group and 5.1% in the placebo group developed high-group prostate cancers.

   How many men need to take finasteride in order to have one excess case of high-grade prostate cancer (number needed to harm [NNH])?

   (A) 1.3
   (B) 12
   (C) 37
   (D) 77
   (E) 94

Questions 37 and 38

A 65-year-old White woman presents to your office and requests to have a screening test for osteoporosis. She has been menopausal for 15 years. She never took hormone replacement therapy. She currently takes 500 mg of calcium a day and walks 2 miles a day. She has no history of fractures.

37. Which of the following tests would be the most appropriate screening test to perform?

   (A) lateral thoracic spine x-ray
   (B) dual energy x-ray absorptiometry (DEXA) of the lumbar spine and proximal femur
   (C) quantitative ultrasound of the phalanges of the hand
   (D) peripheral quantitative computed tomography (CT) of the distal radius
   (E) single x-ray absorptiometry (SXA) of the calcaneus

38. The result of the test that you ordered shows the patient's bone mineral density to be 2.5 standard deviations below the mean bone density of 25-year-old woman. What is the most appropriate management at this point?

   (A) start therapy with an oral bisphosphonate
   (B) increase her calcium supplement to 1000 mg per day
   (C) suggest diet and exercise changes then recheck her bone density in 6 months
   (D) add vitamin D and continue her current calcium supplement
   (E) no intervention as her bone density is considered normal for her age

Questions 39 through 41

A 34-year-old woman with a history of type 1 diabetes mellitus presents to your office for a routine follow-up visit. She is feeling well and has no complaints. Her fasting blood sugars usually run 140–160 and her HgbA1c was recently measured at 8.2. She tells you that she would like to become pregnant but wants to know if there are any risks for her and a baby due to her diabetes.

39. Which of the following statements about the risk to offspring of diabetic mothers is true?

   (A) Approximately 20% of children of diabetic mothers will develop type 1 diabetes.
   (B) Diabetes is associated with an increased risk of stillbirth.

(C) Diabetes is associated with an increased risk of chromosomal anomalies.

(D) The incidence of preterm birth is the same in both diabetics and nondiabetics.

(E) Maternal diabetes delays the development of fetal lung maturity.

40. Which of the following statements regarding the risk of pregnancy to the diabetic mother is true?

(A) Pregnancy significantly exacerbates diabetic nephropathy.

(B) Most diabetic women will develop neuropathic symptoms while pregnant.

(C) About 10% of diabetic women will develop ketoacidosis during pregnancy.

(D) Most diabetic women develop at least one infection during pregnancy.

(E) The occurrence of preeclampsia is directly related to diabetic control

41. Which of the following preconception counseling statements is true?

(A) All diabetics planning to become pregnant should be placed on angiotensin converting enzyme (ACE) inhibitors for renal protection.

(B) Diabetic women should not take folic acid because all commercially available supplements contain sugar.

(C) The goal HgbA1c level during her pregnancy is approximately 9%.

(D) Insulin pump treatment is contraindicated during pregnancy.

(E) Women with good preconception diabetic control have infants with a lower incidence of congenital malformations than women with poor preconception diabetic control.

Questions 42 through 44

42. You would like to design a study to evaluate the prevalence of a certain disease in your patient population. Which study design would be the most appropriate?

(A) case-control study

(B) cohort study

(C) prospective, randomized-controlled trial

(D) cross-sectional study

(E) metaanalysis

43. You find that the specific disease that you are studying is very rare in your patient population. You are interested in determining which risk factors may contribute to the development of this disease.

Which study design would be the most appropriate to further pursue this question?

(A) case-control study

(B) cohort study

(C) prospective, randomized-controlled trial

(D) cross-sectional study

(E) metaanalysis

44. The results of your study in Question 43 find two risk factors associated with the development of the disease that you are studying. Risk factor "X" was found to have an odds ratio for the development of the disease of 2.5 (95% CI: 1.3–4.0). Risk factor "Y" had an odds ratio of 1.9 (95% CI: 1.1–3.3).

Which of the following statements is true?

(A) Both risk factors X and Y are now proven to cause the disease.

(B) Persons with risk factor X will have a worse prognosis than those with risk factor Y.

(C) Risk factor X was more common in your study population than risk factor Y.

(D) Both risk factors occurred more commonly in persons with the disease than in persons who did not have the disease.

(E) For every 100 people with the disease, 25 will have risk factor X and 19 will have risk factor Y.

Questions 45 through 47

45. One of your responsibilities at the community health center is to serve as director of the tuberculosis (TB) screening and prevention program. Which of the following statements about testing for TB is true?

   (A) Multiple puncture (Tine) testing is recommended for children.

   (B) Previous recipients of the BCG vaccine should not receive TB skin testing.

   (C) All adults should be screened for TB every 5 years.

   (D) The test is interpreted by measuring the diameter of any redness at the injection site 48–72 h after the test is placed.

   (E) The intradermal purified protein derivative PPD (Mantoux) method is the preferred skin test for screening.

46. Which of the following test results would be considered positive?

   (A) 10 mm redness and 3 mm induration in a man with HIV

   (B) 10 mm redness and 10 mm induration in a nursing home resident

   (C) 20 mm redness and 8 mm induration in a person with no known risk factors

   (D) 5 mm redness and 5 mm induration in a physician having a routine, annual screening

   (E) 10 mm redness and 5 mm induration in an immigrant from Southeast Asia

47. Which of the following statements regarding the management of an asymptomatic person with a positive TB skin test is true?

   (A) All persons with a positive skin test should have sputum studies for TB before being treated.

   (B) A pregnant woman with a positive skin test should not have a chest x-ray until after she delivers because of the risk of radiation exposure to the fetus.

   (C) A positive reaction in a person who has previously received a BCG vaccine should be considered a false positive and ignored.

   (D) Isoniazid should not be given to an asymptomatic person over the age of 50 because the risk of the medication is higher than the risk of developing active TB.

   (E) Isoniazid daily for 9 months is the preferred treatment for most asymptomatic persons with positive TB skin tests.

48. You see a 2-week-old child for a routine well-baby check-up. The mother is feeding him formula that she prepares by mixing powdered formula with her home tap water that comes from a well. The local health department considers the water to be nonfluoridated. Which of the following suggestions would be appropriate?

   (A) She should start giving her baby a fluoride supplement now.

   (B) Powdered infant formula contains an adequate amount of fluoride, so a supplement will not be required as long as she continues formula feeding.

   (C) A fluoride supplement would be recommended starting at age 6 months.

   (D) She should take a fluoride supplement during subsequent pregnancies for the benefit of the fetus.

   (E) There is no risk to fluoride supplementation, so any dosage may be used.

Questions 49 and 50

A 19-year-old woman comes in for a routine obstetrical follow-up visit at 24 weeks' gestation. She is here with her boyfriend, who is the father of the baby. She is wearing dark sunglasses in the examination room. When you ask her to remove the glasses, you see that she has a bruise around her left eye. Her boyfriend quickly states that she accidentally bumped into a door and she quietly nods in agreement.

49. Which of the following statements about domestic violence is true?

    (A) All states require that physicians report domestic violence to the police.
    (B) Domestic violence is rare in same sex couples.
    (C) A woman cannot make a sexual assault claim against her husband.
    (D) Domestic violence is less likely when one partner is ill or disabled.
    (E) Psychologic intimidation without violence is considered a form of abuse.

50. Which of the following would be the most appropriate intervention at this time?

    (A) Provide the woman with information about domestic violence, including the phone number of shelters and counseling services.
    (B) Confront the boyfriend with your concerns regarding physical abuse.
    (C) No intervention is necessary, as partner violence usually stops while a woman is pregnant.
    (D) Encourage the woman to have ready access to a weapon to defend herself at home.
    (E) Report the boyfriend to Child Protective Services at the time of delivery of the baby, so that they can intervene before child abuse occurs.

Questions 51 through 53

A husband and wife, both aged 30, come to the community health center for advice and evaluation prior to a month-long mission trip to central Africa. Both are in good health. She takes oral contraceptive pills and he is on no prescription medication. Review of their records shows that they have had all of the appropriate vaccinations for their ages, have completed a 3-dose hepatitis B series and had dT boosters 2 years ago. Their mission will involve building a school and health clinic in a rural area of Cameroon.

51. Which of the following immunizations would be recommended prior to the trip?

    (A) measles, mumps, rubella booster
    (B) diphtheria-tetanus booster
    (C) hepatitis B booster
    (D) injectable polio vaccine
    (E) smallpox vaccine

52. What advice would be the most appropriate to provide?

    (A) Swimming in freshwater lakes would be a recommended type of exercise in the hot African climate.
    (B) The mosquito that transmits malaria is most active in the middle of the day.
    (C) The risk of motor vehicle related injuries is much lower because there are fewer cars on the road.
    (D) Due to its potential toxicity, N, N diethyl-m-toluamide (DEET)-containing insect repellents should be avoided.
    (E) Medication for malaria prophylaxis should be started before their trip and continued after they return home.

53. Which of the following statements regarding food and beverage safety is true?

    (A) Carbonated soft drinks served with ice cubes are considered safe to drink.
    (B) Locally grown oranges and bananas are safe to eat.
    (C) Water is safe to drink after filtering through an absolute 1 μm filter.
    (D) Brushing teeth with untreated water is safe as long as it is not swallowed.
    (E) Salads are generally safer to eat than cooked meats.

Questions 54 and 55

A 6-month-old boy is brought to the office for a routine check-up by his mother. They have recently moved to the area and are new to your practice. He is the product of an uncomplicated term pregnancy, has grown and developed appropriately for his age, and is up to date on his immunizations. He has had two cases of otitis media in his life. Neither of his parents has been diagnosed with any chronic medical conditions. Both of his parents smoke cigarettes, but "not in the same room" as the child.

54. Which of the following statements regarding secondhand smoke exposure is true?

(A) Secondhand smoke has a significantly different chemical composition than directly inhaled tobacco smoke.

(B) Secondhand smoke exposure has been associated with the Sudden Infant Death Syndrome (SIDS).

(C) Separating smokers and nonsmokers in the same airspace eliminates the exposure to secondhand smoke.

(D) The amount of carcinogens absorbed by household contacts of smokers is clinically insignificant.

(E) When a cigarette is smoked, most of the smoke is inhaled and very little is released into the environment.

55. Which of the following statements is true?

(A) Children of parents who smoke become smokers less often than children of nonsmokers.

(B) Chemicals from cigarette smoke do not get into breast milk.

(C) More than 95% of the smoke from a cigarette is out of a room within 30 min of smoking cessation.

(D) The United States Environmental Protection Agency (EPA) does not consider secondhand smoke to be a carcinogen.

(E) Parental smoking may be considered as a factor in assessing the "best interest" of a child in child custody hearings.

Questions 56 through 58

A 39-year-old woman presents to the office for the evaluation of a mole on her left arm. It has been present and enlarging over the past 6 months. It itches and occasionally bleeds.

56. Which of the following attributes would be considered high-risk for skin cancer?

(A) diameter of greater than 6 mm

(B) a sharply demarcated, regular border

(C) a uniform coloration

(D) a symmetric, circular shape

(E) a flat lesion

57. Which of the following statements regarding skin cancer is true?

(A) Melanomas are highly associated with cumulative sun exposure.

(B) Squamous cell carcinoma only occurs in sun-exposed areas.

(C) Basal cell carcinomas do not occur in persons of African descent.

(D) Squamous cell carcinomas of the skin have a higher metastatic potential than basal cell carcinomas.

(E) A shave biopsy is recommended for the evaluation of suspicious pigmented lesions.

58. Which of the following statements about skin cancer risks is true?

(A) A cotton T-shirt worn while swimming provides adequate protection from the sun for the chest and back.

(B) Actinic keratoses are potentially premalignant for squamous cell carcinoma.

(C) Tanning booths are recommended for persons desiring a suntan, as they are not associated with a risk of skin cancer.

(D) To protect against skin cancer, a sunscreen needs to inhibit only UV-B rays.

(E) Waterproof sunscreen does not need to be reapplied after swimming.

Questions 59 through 61

A 26-year-old G_2P_1 female comes to your office for her initial obstetric visit. The first day of her last menstrual period was 6 weeks ago. Other than some mild morning sickness, she is feeling fine. Her first pregnancy was 40 weeks in gestation and uncomplicated. She has no significant medical history.

59. Which of the following tests is recommended for the initial obstetric visit?

(A) TSH

(B) blood glucose measurement 1 h after a 50 g glucose load

(C) urine culture

(D) vaginal culture for group B *Streptococcus*

(E) basic metabolic panel (Chem-7)

60. Which of the following tests is recommended as screening for hepatitis B in pregnancy?

(A) hepatitis B surface antibody

(B) hepatitis B surface antigen

(C) hepatitis B core antibody

(D) hepatitis B e antigen

(E) hepatitis B e antibody

61. The result of the test that you ordered in Question 60 is positive. What would be appropriate management for the neonate to reduce the risk of perinatal transmission of the hepatitis B virus?

(A) hepatitis B vaccine within 2 days of birth

(B) hepatitis B immune globulin within 2 days of birth

(C) hepatitis B immune globulin and hepatitis B vaccine within 12 h of birth

(D) deliver the baby by caesarian section

(E) advise the mother not to breast feed

Questions 62 and 63

62. Which of the following statements regarding prostate cancer screening using the PSA blood test is true?

(A) PSA testing has been proven to reduce all-cause mortality in men over 50.

(B) In spite of PSA testing, the disease-specific mortality from prostate cancer has not changed in the past 30 years.

(C) Prostate cancer is the only condition that causes an elevated PSA level.

(D) PSA testing can prevent the development of prostate cancer.

(E) PSA testing can increase the chances of detecting prostate cancer.

63. Which statement regarding PSA screening recommendations is true?

(A) All men over the age of 50 should have a PSA test every year.

(B) There is no harm associated with PSA screening.

(C) Only men with symptoms of prostate enlargement should have PSA screening.

(D) A PSA level of less than 4.0 ng/mL rules out the diagnosis of prostate cancer.

(E) Certain medications may alter PSA level.

Questions 64 through 67

A 49-year-old male postal worker presents to your office for the evaluation of a lesion on his left arm. The lesion started about a week ago as a red pustule but has grown and now has a thick black scab. The lesion is painless. A coworker showed the patient a similar appearing lesion that she developed on her arm for which her doctor prescribed an oral antibiotic. Examination reveals a 5 cm circular black eschar with some surrounding vesicles. A Gram stain of fluid drained from a vesicle reveals chains of gram-positive bacilli.

64. What organism is most likely responsible for this lesion?

(A) methicillin resistant *Staphylococcus aureus*

(B) smallpox virus

(C) *Clostridium tetani*

(D) *Bacillus anthracis*

(E) group A β-hemolytic *Streptococcus*

65. What is the most appropriate management at this point?

(A) topical mupirocin ointment tid for 10 days

(B) oral cephalexin 500 mg qid for a week

(C) oral clindamycin 300 mg tid for 10 days

(D) urgent quarantine of patient's coworkers and family contacts

(E) immediate notification of Public Health authorities

66. The patient asks how he contracted this infection. You tell him

   (A) from direct contact with the coworker who had the similar appearing lesion
   (B) ingestion of contaminated food in the postal facility cafeteria
   (C) a small skin cut or sore was directly contaminated with spores
   (D) inhalation of bacteria from a contaminated ventilation system
   (E) exposure to respiratory droplets from an infected person

67. Which of the following is characteristic of Varicella (chickenpox) but not smallpox?

   (A) The mortality rate is high.
   (B) The lesions are commonly on the palms of the hands and soles of the feet.
   (C) The pox lesions evolve synchronously.
   (D) There is typically a 2–4-day prodrome of fever, malaise, headache, and backache before the development of the rash.
   (E) The vesicles typically occur on an erythematous base (described as *dew drops on a rose petal*)

Questions 68 and 69

A 60-year-old woman presents to your office to discuss her ongoing treatment with hormone replacement therapy that she takes for menopausal symptoms. She was started on estrogen and progesterone replacement at the age of 51 and has been on them since that time. She has read several articles in newspapers and on the Internet stating that hormone therapy is dangerous. You briefly review the results of the Women's Health Initiative study, a randomized-controlled trial comparing health outcomes in women taking combined estrogen-progestin therapy (HRT) versus a placebo. The results are as follows:

Condition	Hazard ratio for women taking HRT	95% Confidence interval
Coronary heart disease (CHD)	1.29	1.02–1.63
Breast cancer	1.26	1.00–1.59
Stroke	1.41	1.07–1.85
Pulmonary embolus	2.13	1.39–3.25
Colorectal cancer	0.63	0.43–0.92
Endometrial cancer	0.83	0.47–1.47
Hip fracture	0.66	0.45–0.98
Deaths from other causes	0.92	0.74–1.14

68. Based on the results listed, you can tell your patient that women taking HRT

   (A) have no difference in endometrial cancer risk
   (B) have no difference in CHD risk
   (C) have no difference in pulmonary embolus risk
   (D) have no difference in stroke risk
   (E) have no difference in hip fracture risk

69. The authors provided composite data on total cardiovascular disease, cancer, fracture, and mortality risks, which are summarized in the chart.

Composite outcome	Hazard ratio for women taking HRT	95% Confidence interval
Cardiovascular disease	1.22	1.09–1.36
Total cancer	1.03	0.90–1.17
Combined fractures	0.76	0.69–0.85
Total mortality	0.98	0.82–1.18

Based on the data presented, which of the following statements is true?

   (A) There is an increase in total cancer risk for women on HRT.
   (B) There is an increase in cardiovascular disease risk for women on HRT.
   (C) There is an increase in combined fracture risk for women on HRT.
   (D) There is a reduction in total mortality for women on HRT.
   (E) The is an overall detriment to the quality of life of women on HRT.

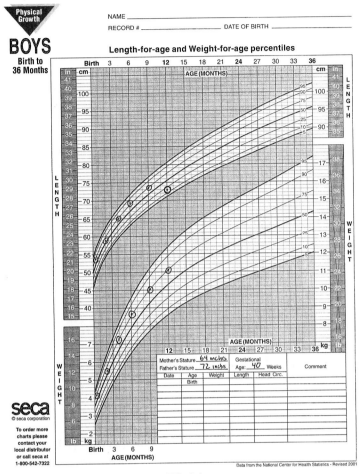

FIG. 6-1

70. A 1-year-old boy is brought to the office for a well-child examination. Your office nurse has plotted his growth on the following chart (see Fig. 6-1). The most appropriate initial management of this abnormality is to

(A) order a CT scan of the head

(B) repeat the measurement

(C) recommend that the mother cut down on the child's caloric intake

(D) review the growth chart of the child's older sibling to look for a similar pattern

(E) ask the mother to bring the child back to the office at monthly intervals to follow his growth more closely

Answers and Explanations

1. **(A)**

2. **(E)**

3. **(E)**

Explanations 1 through 3

The United States Preventative Services Task Force (USPSTF) is an independent panel of experts in primary care and prevention that systematically reviews the evidence of effectiveness and develops recommendations for clinical preventative services. By carefully and systematically reviewing the available literature, the USPSTF makes recommendations on the effectiveness of screening, counseling, immunization, and chemoprevention using the following rating system:

A. The USPSTF strongly recommends that clinicians provide the service to eligible patients.
B. The USPSTF recommends that clinicians provide this service to eligible patients.
C. The USPSTF makes no recommendation for or against routine provision of the service.
D. The USPSTF recommends against routinely providing the service to asymptomatic patients.
I. The USPSTF concludes that the evidence is insufficient to recommend for or against routinely providing the service.

All of the recommendations of the USP-STF are available free of charge at their website www.preventiveservices.ahrq.gov.

In a 50-year-old male who is generally healthy and does not present any apparent high-risk personal or family history, the USPSTF gives a level A recommendation to blood pressure measurement as a screening tool for hypertension in adults over the age of 18, as there is good evidence that screening for, and treating hypertension, can reduce the incidence of cardiovascular disease. There is insufficient evidence to recommend for or against screening for abdominal aortic aneurysm by abdominal palpation or for screening for skin cancer by a whole body skin examination (level I recommendation). This suggests that the evidence is lacking that performing these interventions will reduce the morbidity or mortality associated with these conditions. The USPSTF gives level D recommendations to screening for thyroid cancer by palpation and for screening for testicular cancer by palpation.

Fecal occult blood testing using three self-collected stool cards as a screening test for colon cancer has been given a level A recommendation, with good data to support reduction in colon cancer mortality from periodic screening. There is also evidence to support screening for colon cancer by flexible sigmoidoscopy or colonoscopy, with double-contrast barium enema as a possible alternative as well. Screening for lipid disorders in men over the age of 35 and women over the age of 45 also receives a level A recommendation. In general, the interval for repeat screening for an otherwise low-risk patient with lipid levels within the goal range, based on the National Cholesterol Education Project's Consensus opinion statement, would be 5 years. As this patient had lipid levels within the goal range 1 year ago, it would not be necessary to repeat this blood test at this visit. Screening for cardiovascular disease by the routine use of electrocardiography in asymptomatic, low-risk patients has been given a D recommendation, as there is an absence of evidence of improved health outcomes from this intervention. Screening for lung cancer by chest x-ray and for glaucoma by measurement of intraocular pressure are level I recommendations, with insufficient evidence to recommend for or against these interventions.

Screening for depression, either by a patient-completed questionnaire or physician interview, is a level B recommendation, as there is good evidence that screening improves the identification of depressed patients and treatment results in reduced morbidity. Beta-carotene supplementation to prevent cardiovascular disease or cancer is a level D recommendation, with no evidence of benefit in middle-age or older adults and some evidence of increased risk of harm in certain populations (e.g., heavy smokers). Routine pneumococcal vaccination in adults without high-risk comorbidity, such as diabetes mellitus, is recommended at the age of 65 or older. Tetanus vaccination is recommended at 10-year intervals, in the absence of other risks such as a potentially contaminated wound. Multiple studies have shown that the intake of one to two alcoholic drinks a day in men does not increase morbidity or mortality and may, in fact, lower the risk of cardiovascular disease. *(USPSTF: www.preventiveservices.ahrq.gov)*

4. (D)

5. (D)

6. (D)

Explanations 4 through 6

Screening for osteoporosis in women 65 years old or older is a level B recommendation of the USPSTF, as detection and treatment of osteoporosis may reduce fracture risk. In women who have had a hysterectomy (with removal of the cervix) for reasons other than cervical cancer, pap smear screening of the vaginal cuff is not recommended and cytologic screening can be discontinued. Therapy with either estrogen alone (in women who do not have a uterus) or combined estrogen and progesterone (in women who have a uterus) in postmenopausal women is controversial. Based on findings of the Women's Health Initiative and other studies, the USPSTF gives a level D recommendation to the use of combined estrogen and progesterone therapy and level I recommendation for estrogen therapy alone for the prevention of chronic conditions. Screening for asymptomatic bacteruria in all populations other than pregnant women is given a level D recommendation. No benefit from the intervention has been found and over-treatment with antibiotics may produce harm. While mammography for breast cancer screening has been given a level B recommendation, both self-breast examination and clinical breast examination are level I recommendations, with insufficient evidence to show any benefit in morbidity or mortality. *(USPSTF: www.preventiveservices.ahrq.gov)*

According to the Centers for Disease Control, diseases of the heart make up the most common cause of death in women in this age group. Heart disease is responsible for approximately one-third of all deaths in women aged 65 and older. Malignant neoplasms make up the next largest cause of death, followed by cerebrovascular diseases and chronic lower respiratory diseases. *(CDC. National Vital Statistics Reports, Vol. 7, No. 9, Nov. 2003)*

PPV-23 is recommended for all adults over the age of 65 and at younger ages for individuals at high risk for pneumonia or complications of pneumonia. These include persons with diabetes mellitus, chronic obstructive pulmonary disease, coronary artery disease, and those who have had a splenectomy or are functionally asplenic. The PCV-7 is recommended for the routine vaccination of children. Hepatitis B vaccine is recommended universally for children and for adults who are at high risk for the disease based on profession or lifestyle. Hepatitis A vaccine is recommended for children who live in certain areas of the United States in which the disease is prevalent and may be offered electively to persons traveling to endemic areas. The MMR vaccine is recommended to all children but is not indicated in adults. Rubella vaccination is recommended for women of childbearing age who may become pregnant and who do not have immunity to rubella, in an effort to reduce the risk of congenital rubella infection. *(Centers for Disease Control: www.cdc.gov)*

7. **(E)**

8. **(A)**

9. **(C)**

Explanations 7 through 9

The Third Report of the National Cholesterol Education Program Expert Panel on the Detection, Evaluation, and Treatment of High Blood Cholesterol in Adults (ATP III) was published in May, 2001 by the National Heart, Lung, and Blood Institute of the National Institutes of Health. It is available on-line at: www.nhlbi.nih.gov/guidelines/cholesterol/at p3xsum.pdf. This evidence-based report provides guidelines for the evaluation and management of blood lipid levels for the primary and secondary prevention of heart disease. The basis of the recommendations for management is an overall evaluation of an individual's risk factors for developing cardiovascular disease. Persons at the highest risk for future cardiac events are those with already established coronary artery disease or "coronary artery disease equivalents," which include diabetes mellitus, other forms of atherosclerotic disease or multiple risk factors that confer a 10-year coronary heart disease risk of greater than 20%. Multiple studies have shown that elevated LDL cholesterol levels are a risk for coronary artery disease and that lowering LDL levels can reduce the risk of events. ATP III goals are targeted at LDL levels. For persons with LDL levels above this goal, the options for lowering LDL can include therapeutic lifestyle changes, lipid lowering medications, or a combination of both. In a patient with coronary artery disease, diabetes mellitus, or other CHD equivalents, the LDL goal level is 100 mg/dL. In this population, therapeutic lifestyle changes alone would be recommended for those with LDL levels of 100–130 and medication could be started concomitantly with lifestyle changes for those with LDL above 130, as most persons would require medication to achieve the recommended goal. For the patient in this question with an LDL of 160 mg/dL, therapy with an HMG-CoA reductase inhibitor would be recommended first-line

therapy to try to get his LDL to goal. Therapeutic lifestyle changes alone would be very unlikely to reduce his LDL to less than 100 mg/dL, but are still an important part of his overall lipid management program and should be recommended along with medication therapy. Neither increasing his dosage of metformin nor adding insulin would be recommended as they would not be expected to improve his dyslipidemia significantly and because his diabetic control is appropriate. At his follow-up visit, the patient's lipid levels have met the recommended guidelines; therefore, the recommendation would be to continue with his current therapy. Increasing the dosage of his statin, adding a fibric acid, nicotinic acid, or referring the patient to a dietician would all be appropriate considerations in someone who had not successfully reached his goal lipid levels.

A recent addition to the ATP III provides an option for changing the target LDL goal for those at the highest of risk for coronary events. For persons with known coronary artery disease, or CAD equivalent, and multiple risk factors, such as diabetes or continued smoking, one could consider using an LDL of 70 as a goal. For this patient, with diabetes but no history of CAD or equivalent, the recommended goal would remain an LDL of 100 or less.

10. **(B)**

11. **(C)**

12. **(C)**

13. **(D)**

Explanations 10 through 13

The Seventh Report of the Joint National Committee on the Prevention, Detection, Evaluation, and Treatment of High Blood Pressure (JNC 7) was released in May, 2003 and is available on-line at www.nhlbi.nih.gov/guidelines/hypertension/express.pdf. It provides evidence-based guidelines for the detection, evaluation, and treatment of hypertension, the most common primary diagnosis in the United States. One of the key guidelines presented in this report is the classification of blood pressure for adults. The classification is based on the average of two or more properly measured, seated, blood pressure readings on each of two or more office visits. The proper measurement of blood pressure is critical. Blood pressure should be measured using a properly calibrated instrument in a patient who has been seated quietly in a chair for at least 5 min, with his feet on the floor and arm supported at heart level. The blood pressure cuff should encircle at least 80% of the arm. The systolic blood pressure is the point at which the first of two or more sounds is heard and the diastolic blood pressure is the point before the sounds disappear. In Question 10, where an incidentally noted elevated blood pressure reading is found, it is then necessary to perform blood pressure measurements following the JNC 7 guidelines—two or more readings after the patient has been seated quietly in a chair for 5 or more minutes. Institution of antihypertensive medications would be inappropriate based on one blood pressure reading in this range, as the patient has not been diagnosed as hypertensive as of yet. Aspirin therapy is recommended for most persons over the age of 50 for the primary prevention of CHD events and would be recommended for others at high risk of heart disease. In persons with hypertension, it is recommended to start aspirin after their blood pressure is controlled because the risk of hemorrhagic stroke is increased in uncontrolled hypertension. Risk stratification with an exercise stress test at this point is not supported by evidence showing a reduction of morbidity or mortality and is likely to have many false positive results. Discontinuation of his nasal steroid is unnecessary as it is unlikely to be affecting his blood pressure adversely and should provide good symptomatic relief of his seasonal allergy symptoms.

The blood pressure classifications from the JNC 7 report are as follows:

Blood pressure classification	Systolic BP in mmHg	Diastolic BP in mmHg
Normal	<120	and <80
Prehypertension	120–139	or 80–89
Stage 1 hypertension	140–159	or 90–99
Stage 2 hypertension	≥160	or ≥100

This classification regimen represents a change from previous JNC guidelines with the designation of a prehypertension classification and the combination of the previous stage 2 and stage 3 into a single stage 2 category. By this categorization, the patient in this question has stage 1 hypertension. Recommended evaluation of patients with hypertension includes an ECG, measurement of blood glucose, hematocrit, serum potassium, creatinine and calcium, urinalysis, and a fasting lipid profile. Other testing is not indicated unless suggested by the presence of symptoms or if blood pressure control cannot be achieved.

The management of hypertension involves the institution of lifestyle recommendations and, frequently, the use of antihypertensive medications. Lifestyle modifications can lower blood pressure, enhance the effectiveness of medications, and reduce cardiovascular risks. A low salt diet by itself may lower systolic blood pressure by 2–8 mmHg and is not likely to bring this patient to a goal blood pressure if that is the only modification made. Other lifestyle modifications, including the DASH (dietary approaches to stop hypertension) eating plan and increasing physical activity, could be beneficial as well. When the decision is made to institute pharmacotherapy, the weight of the evidence suggests that thiazide diuretics should be the first-line therapy for most individuals, in the absence of other compelling indications, such as a diabetic patient with nephropathy or a postmyocardial infarction patient.

14. **(C)**

15. **(D)**

16. **(E)**

17. **(D)**

Explanations 14 through 17

Relative risk is the percentage of subjects who achieve an outcome in one experimental group divided by the percentage of subjects who achieve the same outcome in another group. This statistic is used frequently in placebo-controlled trials, where the comparison occurs between the experimental group and the control group. In the study referenced in this set of questions, the comparison is between two groups who were given two different active medications—exemestane and tamoxifen. The outcome studied here is the development of recurrent breast cancer. The data presented state that after the course of treatment, 91.5% of the women in the exemestane group and 86.8% of the women in the tamoxifen group were disease free. Therefore, 8.5% in the exemestane group and 13.2% in the tamoxifen group developed the outcome of recurrent breast cancer. The relative risk is then calculated as 0.085/0.132 = 0.64 = 64%.

The relative risk reduction is the percentage by which the risk in one group has been reduced when compared to the other group. In other words, if the rate of an outcome in one group is 100%, the relative risk reduction is the difference between 100% and the measured relative risk. It is calculated by the formula:

Relative risk reduction = 1 – relative risk

In this example, the relative risk reduction is 1 – 0.64 = 0.36 = 36%.

The ARR, also known as the risk difference, is calculated by subtracting the percentage of subjects who achieve an outcome in one group from the percentage who achieve the outcome in another. In this study, the ARR for those in the exemestane group compared to those in the tamoxifen group is 13.2% – 8.5% = 4.7%.

The NNT is the number of subjects who need to receive an intervention (such as a medication) in order for one of them to have a beneficial outcome. In this study, the beneficial outcome would be one less case of recurrent breast cancer. The NNT is calculated as 1/ARR. In this case, the NNT = 1/0.047 = 21. In other words, 21 women need to be treated with exemestane in order for there to be one fewer case of recurrent breast cancer compared to women treated with tamoxifen. *(Coombes RC, Hall E, Gibson LJ, et al. A randomized trial of exemestane after two to three years of tamoxifen therapy in postmenopausal women with primary breast cancer. N Engl J Med 2004;350:1081–1092)*

18. **(A)**

19. **(D)**

20. **(C)**

21. **(A)**

Explanations 18 through 21

Understanding the concepts of sensitivity, specificity, PPV, and NPV is crucial to interpreting diagnostic test results. Sensitivity is defined as the percentage of people who have a disease who test positive for that disease. Specificity is defined as the percentage of people who are free of a disease who test negative. These two concepts are considered characteristics of the specific test in question and are independent of the prevalence of the disease in the population. The PPV and NPVs of a test are the test's clinical characteristics and these concepts are directly related to the prevalence of the disease in the population. The PPV is the percentage of people who have a positive test result who actually have the disease. Similarly, the NPV is the percentage of people who have a negative test result who do not have the disease. While the definitions may seem subtly different, the implications are significant.

The usual way to calculate sensitivity, specificity, PPV, and NPV is with the 2×2 table, using the following definitions:

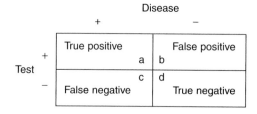

The definitions of sensitivity, specificity, PPV, and NPV would then be:

Sensitivity = a/(a + c)

Specificity = d/(d + b)

PPV = a/(a + b)

NPV = d/(d + c)

The specific information in this question comes from an article describing a study of B-type natriuretic peptide (BNP) for the diagnosis of CHF. The data presented show that 106 persons tested positive using the BNP test. After comparison with the "gold standard," in this case, a review by expert cardiologists, 95 of these 106 were determined to truly have CHF. Therefore, 11 of the 106 were false positives and 95 were true positives. Similarly, 144 persons tested negative using the BNP test. Of these, 142 were confirmed as true negatives and 2 were determined to be false negatives. Putting these numbers into a 2 × 2 table reveals:

Congestive Heart Failure

		+			−
BNP	+	True positive 95	a	b	False positive 11
	−	2 False negative	c	d	142 True negative

The calculations then become:

Sensitivity = a/(a + c) = 95/(95 + 2) = 98%

Specificity = d/(d + b) = 142/(142 + 11) = 93%

PPV = a/(a + b) = 95/(95 + 11) = 90%

NPV = d/(d + c) = 142/(142 + 2) = 99%

(Dao Q, et al. Utility of B-type natriuretic peptide in the diagnosis of congestive heart failure in an urgent-care setting. J Am Coll Cardiol 2001;37:379–385; Slawson D and Shaughnessy A. Becoming an information master. Course materials, 2003)

22. **(D)**

23. **(B)**

24. **(B)**

25. **(B)**

Explanations 22 through 25

Primary care physicians are frequently called on to perform preparticipation examinations on young athletes. These types of encounters can be used to serve a number of purposes, including attempting to identify conditions that may adversely affect the athlete during participation, identify conditions that may predispose the athlete to injury, provide anticipatory guidance on high-risk behaviors common to the age group being addressed, and fulfill legal conditions of the institution involved. Fortunately, the rate of sudden death in young athletes is low.

In those under the age of 35, the most common cause of sudden death is congenital cardiac anomalies. Hypertrophic cardiomyopathy (HCM) is responsible for about one-third of these deaths. Unfortunately, sudden death may be the presenting symptom of HCM. A personal or family history of congenital heart disease, symptoms of chest pain or tightness, palpitations, dyspnea, syncope or near-syncope are important. A family history of HCM or unexplained sudden death in someone under the age of 50 is significant as well. The murmur of HCM may not be present in all persons with this disorder. To identify the murmur, dynamic auscultation is often necessary. The heart should be auscultated while the patient is lying and then standing. As this murmur is accentuated by maneuvers which reduce cardiac preload, the murmur will get louder when the patient stands or performs a Valsalva maneuver and will diminish as the patient lies or squats. As the patient in Question 22 has the concerning historical point of exertional syncope and a family history of an unexplained, early death along with a characteristic murmur on examination, further evaluation is warranted. In the 26th Bethesda Conference report, the American College of Cardiology recommends that persons with HCM should be restricted from all, except possibly for the least strenuous, athletic activity. In this case, restriction of all athletic activity until the patient can be further evaluated by a cardiologist—preferably one with experience in dealing with the evaluation of athletes—would be the most appropriate option of the choices given.

Marfan syndrome is a connective tissue disorder that typically affects the eyes, skeletal system, and cardiovascular system. Persons with Marfan syndrome are typically tall and have arm spans that are greater than their height. Signs include long, slender digits, high-arched palates, and pectus deformities of the chest. Lens dislocations in the eye are common. Detecting Marfan syndrome during a preparticipation examination is important because of the occurrence of aortic root dilation and the risk of sudden death caused by aortic rupture. The patient in Questions 23 and 24 has multiple signs of Marfan syndrome and further evaluation would be indicated. Of the options given, an echocardiogram to evaluate the aortic root and to look for other valvular abnormalities would be indicated. These persons usually require referral to an ophthalmologist as well for a dilated eye examination to evaluate for lens dislocations. Turner syndrome is a syndrome of gonadal dysgenesis, associated with a 45, X karyotype (or another defect of the X chromosome). This syndrome is typically associated with a short stature and multiple anomalies including a webbed neck and "shield" chest. The female athlete triad is a syndrome of disordered eating, amenorrhea, and osteoporosis. It is seen most often in participants in activities that emphasize low body weights, such as gymnastics or ballet. The presence of regular menstrual cycles makes this diagnosis unlikely. Atlanto-axial instability can be associated with Down syndrome. Physicians performing preparticipation examinations on someone with Down syndrome must consider performing lateral cervical spine x-rays with flexion and extension views. This patient does not have any of the classic findings of Down syndrome. Similarly, she does not exhibit any of the classic symptoms of type 1 diabetes— polydipsia, polyphagia, and polyuria. Performing serum glucose testing would therefore not be indicated.

The patient in Question 25 is the most typical type of patient who presents for a preparticipation examination—the healthy adolescent. This may be the only encounter that a physician will have with an adolescent, especially an adolescent male. It is in this population where a physician can use this encounter to address other age appropriate health maintenance issues. Assuming that he has had an appropriate primary series of immunizations, a booster with diphtheria-tetanus toxoid would

be recommended as it has been over 10 years since his last booster. Other vaccinations to consider would be hepatitis B and MMR, if he has not previously been adequately immunized. Varicella vaccine could be considered if he has had neither the vaccine nor the disease by this age. A nonjudgmental discussion of sexual behaviors, drug use, alcohol use, and other high-risk behaviors would also be appropriate. Screening for hepatitis C, however, is not recommended by most authorities, in the absence of symptoms or other known risks. Randomly screening for drug use by urine drug testing is not recommended. Screening athletes who have neither concerning symptoms nor signs with ECGs is not recommended because of the poor predictive values and significant costs involved with mass screening. ECGs should be performed without hesitation in any athlete who has a history, examination finding, or preexisting diagnosis of a potentially high-risk condition. Although some localities may require a urinalysis as part of a preparticipation examination, there is no evidence to recommend universal screening. (*McKeag DB and Sallis RE. Factors at play in the athletic preparticipation examination. Am Fam Physician 2000;61:2617; Kurowski K and Chandran S. The preparticipation athletic evaluation. Am Fam Physician 2000;61:2683–2690, 2696–2698*)

26. **(E)** The landmark 1999 Institute of Medicine report, *To Err is Human: Building a Safer Health System*, estimated that between 44,000 and 98,000 Americans died each year in hospitals as a result of medical errors. Even using the lower number, this represents more deaths than breast cancer, motor vehicle accidents, and AIDS. About 7000 deaths are attributable to medication errors. This number alone is greater than the number of deaths in work-related injuries. Errors in diagnosis, treatment, prevention, communication, equipment failure, and other system failures result not only in significant morbidity and mortality, but also an estimated 17–29 billion dollars in costs. Further, there is a significant loss in trust in the health system by patients and loss in satisfaction by patients, their families, and healthcare providers. Unfortunately, many of these errors that

occurred, and continue to occur, are preventable. Many hospitals, healthcare organizations, and oversight agencies, including the Quality Interagency Coordination Task Force of the Federal Government, are actively pursuing mechanisms of quality improvement to reduce this epidemic. *(Institute of Medicine. To err is human: building a safer health system. Report available online at www.iom.edu/Object.File/Master/4/117/0.pdf)*

27. (A)

28. (E)

Explanations 27 and 28

The odds ratio is a frequently published statistic. The odds of an event occurring are the number of times an event occurred divided by the number of times that it did not. In medical studies it is calculated by dividing the number of subjects who achieved a certain outcome by the number of subjects who did not. An odds ratio is calculated by dividing the odds of an event in one group by the odds of the same event in another group. This is frequently an experimental group and a control group.

In the study presented in this question, the "experimental" group is the induction of labor group and the control is the expectant management group. An odds ratio of less than one means that the outcome in question occurred less often in the experimental group than in the control group. Conversely, an odds ratio of greater than one reveals that the outcome occurred more often in the experimental group than the control group. In the study presented, the odds ratios for both the outcomes of caesarian delivery and perinatal mortality are less than one, suggesting that these outcomes occurred less often in the group of women treated with induction of labor at 41 weeks' gestation compared to those treated with expectant management.

A CI is a range within which the "true" result is likely to be found. A 95% CI states that there is a 95% probability that the true answer exists within these bounds. For statistics, such as odds ratios or relative risks, a 95% CI that includes the number 1 within its bounds is considered not statistically significant. This is because an odds ratio of 1 means that there is no difference in the odds of an event occurring in either group. For the outcome of caesarian delivery, the odds ratio is 0.88 with a 95% CI that does not include 1. Therefore, one can say that there is a statistically significant reduction in the number of caesarian deliveries in the induction group compared to the expectant management group. For the outcome of perinatal mortality, the odds ratio is 0.41 but the 95% CI extends up to 1.18. This result cannot be considered statistically significant. The answer to Question 27 is therefore A.

Statistical power is the ability of a study to determine a difference between two groups if a difference truly exists. It is a function of the magnitude of the difference between the two groups and the number of subjects in the study. For the result of perinatal mortality, the odds ratio is low at 0.41, suggesting that a difference may exist between the two groups. However, the presence of wide CIs around this result suggests that the study is underpowered to detect this difference. For this particular study, it is because the outcome in question—perinatal mortality—occurred (fortunately) rarely. The only realistic way to increase the power of a study is to increase the number of subjects enrolled. (n.b.: This particular meta-analysis had approximately 6000 subjects. The authors estimate that approximately 16,000 would be needed to achieve adequate power to find a statistically significant difference in perinatal mortality.) *(Sanchez-Ramos L, Oliver F, Delke I, Kaunitz AM. Labor induction versus expectant management for postterm pregnancies: A systematic review with meta-analysis. Obstet Gynecol 2003; 101:1312–1318)*

29. (D)

30. (D)

31. (C)

Explanations 29 through 31

Bacterial endocarditis is a rare, but life-threatening, disease. It occurs primarily in persons with underlying structural heart defects who develop bacteremia with organisms that are likely to cause endocarditis. Most cases of endocarditis are not a complication of invasive medical or dental procedures. Because of the risks associated with the disease, efforts should be made to prevent bacterial endocarditis when appropriate. The American Heart Association has published updated, evidence-based recommendations on the prevention of bacterial endocarditis. These guidelines are available at the American Heart Association website (www.americanheart.org). These guidelines outline conditions for which endocarditis prophylaxis is appropriate, procedures for which endocarditis prophylaxis is necessary, and antibiotic regimens that are recommended. Cardiac conditions are stratified into high-risk, moderate-risk, and negligible risk (see Table 6-1). Negligible risk conditions are those in which, although endocarditis may develop, the risk is no greater than in the general population. Of the conditions listed in Question 29, only bicuspid aortic valve would require antibiotic prophylaxis, as it is a moderate-risk congenital cardiac malformation. All of the other conditions listed are considered to be of negligible risk.

Procedures which require antibiotic prophylaxis are those which produce a significant bacteremia with organisms commonly causing endocarditis. For dental procedures, those that tend to cause significant bleeding from hard or soft tissues would necessitate prophylaxis. Of the procedures listed, only the placement of dental implants is likely to do this. In the event that unexpected significant bleeding occurs, antibiotics within 2 h following the procedure would be recommended.

Similarly, surgical procedures that cause bacteremia with organisms associated with endocarditis would necessitate antibiotic prophylaxis. Bacteremia occurs in up to one-fourth of those undergoing a urethral dilation procedure. None of the other procedures listed is likely to cause a significant bacteremia, as long as they are not performed through infected tissues. Therefore, the American Heart Association guidelines would recommend antibiotics prior to urethral dilation and not for the other procedures listed as options. (*American Heart Association: www.americanheart.org/ presenter.jhtml?identifier=1745*)

TABLE 6-1

Endocarditis prophylaxis recommended
High-risk category
Prosthetic cardiac valves, including bioprosthetic and homograft valves
Previous bacterial endocarditis
Complex cyanotic congenital heart disease (eg, single ventricle states, transposition of the great arteries, tetralogy of Fallot)
Surgically constructed systemic pulmonary shunts or conduits

Moderate-risk category
Most other congenital cardiac malformations (other than above and below)
Acquired valvar dysfunction (eg, rheumatic heart disease)
Hypertrophic cardiomyopathy
Mitral valve prolapse with valvar regurgitation and/or thickened leaflets

Endocarditis prophylaxis not recommended
Negligible-risk category (no greater than the general population)
Isolated secundum atrial septal defect
Surgical repair of atrial septal defect, ventricular septal defect, or patent ductus arteriosus (without residua beyond 6 mo)
Previous coronary artery bypass graft surgery
Mitral valve prolapse without valvar regurgitation
Physiologic, functional or innocent heart murmurs
Previous Kawasaki disease without valvar dysfunction
Previous rheumatic fever without valvar dysfunction
Cardiac pacemakers (intravascular and epicardial) and implanted defibrillators

Source: Reproduced, with permission, from American Heart Association, 2004. Available at: http://www.americanheart.org/presenter.jhtml?identifier = 1745.

32.   (B)

33.   (C)

Explanations 32 and 33

The disease tetanus is cause by an exotoxin produced by the anaerobic, gram-positive bacterium *C. tetani*. The spores of *C. tetani* are endemic in soil, particularly in agricultural areas. They can also be found in the intestines and feces of many animals. Human infection usually is the result of the introduction of the spores through a wound, such as a puncture or laceration. The spores can then germinate and toxins are released. Tetanus is characterized by unopposed muscle contractions and spasms. Autonomic nervous system manifestations, seizures, and difficulty swallowing may occur. Recovery may take months, but the disease is often fatal. In the developed world, most cases of tetanus occur in those who either were never vaccinated or who completed a primary vaccine series but have not had a booster in the preceding 10 years. The currently available vaccine is a toxoid which consists of a formaldehyde-treated toxin. It is available as a single antigen vaccine, combined with diphtheria (pediatric DT or adult Td) or combined with both diphtheria and acellular pertussis vaccine (DTaP). Whenever possible, tetanus toxoid should be given in combination with diphtheria toxoid to provide periodic boosting for both antigens. There is little reason to use single antigen tetanus toxoid alone.

Management of a potentially contaminated wound initially involves local wound care. Necrotic tissue should be debrided, foreign material removed, and the wound irrigated. The need for active and/or passive immunization against tetanus depends on the wound and the patient's history of immunization. A person who has completed a primary series of three or more doses of tetanus toxoid vaccine will not require passive immunization with tetanus immune globulin (TIG), but may require a booster of dT. For a clean, minor wound, a Td booster would be indicated if it has been more than 10 years since the patient's most recent booster. For all other wounds, a booster would be indicated if it has been 5 years since the most recent booster. In a person who has not completed a primary series, who is completely unimmunized, or in whom the vaccine status is unknown, initiating passive immunization with Td is indicated for all wounds. If the wound is clean and minor then TIG would not be recommended. For all other wounds, both Td and TIG would be indicated, as the initial doses of Td may not produce immunity and TIG can provide immediate, temporary immunity. Antibiotic prophylaxis against tetanus is not useful. As the patient in Question 32 has no history of having completed a primary vaccine series and has a contaminated wound, the most appropriate management would be to provide both Td and TIG.

Following the initial management in the emergency room, efforts should be made to ensure that an appropriate primary series of tetanus vaccination is completed. For adults and for children age 7 or older with no history of having received a primary series, the recommended Td schedule is to provide a three-dose primary series with an initial dose, a second dose

in 4 weeks, and a third dose in 6–12 months. Following completion of the primary series, a booster would be recommended every 10 years. Options A and B in Question 33 do not provide for an adequate primary series. Option D is the recommended, routine vaccination schedule for infants. Option E is not indicated as TIG provides only temporary immunity and should only be used in the prophylaxis of wounds in those who are under-immunized or in the treatment of persons with tetanus disease. *(Centers for Disease Control: www.cdc.gov/nip/publications/pink/tetanus.pdf)*

34. **(A)** There is an increased risk of influenza-related complications in pregnant women who contract influenza, therefore the influenza vaccine is recommend for all pregnant women who will be beyond the first trimester during influenza season. The live, attenuated influenza vaccine is contraindicated during pregnancy but the inactivated influenza vaccine is recommended. The hepatitis B vaccine contains only noninfectious hepatitis B surface antigen particles and poses no real or theoretical risk of fetal infection, whereas the disease hepatitis B may cause severe illness for the pregnant woman and chronic disease for the newborn. For these reasons, neither pregnancy nor lactation is a contraindication to vaccination with hepatitis B vaccine. All pregnant women should routinely be tested for immunity to the rubella virus and should be immunized postpartum if they have no measurable immunity. The rubella vaccine, like other live-virus vaccines, is contraindicated during pregnancy due to the theoretical risk of causing fetal infection. In reality, studies of women who were pregnant or soon became pregnant after receiving rubella vaccination showed that the risk is extremely small. A registry of 226 susceptible women who received the rubella vaccine between 3 months before and 3 months after conception showed no evidence of congenital rubella syndrome. Women who inadvertently receive this vaccine should be counseled about the theoretical risk involved, however this would not be considered a reason to terminate a pregnancy. Finally, Td toxoid is routinely indicated for pregnant women. A woman with no documented booster

within 10 years should receive one and a woman with no documented primary series should start or complete her primary series. Some authorities do recommend waiting until the second trimester to administer a Td in order to minimize any theoretical concerns regarding teratogenicity. *(Centers for Disease Control: www.cdc. gov/nip/publications/preg_guide.htm)*

35. (C)

36. (D)

Explanations 35 and 36

The NNT is calculated by first determining the ARR for a specific outcome between two groups in a study. The ARR, or risk difference, is calculated by subtracting the percentage of subjects who develop an outcome in the treatment group from the percentage who develop the outcome in the control group. In Question 35, the outcome considered is the development of prostate cancer. This occurred in 24% of the control group and 18% of the finasteride group. The ARR is calculated as 24% − 18% = 6% or 0.06. The NNT is calculated as: NNT = 1/ARR. In this example, the NNT = 1/0.06 = 16.67, approximately 17. This suggests that for every 17 men who took finasteride there was one fewer case of prostate cancer.

The NNH is calculated in exactly the same manner as the NNT. The only difference is that the outcome is adverse. In this study, high-grade prostate cancers occurred more often in the finasteride group than the placebo group; 6.4% of men who took finasteride and 5.1% who took a placebo developed high-grade prostate cancer. The risk difference, in this case an absolute risk increase, is 6.4% − 5.1% = 1.3% or 0.013. The NNH = 1/absolute risk increase = 1/0.013 = 77. *(Thompson IM, et al. The influence of finasteride on the development of prostate cancer. N Engl J Med 2003;349:215–224)*

37. (B)

38. (A)

Explanations 37 and 38

DEXA is the most widely used test for the screening and diagnosis of osteoporosis. It is sensitive for the loss of bone density, exposes the patient to a relatively low dose of radiation, and is widely available at a reasonable cost. It is the mode of evaluation that has been used in most of the studies of the evaluation and management of osteoporosis. The American College of Radiology Guidelines state that DEXA of the lumbar spine and proximal femur as the most appropriate screening test for osteoporosis in postmenopausal women who are not on any therapy. Quantitative CT scanning is also highly sensitive but is less widely available, more expensive, and exposes the subject to higher radiation doses. Lateral thoracic spine radiographs can diagnose or confirm the presence of osteoporotic fractures but are not appropriate as a screening test for bone density. Quantitative ultrasonography, usually of the calcaneus or digits, is becoming more widely available at low costs, but has the disadvantage of being unable to directly evaluate the areas where most ostoporotic fractures are likely to occur—hip, spine, and radius. Single energy x-ray absorptiometry has not correlated as well to fracture risk as dual energy techniques and is, therefore, less appropriate than DEXA.

The T-score is a comparison of the subjects' bone density to that of the mean bone density of 25-year-old women, when bone density is predicted to be at or near its maximum. The T-score represents the number of standard deviations away from the mean value that a specific bone density represents. The World Health Organization defines osteoporosis as a T-score of less than −2.5; that is to say, a bone density of 2.5 standard deviations less than that of the mean bone density of a 25-year-old woman. Osteopenia is defined as a T-score of between −1 and −2.5, and a T-score greater than −1 is considered normal. Of the options listed in Question 38, treatment with a bisphosphonate, which has been shown both to increase bone density and reduce fracture incidence, would be indicated as we are treating a patient with established osteoporosis. Increasing the intake of both calcium and vitamin D are also important but not adequate as sole interventions. Most authorities recommend 1200–1500 mg calcium intake per day for postmenopausal women. Exercise, particularly weight bearing exercise, is also important in the management of patients with osteoporosis both to maintain bone density but also to improve strength, coordination, and balance in an effort to reduce fall risk. It should be part of an overall management plan. When osteoporosis is treated, most authorities recommend waiting approximately 2 years for repeat bone density testing. (*American College of Radiology (ACR), Expert Panel on Musculoskeletal Imaging. Osteoporosis and bone mineral density. Reston, VA: American College of Radiology (ACR), 2001, p. 17 (ACR Appropriateness Criteria); University of Michigan Health System. Osteoporosis: prevention and treatment. Ann Arbor, MI: University of Michigan Health System, 2002, Mar. 12*)

39. (B)

40. (D)

41. (E)

Explanations 39 through 41

Pregestational diabetes is associated with numerous risks to both the mother and the fetus. Stillbirths are more common in pregnancies to diabetic women and stillbirths without an identifiable cause, called "unexplained" stillbirths, are a well-described phenomenon. Similarly, preterm births are more common in diabetics than nondiabetics. While congenital malformations are more common in pregnancies to diabetic women, fetal chromosomal abnormalities are not more common. Children of women with diabetes have an approximately 1–3% incidence of developing type 1 diabetes. While earlier obstetrical teaching suggested that maternal diabetes delayed fetal lung maturation, more recent studies do not support this. Gestational age is likely the most significant factor in the development of respiratory distress.

While there are significant maternal risks from the interaction of diabetes and pregnancy, with the possible exception of diabetic retinopathy, the long-term course of diabetes does not appear to be affected by pregnancy. Pregnancy neither exacerbates nor modifies diabetic nephropathy and the development of diabetic peripheral neuropathy during pregnancy is uncommon. While preeclampsia is a significant risk and the perinatal mortality rate is 20 times higher in preeclamptic diabetic women compared to normotensive women, the occurrence of preeclampsia does not appear to be related to diabetic control. Diabetic ketoacidosis is a serious complication with an approximately 20% rate of fetal loss. However, it is estimated to occur in 1% of pregnancies of diabetic women. Infections occur in approximately 80% of pregnancies in insulin-dependent diabetics, with candida vaginitis, urinary tract infections, and respiratory infections being common.

Preconception counseling in diabetic women who desire to become pregnant is a critical issue that often is best served by a team that includes the obstetrician, primary care physician, endocrinologist, and diabetic educators. When possible, attempts should be made to attain optimal diabetic control. Women with good diabetic control have been shown in observational studies to have a lower rate of having infants with congenital anomalies than women with poorer diabetic control. Optimal diabetic control has been defined as glycated hemoglobin levels within or near the upper limit of the normal range. This can be obtained with multiple daily insulin injections or, in selected patients, a continuous infusion via an insulin pump. All women—diabetic or not—should be counseled to take folic acid prior to conception in order to lower that rate of neural tube defects. ACE inhibitors are contraindicated during pregnancy and should, whenever possible, be discontinued prior to conception. (*Cunningham FG, Gant NF, et al. Williams Obstetrics, 21st ed. New York, NY: McGraw-Hill, 2001, pp. 1367–1376*)

42. (D)

43. (A)

44. (D)

Explanations 42 through 44

All types of study designs have potential benefits and drawbacks and it is important to understand this when designing research or reviewing research reports. A cross-sectional study is one in which information is gathered from a certain population at one point in time with no follow-up period. This type of study is very useful for the determination of the prevalence of a disease or risk factor in a population at a certain point in time. Cross-sectional studies cannot determine cause and effect because there are no interventions being made and there is no follow-up. A case-control study is very useful and efficient at studying diseases that occur rarely. In a case-control study persons with a disease are identified and then information is determined by looking back in time (i.e., retrospective review). A population of those without the disease (controls) is also defined and studied in the same way. The prevalence of a risk factor in the cases and controls can then be determined and compared. A case-control study cannot prove cause and effect, but it can be a powerful tool to determine risk factors that can generate hypotheses for further study. A cohort study is one in which a population is defined and then followed over time. A cohort study may be either prospective or retrospective. Cohort studies can be used to describe the incidence of diseases over time or to determine associations between predictors and outcomes. Cohort studies are inefficient for the study of rare outcomes, as a very large sample size would be required in order to find a few events. A prospective, randomized-controlled trial is the gold standard study for determining the effect of a treatment or intervention. It is not the type of study that would be used to determine the prevalence of a disease in a population or to determine what risk factors are associated with the development of a disease. A metaanalysis is a systematic review of completed research studies. By evaluating similarly done studies, the metaanalysis technique can allow for an evaluation of a body of literature and can be used to increase the overall statistical power by creating a larger sample by combining studies.

The odds ratios given in Question 44 show that both risk factors X and Y occurred more often in those with the disease (cases) than they did in those without the disease (controls). Neither of the CIs given cross 1, therefore, these are statistically significant findings. We cannot use this type of study to definitively prove cause and effect, therefore option A is false. While risk factor X had a higher odds ratio for the development of the disease than risk factor Y, no prognostic data are supplied and none can be inferred from the information given, therefore B is false. The odds ratios as given in this case compare the prevalence of a risk factor in the case group with the control group, not the prevalence of one risk factor compared to another. For this reason, we cannot say which risk factor is more common in the population and option C is false. No absolute numbers are presented in this question and therefore we cannot determine how often each of the risk factors occurs in our population, so E is false as well. *(Hulley SB, Cummings SR, et al. Designing Clinical Research, 2nd ed. Philadelphia, PA: Lippincott Willams & Wilkins, 2001)*

45. **(E)**

46. **(B)**

47. **(E)**

Explanations 45 through 47

Current guidelines for TB control emphasize testing of those who are at high risk for the development of TB and who would benefit from the treatment of a latent TB infection, if detected. Based on that principle, testing is encouraged in those who are at high risk and discouraged among those who are at low risk. Further, anyone who is at high risk for the development of TB and who tests positive should be offered treatment, regardless of age. The preferred testing modality for asymptomatic persons of all age is the intradermal (Mantoux) method of testing with purified protein derivative. Multiple puncture tests (e.g., Tine) are not sufficiently accurate and should not be used. The test should be read at 48–72 h and the diameter of induration, not redness, should be measured and recorded. Previous BCG vaccination is not a contraindication to skin testing and a positive skin reaction should be used as an indication of TB infection when the tested person is at increased risk for infection or has medical conditions that increase the risk of the disease.

Three cutoff points for the determination of a positive test are currently in use: ≥5 mm of induration is used for those who are at the highest risk of disease, such as those immunosuppressed from HIV or medications, or those recently exposed to TB; ≥10 mm induration is used as a positive result for persons who have an increased probability of infection (such as immigrants from endemic areas), who have clinical conditions that increase the risk for TB (such as injection drug users) or who are residents or employees in high risk settings (nursing homes, hospitals, prisons, and so on); ≥15 mm is used as a cutoff for those who have no known risk factors. In Question 46, ignoring the amount of redness and using only induration as the criteria for positive or negative, the nursing home resident (option B) is the only one with a positive test.

All persons who test positive by a skin test should then have a chest x-ray to evaluate for evidence of pulmonary TB. In an asymptomatic person, sputum studies are not necessary to determine the need for treatment. Pregnant women should still get a chest x-ray, with appropriate abdominal shielding, as soon as feasible. As stated above, a history of BCG vaccination should not deter from the need for further evaluation and treatment of a positive test result. Age should also not be a determining factor in treating someone who is at risk for the development of TB. Currently there are four acceptable treatment recommendations for latent TB infections. Daily isoniazid for 9 months is the most widely used regimen and has the highest level of recommendation because of its effectiveness, relative safety, ease of administration, and low cost. Twice-weekly isoniazid may also be used but should only be given as directly observed therapy, due to the fact that a missed dose of this regimen repre-

sents a substantial risk of undertreatment. Rifampin alone or rifampin plus pyrazinamide are alternative regimens for use in certain, specified situations. *(Centers for Disease Control: www.cdc.gov/mmwr/PDF/rr/rr4906.pdf)*

48. **(C)** The widespread use of fluoride has been a major factor in the decline in the prevalence and severity of tooth decay in the United States. In most communities public water supplies are fluoridated. Supplementation is recommended by the Centers for Disease Control, American Academy of Pediatrics, American Academy of Family Practice, and other authorities, for those who do not have access to fluoridated water. Fluoride supplementation can occur from both ingestion and from topical supplementation, such as in fluoride-containing toothpaste. Current guidelines recommend no supplementation until 6 months of age and then a dietary fluoride supplement of 0.25 mg per day from the age of 6 months to 3 years, 0.5 mg per day for ages 3–6 years, and 1.0 mg per day for ages 6–16 years for those persons who do not have access to fluoridated water. Current powdered infant formulas do not provide a significant amount of fluoride because of the risk of a child receiving too much fluoride if the formula is mixed with fluoridated water. The chronic ingestion of high levels of fluoride can result in fluorosis, a state of hypomineralization of tooth enamel. Studies have shown that fluoride supplements taken by pregnant women do not benefit their offspring. *(Centers for Disease Control: www.cdc.gov/mmwr/PDF/RR/RR5014.pdf)*

49. **(E)**

50. **(A)**

Explanations 49 and 50

Domestic violence is an abuse of power in a relationship in which a more powerful person exerts inappropriate control or domination over a less powerful person. Abuse is not only physical, but also can be emotional, sexual, or economic. Intimidation and psychologic abuse also occur and are used sometimes by batterers in place of physical violence. Domestic, or partner, violence occurs in all types of relationships, regardless of the gender of the partners. The risk of violence increases in many situations, which exaggerate the disparity in power in the relationship, such as illness or disability in one of the partners. Pregnancy, especially unintended pregnancy, may also increase the risk of battery. Laws regarding the reporting of domestic violence vary from state to state. Many states do not require the reporting of domestic violence when the abused is a competent adult. Marriage, in and of itself, does not prevent a partner from making a sexual abuse charge against the other partner.

Management in the setting of partner violence can be difficult. Providing information and referrals to appropriate shelters and services is critical. Assisting with the development of emergency plans may be of benefit as well. Asking about the availability of weapons in the home is important, as up to half of female murder victims are killed by a current male partner or ex-partner. At this time, reporting to the Child Protective Services is inappropriate, as they cannot intervene. After the baby is born, however, any sign of child abuse should be immediately reported. *(Eyler AE and Cohen M. Case studies in partner violence. Am Fam Physician 1999;60:2569–2576)*

51. (D)

52. (E)

53. (B)

Explanations 51 through 53

Encounters with persons traveling to other countries are common in primary care or community health settings. The advice and interventions provided are dependent on where the person is going, what he will be doing, and for how long he will be there. The most accessible and up-to-date source of this information in the United States is at the Centers for Disease Control website, which provides detailed recommendations on vaccinations, health and safety risks involved in overseas travel. In this series of questions, the travelers are going to the region of central Africa and, more specifically, to a rural area of

Cameroon. This is an area of the world where polio remains a risk. As most Americans have not been vaccinated against polio since childhood, booster immunization against polio is recommended. The injectable polio vaccine is recommended as it does not carry with it the risk of vaccine-induced disease that the oral (live virus) vaccine does. Smallpox has been eliminated as a naturally occurring disease, although it remains of importance in bioterrorism discussions. The smallpox vaccine is not necessary for travel to any part of the world, but is used by the military or medical first-responders who may be exposed in the event of a biowarfare attack. The traveling couple is up-to-date on their dT status with boosters within the past 2 years. They have completed a series of both MMR and hepatitis B, which is felt to confer lifetime immunity.

Malaria prevention is an important consideration for travel to many areas of the developing world. Different regimens may be used depending on the area to which the travel will occur. All regimens, however, require the institution of prophylaxis prior to travel and the continuation of prophylaxis for up to 4 weeks after completion of travel. This is due to the life cycle of organisms that cause the disease. Prevention of malaria also involves attempts to reduce one's risk of exposure to the *Ixodes* mosquito which can transmit the disease. This mosquito tends to be more active early in the morning and at dusk, and less active in the middle of the day. Wearing long sleeved clothing, using mosquito nets, and insect repellent is important. DEET-containing insect repellents are recommended as the most effective products available and are safe when used appropriately. The most common cause of injury during travel is motor vehicle accidents. The risk of injury is higher in many developing countries than in the United States due to poor roads, poor vehicle maintenance, lack of seat belts, and other issues. Very cautious driving and avoidance of driving after dark may help to reduce the risk somewhat. While swimming is an ideal exercise in such hot climates as central Africa, freshwater lake swimming should be avoided due to the risk of exposure to schistosomiasis. The *Schistosoma* species that cause this disease are endemic in standing freshwater bodies. Swimming or bathing in salt water or chlorinated swimming pools is safer.

Traveler's diarrhea and exposure to food-borne pathogens is a common cause of illness during travel to developing countries. The guideline with food is to cook it, peel it, purify it, or forget it. Fruits that can be peeled, such as oranges or bananas, are generally safe to eat. Carbonated beverages are also safe. However, ice cubes made from local water supplies are a common, and sometimes ignored, source of infection. Water purification can be accomplished by boiling or by filtering through an absolute 1 μm filter and then purifying with iodine. Filtering alone does not provide adequate protection. Salads that are not made of carefully cleaned vegetables should be avoided and salad dressings may also be contaminated. Meats that are well cooked and served hot would be considered less likely to transmit an infection. Finally, brushing one's teeth with unpurified water carries a significant risk of transmission of waterborne illness and should be avoided. Purified water or bottled water should be used instead. (*Centers for Disease Control: www.cdc.gov*)

54. **(B)**

55. **(E)**

Explanations 54 and 55

Environmental tobacco smoke or "secondhand smoke" consists of both "mainstream smoke," which is exhaled by the smoker and "sidestream smoke," which comes from the burning cigarette between puffs. About half of the smoke from a cigarette is sidestream smoke, which consists of the same chemicals as the mainstream smoke that is inhaled by the user. Nonsmokers exposed to secondhand smoke absorb nicotine, carcinogens, and other chemicals from the smoke just as the smoker does. While the concentration of the chemicals absorbed is less than in a smoker, the levels absorbed increase as exposure increases and there are significant health risks involved. The

Environmental Protection Agency considers secondhand smoke to be a class A carcinogen— a substance that causes cancer in humans. Among the health risks are increased incidences of asthma, respiratory infections, otitis media, and SIDS in children exposed to secondhand smoke. Nursing mothers can pass harmful chemicals from cigarette smoke in breast milk.

While separating smokers and nonsmokers in the same airspace may reduce the exposure to secondhand smoke, the exposure is not eliminated. It is estimated to take 3 h to remove 95% of the cigarette smoke from a room once smoking is completed, so there is still significant risk for exposure even though the nonsmoker is not in the same room. Courts in the United States and Canada have considered the smoking behaviors of parents as factors in determining the "best interests" of a child during custody hearings. Finally, parental smoking is an important predictor of the smoking behaviors of their children as they become adolescents. (*National Cancer Institute: cis.nci.nih.gov/ fact/3_9.htm; American Academy of Pediatrics: www.aap. org/advocacy/chmhets.htm*)

56. **(A)**

57. **(D)**

58. **(B)**

Explanations 56 through 58

The mnemonic "ABCDE" is often used to remember some of the attributes of skin lesions that would make them more suspicious for being malignancies. "A" is for asymmetry; "B" for border that is irregular or indistinct from the surrounding skin; "C" for color such as dark black or variations in colors within the same lesion; "D" for diameter greater than 6 mm, or larger than the size of a pencil eraser; "E" for elevation of lesion with surface irregularity. Of the choices in Question 56, the presence of a diameter of greater than 6 mm would be considered a higher-risk attribute.

Primary skin malignancies are divided into three major categories—basal cell carcinoma, squamous cell carcinoma, and melanoma. Basal cell carcinomas may grow large and be locally destructive, but they have the lowest metastatic potential of the three types of skin cancer. Basal cell carcinomas are more common in persons with fair-complexions but they occur in all skin types and colors. Squamous carcinomas of the skin have a metastatic potential greater than basal cell carcinomas and less than malignant melanomas. Squamous carcinomas most commonly occur in sun-exposed areas but are also associated with other etiologies, such as human papilloma virus (HPV), and can occur anywhere on the body. Malignant melanoma has the highest metastatic potential of the primary skin malignancies. Obtaining a tissue sample for pathologic studies of suspicious skin lesions is critical for diagnosis and planning of appropriate treatment of melanoma. The thickness of the lesion is an important factor in these decisions. Therefore, shave biopsy would be inappropriate for the evaluation of a pigmented lesion. Complete excisional biopsy would be preferable, or, when that is not possible, full-thickness punch biopsy is an acceptable alternative. While sun exposure is an important risk factor for all types of skin cancers, for melanomas there is some evidence that intermittent, intense sun exposure and sunburning is more of a risk than cumulative sun exposure.

Actinic keratoses are sun-induced skin lesions that are considered risks for the development of squamous carcinomas. They can be treated with local destructive methods, such as cryosurgery or the topical chemotherapeutic agent 5-fluorouracil. Protection of susceptible skin from excessive sun exposure from childhood is important in reducing the risk of developing skin cancer. Precautions such as wearing broad-brimmed hats, long sleeved clothing, and avoidance of intense midday sunlight are helpful. Using chemical sunscreens with SPF of greater than 15 with frequent reapplication is also beneficial. Even "waterproof" sunscreens need to be reapplied after bathing or swimming. A wet cotton T-shirt provides very little, if any, protection from ultraviolet light exposure. Both the UV-A and UV-B rays play roles in skin damage from the sun and it is important to use sun protection products, which block both types of rays. Sun tanning booths are also considered risks for the induction of skin damage and skin cancer as they expose skin to potentially damaging ultraviolet rays. (*Fitzpatrick TB, Johnson RA, Wolff K, Suurmond D. Color Atlas and Synopsis of Clinical Dermatology, 4th ed. New York, NY: McGraw Hill, 2001*)

59.   (C)

60.   (B)

61.   (C)

Explanations 59 through 61

At the initial prenatal visit, a complete history and physical examination is performed along with a panel of laboratory studies. Routinely, a complete blood count, blood type, and Rh group with antibody screen, rubella antibody, RPR, HIV, pap smear, cervical swab for gonorrhea and chlamydia, urinalysis, and urine culture are performed. Pregnancy is one of the few conditions in which treatment of asymptomatic bacteruria would be recommended. Neither a basic metabolic panel nor a TSH measurement would be indicated unless the patient had an underlying medical condition that warranted further evaluation. Screening for gestational diabetes with a glucose measurement after ingestion of 50 g of glucose is performed in many pregnancies, but not until 24–28 weeks' gestation. Routine screening for vaginal or rectal colonization with group B *Streptococcus* is also performed, but not until 34 weeks of gestation or later.

It is recommended that all pregnant women be screened for hepatitis B at their initial prenatal visit by obtaining a hepatitis B surface antigen. This helps to determine if the woman has hepatitis B that could put her baby at risk for the infection. Hepatitis B surface antibody may be a sign of previous infection or of previous vaccination with the hepatitis B vaccine. The presence of core antibody and e antibody may be signs of previous infection. Testing for the e antigen is not useful for initial screening purposes but may be warranted if the patient were found to have chronic hepatitis B infection.

If the mother tests positive for hepatitis B surface antigen during her pregnancy, then the neonate should receive both hepatitis B immune globulin and the initial dose of the hepatitis B vaccine series. This combination has been shown to reduce risk of perinatal transmission from approximately 10% if the woman is surface antigen positive to less than 3%. There are currently no data to show that delivering a baby by caesarian section will reduce the risk of perinatal transmission of the infection. Breastfeeding has not been shown to increase the rate of transmission of infection to a nursing infant. (*Lin KW and Kirchner JT. Hepatitis B. Am Fam Physician 2004;69:75–82, 86*)

62. (E)

63. (E)

Explanations 62 and 63

Screening for prostate cancer with the PSA test is a controversial area. Some advocate routine screening of most men over the age of 50 while others recommend selective screening or no routine screening at all. The United States Preventative Services Task Force gives prostate cancer screening an "I" recommendation, stating that there is insufficient evidence to recommend for or against this intervention. Prostate cancer is the second most common cause of cancer death in men (behind lung cancer). PSA screening does not help to prevent prostate cancer but it does increase the likelihood of detection of prostate cancer. However, many prostate cancers are slow growing and many with prostate cancer die of other causes. PSA screening has not been shown to reduce all causes of mortality. While the mortality from prostate cancer has been decreasing over the years, the reason for this is not yet clear. PSA screening may play a role in this, but improvements in the treatment of prostate cancer may also be responsible. The PSA also has significant rates of false positive and false negative readings. Benign conditions

such as prostatic hyperplasia or prostatitis can elevate PSA readings and prostate cancer can exist in men with normal PSA readings.

Another factor that can interfere with PSA readings is the presence of medications. Finasteride, which is widely used in the treatment of benign prostatic hyperplasia, can lower PSA readings, even in the presence of prostate cancer. If PSA screening is chosen by the patient and his physician, selection of appropriate patients for screening is important. The presence of symptoms related to the prostate may influence one's decision to perform a PSA test. However, many prostate cancers are asymptomatic, so the absence of symptoms may not be a reason to withhold testing. Most authorities would not recommend the routine screening of men with significant comorbidities that would result in them having a life expectancy of fewer than 10 years. One of the reasons for the controversy surrounding PSA screening is the risk of harm of testing. Elevated PSA levels frequently result in further—sometimes invasive—testing and may result in the detection of cancers that may or may not have become clinically significant. The treatment of these cancers with surgery, radiation, medical therapy, or combinations, does have significant risks, side effects, and potential harm. Further studies are currently underway to help us to be better able to address the controversies involved in PSA testing. (*USPSTF: www.preventiveservices.ahrq.gov*)

64. (D)

65. (E)

66. (C)

67. (E)

Explanations 64 through 67

Bacillus anthracis causes three diseases in humans: cutaneous, inhalation, and gastrointestinal anthrax. Cutaneous anthrax is the most common of the naturally occurring anthrax diseases. The spores of the gram-positive bacillus can survive for years in soil. The disease cutaneous anthrax occurs when the spores contaminate a wound on the skin of the victim and then start to grow. This disease occurs most commonly in agricultural areas where the soil becomes contaminated by the presence of animals. Initially a painless papule develops, followed by vesicles which then ulcerate and a black eschar forms. In the setting of cutaneous anthrax in a postal worker who has a coworker with an apparently similar disease, bioterrorism must be suspected. This type of attack occurred in the Fall of 2001, when anthrax spores were sent through the U.S. Postal system and over 20 persons were infected. In this setting, the most appropriate initial management is to immediately contact the appropriate Public Health authorities, usually the local or state health department. Appropriate treatment will also need to be instituted, under the guidance of the public health specialists, as untreated cutaneous anthrax may carry a 20% mortality rate. Antibiotic therapy would usually be with ciprofloxacin, penicillin, or doxycycline. Anthrax does not spread from person to person, so quarantine is not necessary. Inhalation anthrax is caused by the direct inhalation of spores into the lungs and gastrointestinal anthrax, the least common of the anthrax syndromes, is caused by ingestion.

Smallpox does not occur naturally anywhere in the world. Therefore, any suspicion of smallpox must be assumed to be a bioterror event and must be reported immediately to public health officials. Physicians should be able to recognize the signs and symptoms of smallpox and be able to distinguish them from the common occurrence of chickenpox. Chickenpox lesions tend to occur in clusters and evolve asynchronously. They are often described as "dew drops on a rose petal" as they are vesicles occurring on an erythematous base. The lesions tend to start on the trunk and rapidly spread outward. The rash will be associated with a fever but there are usually few to no prodromal symptoms. Because of the asynchronous growth and outbreaks, a patient will typically have lesions in different stages of evolution. In contrast, smallpox lesions tend to occur synchronously and the lesions tend to be uniform. The rash frequently occurs on the palms and soles. It typically starts on the face and arms and then spreads to the trunk and legs. The development of the rash tends to be slower than that of chickenpox. There is often a dramatic prodrome of high fever, malaise, headache, and backache for 2–4 days prior to the onset of the rash. Smallpox carries an approximately 30% mortality, while mortality associated with chickenpox is very low. (*O'Brien KK, Higdon ML, Halverson JJ. Recognition and management of bioterrorism infections. Am Fam Physician 2003;67: 1927–1934*)

68. (A)

69. (B)

Explanations 68 and 69

The hazard ratio statistic as presented is a comparison of the rate of development of an outcome in the treatment group divided by the rate of development of the same outcome in the control group. It is a "hazard" ratio because all of the outcomes measured are adverse. A hazard ratio of 1.00 means that there is no difference in the rate of development of the outcome between the two groups. Further, if the 95% CI crosses 1.00 then there is no statistically significant difference between the two groups. From the data presented, the hazard ratio for the development of endometrial cancer is 0.83, suggesting that there may be a reduction in the risk of endometrial cancer for women on HRT. However, the 95% CI crosses 1, therefore we cannot consider this result to be statistically significant. For the other outcomes listed, the 95% CIs do not cross 1.00, thus representing statistically significant increases in the risk of CHD, pulmonary embolism, and stroke and a statistically significant reduction in the risk of hip fracture.

In Question 69, the data reveal statistically significant rates of combined cardiovascular disease and fracture risk between the two groups. The risk of cardiovascular disease is increased but the combined fracture risk is reduced in women on HRT. The combined cancer risk and total mortality do not reach the level of statistical significance. There are no data presented on quality of life in the chart, so we cannot state that option E is true. (*Women's Health Initiative Investigators. Risks and benefits of estrogen plus progestin in healthy post-menopausal women. JAMA 2002;288:321–333*)

70. **(B)** The most common reason for an unusual or unexpected finding on a pediatric growth chart is erroneous measurement. Whenever such an occurrence is noted, the first intervention should be to repeat and confirm the measurement. All of the other options may be appropriate for further evaluation and management if the abnormality noted is confirmed to be real.

BIBLIOGRAPHY

ACR Appropriateness Criteria. *Osteoporosis: Prevention and Treatment*. Ann Arbor, MI: University of Michigan Health System, 2002.

American Academy of Pediatrics: www.aap.org/advocacy/chmhets.htm.

American College of Radiology (ACR), Expert Panel on Musculoskeletal Imaging. *Osteoporosis and Bone Mineral Density*. Reston, VA: American College of Radiology (ACR), 2001, p. 17.

American Heart Association, 2004. Available at: www.americanheart.org/presenter.jhtml?identifier = 1745.

CDC. National Vital Statistics Reports, Vol. 7, No. 9, 2003.

Centers for Disease Control: www.cdc.gov.

Centers for Disease Control: www.cdc.gov/mmwr/PDF/rr/rr4906.pdf.

Centers for Disease Control: www.cdc.gov/mmwr/PDF/RR/RR5014.pdf.

Centers for Disease Control: www.cdc.gov/nip/publications/pink/tetanus.pdf.

Centers for Disease Control: www.cdc.gov/nip/publications/preg_guide.htm.

Coombes RC, Hall E, Gibson LJ, et al. A randomized trial of exemestane after two to three years of tamoxifen therapy in postmenopausal women with primary breast cancer. *N Engl J Med* 2004;350:1081–1092.

Cunningham FG, Gant NF, et al. *Williams Obstetrics*, 21st ed. New York: McGraw-Hill, 2001, pp. 1367–1376.

Dao Q, et al. Utility of B-type natriuretic peptide in the diagnosis of congestive heart failure in an urgent-care setting. *J Am Coll Cardiol* 2001;37:379–385.

Eyler AE and Cohen M. Case studies in partner violence. *Am Fam Physician* 1999;60:2569–2576.

Fitzpatrick TB, Johnson RA, Wolff K, Suurmond D. *Color Atlas and Synopsis of Clinical Dermatology*, 4th ed. New York: McGraw Hill, 2001.

Hulley SB, Cummings SR, et al. *Designing Clinical Research*, 2nd ed. Lippincott Willams & Wilkins, 2001.

Institute of Medicine. *To Err is Human: Building a Safer Health System*. Report available online at www.iom.edu/Object.File/Master/4/117/0.pdf.

Kurowski K and Chandran S. The preparticipation athletic evaluation. *Am Fam Physician* 2000;61:2683–2690, 2696–2698.

Lin KW and Kirchner JT. Hepatitis B. *Am Fam Physician* 2004;69:75–82, 86.

McKeag DB and Sallis RE. Factors at play in the athletic preparticipation examination. *Am Fam Physician* 2000;61:2617.

National Cancer Institute: cis.nci.nih.gov/fact/3_9.htm.

O'Brien KK, Higdon ML, Halverson JJ. Recognition and management of bioterrorism infections. Am Fam Physician 2003;67:1927–1934.

Sanchez-Ramos L, Oliver F, Delke I, Kaunitz AM. Labor induction versus expectant management for postterm pregnancies: A systematic review with meta-analysis. *Obstet Gynecol* 2003;101:1312–1318.

Slawson D and Shaughnessy A. *Becoming an Information Master*. Course materials, 2003.

Thompson IM, et al. The influence of finasteride on the development of prostate cancer. *N Engl J Med* 2003;349:215–224.

USPSTF: www.preventiveservices.ahrq.gov.

Women's Health Initiative Investigators. Risks and benefits of estrogen plus progestin in healthy postmenopausal women. *JAMA* 2002;288:321–333.

CHAPTER 7

Pathology
Questions

Questions 1 and 3

A full-term baby boy was noted in the immediate neonatal period to fail to pass meconium. Progressive abdominal distention was noted. Multiple laboratory and clinical tests lead to a decision to perform a rectal biopsy.

1. What is the most important histologic finding that you expect to see in the rectal biopsy?

   (A) ischemic necrosis of the bowel mucosa
   (B) acute ulcerative colitis
   (C) granulomatous inflammation
   (D) absence of ganglion cells in the rectal mucosa and submucosa
   (E) a malignant tumor

2. What special stains would you use that would be helpful to confirm the finding of ganglion cells?

   (A) periodic acid-Schiff (PAS)
   (B) mucicarmine
   (C) elastic stain
   (D) trichrome stain
   (E) acetylcholinesterase

3. The treatment of choice for Hirschsprung disease is

   (A) laxatives
   (B) colonoscopy with relief of the obstruction
   (C) surgical therapy
   (D) antiperistaltic drugs
   (E) chemotherapy

Questions 4 through 6

A 3$\frac{1}{2}$-year-old female presented with a left upper quadrant abdominal mass. The child had no previous history of medical illnesses. An ultrasound examination revealed a markedly deformed left kidney with 12 cm nonhomogenous soft tissue mass arising from the upper pole. Medial displacement of the bowel loops was also noted.

4. What would be the most likely diagnosis in this case?

   (A) hydronephrotic kidney
   (B) Wilms tumor
   (C) tuberculosis
   (D) congenital malformation
   (E) papillary transitional cell carcinoma of the renal pelvis

5. Characteristically Wilms tumors are histologically recognizable for

   (A) classic triphasic combination of blastema, stromal, and epithelial cells
   (B) epithelial elements alone
   (C) blastemic elements
   (D) focal keratinization
   (E) glandular formation

6. The survival rate of this tumor with chemotherapy, radiation therapy, and surgery is

   (A) 10%
   (B) 30%
   (C) 60%
   (D) 90%
   (E) no long-term survival can be achieved with this tumor

Questions 7 through 9

A 23-year-old female sought medical help because of a painless asymmetrical enlargement of the lower neck. The patient had no history of dyspnea, dysphagia, hoarseness, or previous radiation exposure. On physical examination, besides the enlarged asymmetrical thyroid gland, there was also a palpable lymphadenopathy. A lymph node biopsy (see Fig. 7-1) was performed. H&E stained slide shows the lesion.

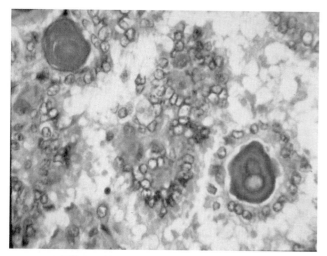

FIG. 7-1 (*Courtesy of Edison Catalano, MD.*)

7. What is the most appropriate diagnosis?

   (A) medullary carcinoma of the thyroid
   (B) follicular carcinoma
   (C) papillary carcinoma
   (D) anaplastic carcinoma
   (E) small cell anaplastic carcinoma

8. What is often present in this lesion within the papillary core?

   (A) necrosis
   (B) mitotic activity
   (C) apoptotic bodies
   (D) psammoma bodies
   (E) venular thrombosis

9. What are the typical nuclear findings of this tumor?

   (A) ground glass appearance with intranuclear inclusions
   (B) abnormal mitosis
   (C) scant cytoplasm
   (D) glandular formations
   (E) squamous metaplasia

10. The photomicrograph shown in Fig. 7-2 is of a bone biopsy. The most likely diagnosis is

   (A) benign neoplasm
   (B) cellular hyperplasia
   (C) osteogenic sarcoma
   (D) metastatic lesion
   (E) chronic leukemia

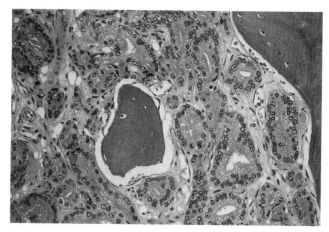

FIG. 7-2

11. The changes seen in the kidney shown in Fig. 7-3 most likely were produced by

(A) postrenal obstruction

(B) renal infarct

(C) hypertension

(D) renal cell carcinoma

(E) abuse of analgesics

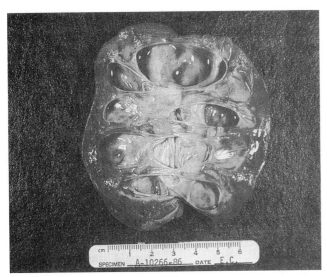

FIG. 7-3

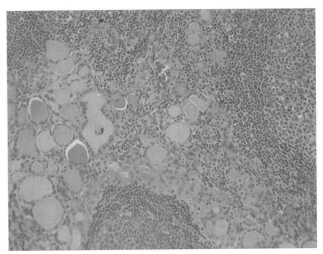

FIG. 7-4 (*Courtesy of Edison Catalano, MD.*)

Questions 12 through 14

A middle-aged female presents with a painless enlargement of the lower aspect of the neck. With appropriate testing this is proven to be thyroid enlargement. Thyroid function tests were normal. A surgical intervention was performed for diagnostic purposes. Figure 7-4 depicts a representative area of how most of the thyroid gland histologic features were seen.

12. With what is this lesion commonly associated?

(A) HLA-DR1

(B) HLA-DR5

(C) HLA-DR4

(D) HLA-DR3

(E) HLA-DR2

13. The thyroid parenchyma in this disease is characterized by

(A) leukocytic infiltrate

(B) plasma cell infiltrate

(C) lymphocytic infiltrate with germinal centers

(D) eosinophils and plasma cells

(E) dendritic cells

14. What are the clinical thyroid function test characteristics of the last stages of this disease?

(A) thyrotoxicosis

(B) normal thyroid function tests

(C) some degree of hypothyroidism

(D) invasion of the recurrent laryngeal nerve

(E) hoarseness

15. Pulmonary tuberculosis is most frequently encountered in

    (A) U.S. Whites
    (B) U.S. Blacks
    (C) Scandinavians
    (D) Black Africans
    (E) Japanese

16. Polyarteritis nodosa (PAN) typically involves

    (A) large elastic arteries
    (B) small or medium-size muscular arteries
    (C) arterioles
    (D) capillaries
    (E) venules

17. The most likely cause of the pathologic findings in the spleen shown in Fig. 7-5 is

    (A) amyloidosis
    (B) metastatic carcinoma
    (C) septic infarct
    (D) Hodgkin disease
    (E) traumatic rupture

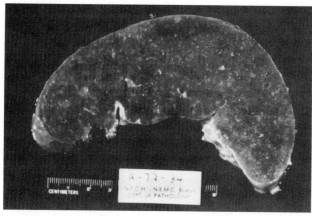

FIG. 7-5

Questions 18 through 20

A 72-year-old male presented with nonspecific symptoms of easy fatigability, weight loss, and anorexia. On physical examination, generalized lymphadenopathy and hepatosplenomegaly were present. On the peripheral blood, he was found to have a marked lymphocytosis and in the serum, a small monoclonal spike was present.

18. What would be the most likely histology seen in a lymph node biopsy?

    (A) reactive germinal centers
    (B) diffuse effacement of the normal architecture by a small lymphocytic population
    (C) diffuse architecture effacement with large cells with prominent nucleoli
    (D) a pleomorphic background composed of eosinophils, plasma cells, and small lymphocytes
    (E) a total replacement of the node by plasma cells

19. This disease is most prevalent in which age group?

    (A) teenagers
    (B) 20–30 age group
    (C) 30–40 age group
    (D) over 50 years
    (E) it may appear at any age

20. The clinical behavior of this disease is

    (A) rapidly progressive
    (B) never relapses
    (C) can be completely eradicated by chemotherapy
    (D) the median survival is 4–6 years
    (E) never responds to chemotherapeutic agents

21. Which of the following non-Hodgkin's lymphoma are considered high grade in the working formulation classification?

    (A) Burkitt's lymphoma
    (B) follicular small cell cleaved lymphoma
    (C) diffuse small and large cell cleaved lymphoma
    (D) small lymphocytic lymphoma
    (E) mucosal associated lymphoid tissues (MALT) lymphoma

22. Which of the following represents irreversible morphologic changes associated with cell death?

(A) hydropic swelling
(B) fatty metamorphosis
(C) apoptosis
(D) hypertrophy
(E) atrophy

23. Which of the following is most likely to be associated with systemic effects caused by products of the tumor?

(A) osteogenic sarcoma
(B) follicular adenoma of thyroid
(C) papillary carcinoma of thyroid
(D) pheochromocytoma
(E) anaplastic carcinoma of thyroid

24. Which is the most common benign tumor of the breast?

(A) lipoma
(B) fibroadenoma
(C) hemangioma
(D) intraductal papilloma
(E) phylloides tumor, benign

25. In inflammatory carcinoma of the breast, what are the most prominent histologic changes?

(A) carcinoma with dense fibrous stroma
(B) carcinoma with a lymphatic stroma
(C) groups of carcinoma cells filling dermal vascular channels
(D) neutrophils in the skin overlying the carcinoma
(E) single carcinoma cells infiltrating the dermis

26. Duct dilatation, fibrosis, apocrine metaplasia, epitheliosis, and cyst formations are some of the histologic changes seen in

(A) acute mastitis
(B) fibroadenoma
(C) lobular carcinoma –in situ
(D) fibrocystic breast disease
(E) atypical ductal hyperplasia

Questions 27 through 29

A 67-year-old female was admitted to the hospital because of chronic fatigue and low back pain. An x-ray of the vertebral column showed diffuse osteoporosis and compression fractures of L1 and L2 vertebral bodies. The complete blood count (CBC) was within normal limits. The peripheral blood smear showed rouleaux formation. The immunoelectrophoresis showed a monoclonal spike of more than 3 g. A bone marrow biopsy was performed and showed an increase of more than 20% in plasma cells (see Fig. 7-6).

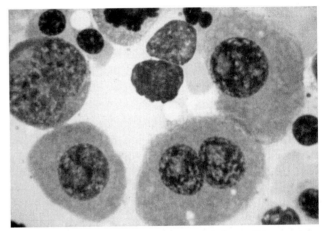

FIG. 7-6 (*Courtesy of Edison Catalano, MD.*)

27. Radiograph of the bone and skeletal system in multiple myeloma will more characteristically show

(A) fractures
(B) osteoblastic lesions
(C) destructive bone lesions throughout the skeletal system
(D) the skeletal system will remain intact
(E) changes that resemble Paget disease

28. In this particular patient what would be the electrophoretical characteristic changes?

(A) increases levels of IgG and light chains in the urine
(B) IgM spike
(C) IgA elevation
(D) increase in albumin
(E) polyclonal electrophoretic pattern

29. Microscopically the bone marrow examination will reveal

    (A) normocellular marrow with normal hematopoiesis
    (B) an increase in myeloid elements
    (C) increase in megakaryocytes
    (D) increase in mature lymphocytes
    (E) increase in plasma cells, usually more than 30% of the total cells

30. What type of cell is necessary to make the diagnosis of Hodgkin's disease?

    (A) Reed-Sternberg cells
    (B) lacunar cells
    (C) eosinophils
    (D) plasma cells
    (E) dendritic cells

31. Which type of Hodgkin's disease has the worst prognosis?

    (A) lymphocytic depletion type
    (B) lymphocytic predominance type
    (C) nodular sclerosing type
    (D) mixed cellularity type
    (E) there is no difference

32. Which is the most common pathologic finding in lymph nodes that are close to a malignant neoplasm?

    (A) acute lymphadenitis
    (B) follicular hyperplasia
    (C) paracortical hyperplasia
    (D) granulomatous inflammation
    (E) sinus histiocytosis

33. Which of the following is the lowest grade type of lymphoma?

    (A) Burkitt's lymphoma
    (B) diffuse small cleaved cell lymphoma
    (C) large cell immunoblastic lymphoma
    (D) lymphoblastic lymphoma
    (E) small lymphocytic lymphoma

Questions 34 through 36

34. A 62-year-old male, who has been smoking two packs of cigarettes a day for the past 35 years, was found to have a 2.5 cm peripheral solitary nodule in the left upper lobe of lung. Thoracotomy with biopsy was performed and a picture of the biopsy findings is depicted in Fig. 7-7. With the clinical information and the biopsy findings what would be the most likely diagnosis?

    (A) pulmonary infarct
    (B) adenocarcinoma
    (C) small cell anaplastic carcinoma
    (D) tuberculosis
    (E) granulomatous inflammation

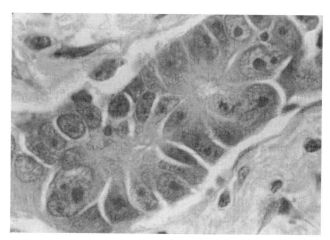

FIG. 7-7 (*Courtesy of Edison Catalano, MD.*)

35. In adenocarcinomas of the lung, frequently the neoplastic cells show in the cytoplasm large amounts of

    (A) mucin
    (B) glycogen
    (C) lipofusin pigment
    (D) iron
    (E) fat droplets

36. In what type of bronchogenic carcinoma are peripheral solitary nodules of the lungs most frequently found?

(A) squamous cell carcinoma
(B) adenocarcinoma
(C) small cell carcinoma
(D) large cell carcinoma
(E) carcinoid tumor

37. A 32-year-old female was seen by her family physician because of an enlarged and pigmented lesion of her back. On examination, the lesion measures 2×1.5 cm and it is variegated by hues of brown, black, and pink areas. The central area appears to ulcerate. A biopsy of the area was performed. What would be the most likely diagnosis?

(A) malignant melanoma
(B) keratoacanthoma
(C) drug eruption
(D) squamous cell carcinoma
(E) dermatofibroma

Questions 38 through 40

38. A 65-year-old postmenopausal woman relates a complaint of being excessively tired for 6 months. Her laboratory results were remarkable for a microcytic anemia and elevated carcinoembryonic antigen (CEA). A barium enema followed by a biopsy revealed a mass of the right colon. After the initial biopsy, a right colectomy was performed (see Fig. 7-8). What would be the most likely diagnosis?

(A) adenomatous polyp
(B) lipoma of the cecal valve
(C) adenocarcinoma of the right colon
(D) eschemic colitis
(E) Crohn disease

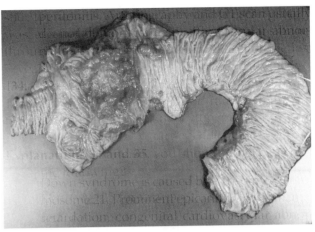

FIG. 7-8 (*Courtesy of Edison Catalano, MD.*)

39. Adenocarcinoma of the colon is more frequently associated with which of the following?

(A) Crohn's disease
(B) diverticulosis
(C) hamartomatous polyp
(D) pseudomembranous colitis
(E) ulcerative colitis

40. Cytoplasmic granules that stain positive on immunoperoxidase technique for neuron-specific enolase and chromogranin are characteristics of which of the following?

(A) adenomatous polyp
(B) lymphoma
(C) adenocarcinoma
(D) squamous cell carcinoma
(E) carcinoid tumor

41. Which of the following is the most common characteristic of a serous cystadenocarcinoma of the ovary?

(A) It causes pseudomyxoma peritonei.
(B) It is composed of transitional epithelial cells.
(C) It is frequently bilateral.
(D) It is most common in children and young adults.
(E) It often metastasizes to the brain.

42. A 28-year-old female shows clinical manifestations related to secretion of excess androgenic hormones and persistent anovulation. What would be the most likely finding in the ovary?

   (A) endometriosis
   (B) polycystic ovary
   (C) endometrioid carcinoma of the ovary
   (D) granulosa cell tumor of the ovary
   (E) mature cystic teratoma

43. In IgA nephropathy (Buerger disease) electron deposits are found most prominently in which of the following compartments?

   (A) the walls of the small veins
   (B) the walls of the arterials and small arteries
   (C) tubular basement membranes
   (D) glomerular capillary basement membrane
   (E) mesangium

44. A 60-year-old male developed painless hematuria. On further clinical evaluation, a CT scan showed a 7 cm mass on the lower pole of the right kidney. What would be your most likely diagnosis in this case?

   (A) neuroblastoma
   (B) medullary fibroma
   (C) Wilms tumor
   (D) transitional cell carcinoma
   (E) renal cell carcinoma

45. Which of the following testicular tumors is grossly and microscopically characterized by hemorrhage, necrosis, and mostly composed of cytotrophoblastic and syncytiotrophoblastic cells?

   (A) embryonal carcinoma
   (B) seminoma
   (C) teratoma
   (D) choriocarcinoma
   (E) yolk sac tumor

46. An 18-year-old male developed chills, fever, and a painful swollen knee. What test would be most appropriate in order to help in making the diagnosis?

   (A) culture of joint fluid from the affected knee
   (B) Lyme disease test
   (C) magnetic resonance imaging
   (D) serum protein electrophoresis
   (E) study of crystals in the synovium

Questions 47 and 48

47. What is the most common location of 60% of osteogenic sarcomas?

   (A) skull
   (B) spine
   (C) pelvic bones
   (D) metaphyseal ends of distal femur and proximal tibia
   (E) sternum

48. What group is most affected by osteosarcoma?

   (A) 5–10 years, female
   (B) 10–20 years, male
   (C) 40–60 years, female
   (D) 75 and older, male
   (E) anyone regardless of age or sex

49. Which of the following malignant tumors shows at least 85% translocation of chromosomes 11 and 22?

   (A) osteosarcoma
   (B) osteoblastoma
   (C) metastatic carcinoma
   (D) multiple myeloma
   (E) Ewing sarcoma

50. Which of the following bone neoplasms is most likely to have osteoclasts?

   (A) chondrosarcoma
   (B) giant cell tumor
   (C) osteosarcoma
   (D) osteochondroma
   (E) osteoid osteoma

Questions 51 through 53

A 23-year-old male, known IV drug abuser, presents to the emergency room with a cough and fever. On examination, his temperature is 101°F, his respiratory rate is 30, his pulse is 105, and BP is 100/70. He has diffuse wheezes on auscultation of his lungs. A chest x-ray reveals a "ground-glass" appearing infiltrate. Along with appropriate treatment of his current infection, you order an HIV test.

51. Which cells are markedly depleted in HIV infection?

   (A) pre-B lymphocytes
   (B) mature plasma cells
   (C) cytotoxic-suppressor T lymphocytes
   (D) helper/inducer T cell lymphocytes
   (E) cells of the monocyte/macrophage lineage

52. In an HIV-infected individual, the monocytes/macrophages will

   (A) form caseating granulomas
   (B) be immediately killed by the HIV
   (C) become a highly malignant neoplasm
   (D) directly lyse T4 lymphocytes
   (E) serve as a reservoir and carriers of the HIV

53. By what mechanism does lymphoid hyperplasia occur in patients with HIV?

   (A) productive infection of T4 lymphocytes by HIV
   (B) destruction of polymorphonuclear leukocytes
   (C) productive infection of the T8 lymphocytes by HIV
   (D) productive infection of monocytes/macrophages by HIV
   (E) direct activation of B lymphocytes by HIV

Questions 54 through 56

54. What is required for a killer cell to lyse another cell?

   (A) It must be coated with IgE.
   (B) It must be coated with IgM.
   (C) It must be coated with IgG.
   (D) It has bound histamine.
   (E) It expresses CD3.

55. What action is more pertinent of interleukin-2?

   (A) It increases chemotaxis of eosinophils.
   (B) It promotes B cell differentiation.
   (C) It increases immunoglobulin secretions.
   (D) It activates macrophages.
   (E) It induces T cell proliferation.

56. An increase in interferon gamma in delayed hypersensitivity will promote

   (A) expression of alpha II macroglobulin on all cells
   (B) killing of microorganisms and neoplastic cells by macrophages
   (C) chemotaxis and phagocytosis by neutrophils
   (D) activation of the alternate complement pathway
   (E) prostacyclin secretion by endothelial cells

57. A 49-year-old female noticed that, in the morning, the small joints of her hands are swollen, painful, and stiff. Her rheumatoid factor is reportedly strongly positive. Citruline tests (CCP) are also positive. What disease does the patient most likely have?

   (A) degenerative joint disease
   (B) rheumatoid arthritis
   (C) spondyloarthritis
   (D) tennis elbow
   (E) septic arthritis

58. Goodpasture's syndrome is characterized by autoantibodies to

   (A) platelet surface antigens
   (B) basement membrane
   (C) parietal cell antigens
   (D) colonic mucosal cells
   (E) macrophage receptors

59. A hemorrhagic infarct would most likely occur in which site?

   (A) spleen
   (B) kidney
   (C) anterior left cardiac ventricle
   (D) posterior left cardiac ventricle
   (E) lung

Answers and Explanations

1. **(D)**

2. **(E)**

3. **(C)**

Explanations 1 through 3

Hirschsprung disease usually manifests in the immediate neonatal period by failure to pass meconium, followed by obstructive constipation. Abdominal distention develops and, in general, a large segment of the colon is involved and distended. The incidence of Hirschsprung disease is 1 in 5000 live births, with an 80% male predominance in nonfamilial cases. There is no apparent difference in occurrence among races. A number of abnormalities have been associated with Hirschsprung disease, including Down syndrome (2–3% of the cases), congenital heart disease, colonic atresia, and malrotation. The tissue diagnosis is made on the basis of an absence of ganglion cells in the submucosa and the myenteric plexus on a full thickness rectal biopsy. Some surgeons prefer suction biopsy to full thickness biopsy because it is easy to obtain the specimen and they can avoid scarring and fibrosis in the area. The other four choices are not applicable and can be ruled out on the basis of clinical history and an extremely low incidence of other pathologic conditions at the perinatal age.

When suction biopsies are performed, the tissue sample for acetylcholinesterase stain should be frozen as soon as possible. All of the other stains would not be helpful to identify ganglion cells. As soon as the diagnosis is confirmed with the rectal biopsy, a surgical procedure should be undertaken that consists of a resection of the aganglionic section of colon. All the other options are not the treatment of choice for this disease. *(Cotran, 6th ed., pp. 805–806)*

4. **(B)**

5. **(A)**

6. **(D)**

Explanations 4 through 6

Wilms tumor is the most common primary renal tumor in childhood, usually diagnosed between the ages of 2 and 5. The risk of Wilms tumor is increased in association with at least three recognizable groups of congenital malformations exhibiting alteration in at least two distinct chromosomal loci. A few familial cases of Wilms tumor not associated with identifiable lesions or mutations involving either the WT-1 or the WT-2 gene suggest that there may be another locus that plays a role in some tumors, but that still remains unknown. Wilms tumor presents as a large solitary mass and in 10% of cases may be bilateral. Microscopically, the Wilms tumor is characterized by recognizable attempts to recapitulate different stages of nephrogenesis. The classic triphasic combination of blastemic, stromal, and epithelial cell types is observed in the majority of the lesions. Occasional skeletal muscle differentiation can be seen, as well as squamous, mucinous epithelium, cartilage, or bone. The combined therapy of chemo, radiation, and surgery has dramatically improved the results of long-term survival in these patients, up to 90%. *(Cotran, 6th ed., pp. 487–489)*

7. **(C)**

8. **(D)**

9. **(A)**

Explanations 7 through 9

Papillary carcinoma of the thyroid is the most common form of thyroid cancer. Most cases are seen between the second and third decade of life and are associated with previous radiation therapy. Many times the first manifestation is a metastasis to the regional neck nodes. The histologic characteristics of papillary carcinoma are branching papillae with single or multiple layers of cuboidal to columnar cells. The characteristic appearance of the nucleus is rather clear, ground-glass (orphan Annie) nuclei. Characteristic intra-cytoplasmic inclusions, and occasional grooves, are seen. Psammoma bodies are often present in the papillae. The most common variant of papillary carcinoma is the follicular variant, in which the tumor cells form follicular architecture; however, the nuclear changes, as well as focal areas of papillary structures, are enough to make the differential diagnosis from follicular carcinoma. (Cotran, 6th ed., pp. 1143–1144)

10. **(D)** The photomicrograph accompanying the question shows bone marrow spaces replaced by a well-differentiated adenocarcinoma. The bone spicules are normal. The glandular structures replacing the interspicular spaces and replacing the marrow elements are diagnostic of metastatic adenocarcinoma. (Cotran, 5th ed., pp. 268–271)

11. **(A)** The photograph that accompanies the question demonstrates severe hydronephrosis, which is due to obstruction of the flow of urine. The obstruction may be located at any site along the urinary outflow tract and may be partial or total, unilateral or bilateral. Because glomerular filtration may continue for some time after the development of the obstruction, the renal pelvis and calices become dilated by continued urine production. The resultant backpressure produces atrophy of the renal parenchyma with obliteration of the pyramids. The degree of hydronephrosis depends on the extent and rapidity of the obstructive process. (Cotran, 5th ed., p. 988)

12. **(B)**

13. **(C)**

14. **(C)**

Explanations 12 through 14

Hashimoto's thyroiditis is a very common cause of hypothyroidism in the parts of the world where iodine levels are insufficient. The clinical picture is characterized by a gradual enlargement of the thyroid gland with autoimmune destruction. There is a great female to male predominance, with a ratio of 10–20:1. Clusters of families are seen which are associated with HLA-DR5 on the major histocompatibility complex (MHC). A few cases are also characterized by HLA-DR3. The pathogenesis is attributed to cellular and humoral immunity which produces thyroid tissue injury. The morphology of the thyroid gland is characterized by typical destruction of the thyroid parenchyma with dense lymphocytic infiltrate and many secondary germinal centers. Occasional scattered Hurthle cells are also seen. Depending on the stage of the disease, extensive areas of fibrosis may also be present. The clinical course of Hashimoto's thyroiditis is usually an initial period of time in which the patient may be euthyroid followed by hypothyroidism. (Cotran, 6th ed., pp. 1134–1135)

15. **(D)** Although pulmonary tuberculosis is worldwide, changes in public health awareness and treatments have reduced the incidence of the disease in many of the developed Western countries, although sporadic cases still occur, particularly in the poorer areas of these countries. Blacks in the United States have a higher rate of tuberculosis than U.S. Whites. The disease is very much reduced in modern times in Scandinavians and in Japanese. However, Black Africa is certainly the area where tuberculosis still remains one of the major causes of morbidity and mortality. It has been said that tuberculosis is the great tropical disease of Africa and still represents a major life-threatening disease to its inhabitants. (Cotran, 5th ed., p. 349)

16. **(B)** PAN typically involves small- to medium-sized muscular arteries. In contrast, large arteries and the aorta are involved in Takayasu's arteritis. Small arteries and arterioles are involved in a number of other diseases, including systemic lupus erythematosus. Active

lesions in PAN demonstrate a neutrophilic infiltration of the involved vessel wall with thrombosis and segmental, fibrinoid necrosis. Intermittent healing produces fibrosis of the arterial wall and intimal thickening, which may lead to obstruction and infarction. Aneurysmal dilations may arise as a result of asymmetrical involvement. Although the lesions in PAN resemble other immune-mediated vascular lesions, the exact etiology of the disorder has not been elucidated. PAN generally affects middle-aged men and has a poor prognosis, although steroids may be beneficial. *(Cotran, 5th ed., pp. 520–521)*

17. **(A)** Amyloidosis is caused by the deposition of an abnormal proteinaceous material between cells. The majority of the cases are idiopathic, but a small percentage is secondary to chronic infection or inflammation, plasma cell dyscrasias, or immune diseases. One of the characteristic presentations of amyloidosis is splenic infiltration and splenomegaly caused by deposition of amyloid in the follicular regions. Grossly, the spleen has a diffuse, pink, glassy, waxy appearance with obliteration of the white pulp. Amyloid infiltration can also affect the kidneys, liver, and heart. Clinical symptoms are usually due to functional impairment of the diseased organ. The diagnosis of amyloidosis is made by tissue biopsy or, more recently, by fat-pad biopsy looking for amyloid deposits. With Congo red stain, amyloid appears red; with polarization, it shows an apple-green birefringence, which is diagnostic of amyloid. *(Cotran, 5th ed., pp. 251–257)*

18. **(B)**

19. **(D)**

20. **(D)**

Explanations 18 through 20

Chronic lymphocytic leukemia is a disease that presents generally over the age of 50 with a male predominance. For a long time many of these patients remain asymptomatic and, when they do present, the symptomatology is nonspecific, with generalized lymphadenopathy and hepatosplenomegaly. The peripheral lymphocyte count is generally high and composed of small lymphocytes. A low percentage of patients develop autoantibodies directed against red cells or platelets, which produces autoimmune hemolytic anemia or thrombocytopenia. Although the disease progresses and relapses in spite of the chemotherapy treatment, the overall median survival is 4–6 years, but this appears to be very variable. Some patients may survive longer than 10 years. All of the parameters for a worse prognosis have to be measured before a final statement of prognosis can be made. The lymph node architecture is diffusely effaced by a population of small lymphocytes, which contain nondiscernible cytoplasm and inconspicuous nucleoli. Mitotic activity is rare, focal proliferation centers with an increase in the number of mitotic activity cells are seen. *(Cotran, 6th ed., pp. 658–659)*

21. **(A)** Burkitt's lymphoma is a neoplasm of B cell lymphocytes that is classified as a high-grade lymphoma of the small, noncleaved cell type, according to the National Cancer Institute's new working formulation classification system for non-Hodgkin's lymphomas. The search for the cause of Burkitt's lymphoma has revealed an association with the Epstein-Barr virus (EBV) in many cases. In endemic African Burkitt lymphoma, 80–90% of tumors contain copies of the EBV DNA genome. However, in the sporadic, and less frequent, nonendemic cases of Burkitt's lymphoma, there has been an infrequent association with EBV (15–20% of cases). The search for a chromosomal abnormality has revealed an 8-14q translocation in many cases. However, this translocation is not apparent in 10–20% of cases nor is it identified in all tumor cells in any given Burkitt's lymphoma. Despite many hypotheses, the cause of Burkitt's lymphoma remains unclear. *(Cotran, 5th ed., pp. 662–663)*

22. **(C)** Apoptosis occurs when a cell dies through activation of an internally controlled suicide program. It is a subtly orchestrated disassembly of cellular components designed to eliminate unwanted cells during embryogenesis and various physiologic processes. Apoptosis should be distinguished from coagulative necrosis for

several histologic, as well as electron microscopy, changes. Those are: (1) cell shrinkage; (2) chromatin condensation; (3) formation of cytoplasmic blebs and apoptotic bodies; (4) phagocytosis of apoptotic cells or bodies. Hydropic swelling is a form of reversible cell injury due to accumulation of fluid within the cisternae of the endoplasmic reticulum. Subcellular alterations also occur in the cell in response to sublethal stimulae, such as accumulation of lipid in the cytoplasm (fatty metamorphosis). Hypertrophy, as well as atrophy, are adaptive responses of cells, either with an increase or decrease in cell function. (Cotran, 5th ed., pp. 2–4, 18–25)

23. **(D)** Although many tumors can produce systemic effects by means of products of the tumor cells, pheochromocytoma is by far the best choice of the ones listed. In a high proportion of cases it produces adrenalin and noradrenaline-like substances that cause dramatic changes in the vasculature and in blood pressure. It is often the symptoms produced by these substances, the by-products of which can also be measured in the urine, that first bring to light the presence of the tumor. Osteogenic sarcoma does not produce such effects and neither does anaplastic carcinoma of the thyroid. Follicular adenoma of the thyroid may occasionally be associated with increased uptake of radioactive iodine, but does not produce the thyrotoxicosis characteristically seen in some cases of follicular thyroid carcinoma. Papillary carcinoma of the thyroid rarely produces such effects. (Cotran, 5th ed., pp. 1164–1166)

24. **(B)** Fibroadenoma is the most common benign neoplasm of the breast and is composed of two types of tissue. A mesenchymal element most commonly composed of edematous or collagenized fibrous tissue and an epithelial component, which consists of compressed, and sometimes hyperplastic, irregular ductal lumens. They are usually found in young women and may be hormonally reactive during pregnancy or menopause. (Cotran, 6th ed., pp. 1102–1103)

25. **(C)** When a tumor of the breast invades the lymphatics, as well as the venules, of the skin, it clinically produces a skin reaction that is reddish in color and, for that reason, is called inflammatory carcinoma of the breast. This dermal lymphatic invasion correlates with the prognosis, which, in this particular case, is poor despite the triple therapy modality (radiation, chemotherapy, and surgery). (Cotran, 6th ed., pp. 1113–1114)

26. **(D)** Fibrocystic disease is a common benign disease of the breast that usually affects women between the ages of 25 and 45 years. It is thought to be related to hormone levels. The process is usually bilateral, but one breast is often more affected than the other. The microscopic appearance of fibrocystic disease varies. Changes may include duct dilatation with cyst formation, apocrine metaplasia, fibrosis, chronic inflammation, duct hyperplasia, papillomatosis, and lobular distortion. Acute mastitis is seen most frequently in the earliest week of nursing and is secondary to bacterial infections developing in cracks or fissures of the nipples, most frequently by *Staphylococcus*. Fibroadenoma of the breast is the most common benign tumor of the female breast and, as its word implies, is composed of both fibrous and glandular tissues. Neither lobular carcinoma nor atypical ductal hyperplasia are features of fibrocystic disease. (Cotran, 5th ed., pp. 1098–1100)

27. **(C)**

28. **(A)**

29. **(E)**

Explanations 27 through 29

Multiple myeloma is a plasma cell dyscrasia that is characterized by involvement of the skeleton in multiple sites. The characteristic x-ray shows punched-out bone lesions that are very easily seen in the calvarium. Extension of the disease to lymph nodes and extranodal sites, such as skin, can be seen. The bone marrow biopsy and smears reveal an increased number of plasma cells, which usually constitute greater than 20% of all of the cells. The cells either diffusely infiltrate and replace the marrow elements or can be seen scattered throughout the hematopoietic elements. The neoplastic plasma cells have a perinuclear halo of an eccentrically placed nucleus which allows the recognition. In 99% of patients with multiple myeloma, electrophoretic analysis reveals increased levels of IgG in the blood, light chains (Bence-Jones proteins) in the urine, or both. The monoclonal IgG produces a high spike when seen in the serum or in the urine, subject to electrophoresis. In general, the quantitative analysis of the monoclonal IgG is more than 3 g. The clinicopathologic diagnosis of multiple myeloma rests on radiographic and laboratory findings. Marrow examination may reveal increased plasma cells or sheet-like aggregates that may completely replace the normal elements. The prognosis for this condition is variably, but generally poor. *(Cotran, 6th ed., pp. 664–666)*

30. **(A)** The Reed-Sternberg cell can be classified as the classic type, the mononuclear variant, the lymphocytic histiocytic variant, lacunar and pleomorphic variant. The classic Reed-Sternberg cell is a binucleated cell that contains an ovoid-shaped nucleus with regular contours and prominent eosinophilic nucleoli. Cytoplasm is abundant and eosinophilic. On cytogenetic studies, the Reed-Sternberg cells are either aneuploid or frequently hypertetraploid. The classic Reed-Sternberg cell is thought to be an end-stage cell that does not divide. The mononuclear variants of the Reed-Sternberg cells (so-called Hodgkin's cells) could be identified in any type of Hodgkin's disease, but they are not diagnostic of Hodgkin's. *(Cotran, 6th ed., pp. 670–675)*

31. **(A)** Lymphocytic depletion type Hodgkin's disease represents the most aggressive form of Hodgkin's disease. In general, it presents in middle-aged to elderly males. At the time of diagnosis, it is usually in the advanced stage (either III or IV) with "B" symptoms. The cure rate for lymphocytic depleted Hodgkin's disease is approximately 40–50%. Morphologically, it is characterized by an abundance of Reed-Sternberg cells where the lymphocytes are very scattered and sparse, hence its denomination. *(Cotran, 6th ed., pp. 670–675)*

32. **(E)** Sinus histiocytosis represents hyperplasia of the endothelial lining of the sinusoids, which become dilated and contain many histiocytes. This reaction, which is also called reticular hyperplasia, becomes very prominent in lymph nodes when they are draining a cancerous process. This is particularly common in the axillary nodes when cancer of the breast has been detected. It is thought to represent an immune response to the host against the tumor products. *(Cotran, 6th ed., p. 650)*

33. **(E)** Small lymphocytic lymphoma is a neoplastic proliferation of small mature lymphocytes that, morphologically and phenotypically, are indistinguishable from chronic lymphocytic leukemia. The morphology of this process is a replacement of the normal lymph node architecture by a diffuse proliferation of the small lymphocytes with very condensed chromatin pattern and indiscernible cytoplasm. Occasionally, we may see areas in which the cells become slightly enlarged and these centers are called proliferating centers. The clinical features show that most of the patients are elderly and have been asymptomatic for a long time. They generally present with lymphadenopathy and splenomegaly. The prognosis of this neoplasm is variable, but patients that present with a small tumor burden may survive for more than 10 years. Transformation of this process into a more aggressive B cell lymphoma is seen in about 10% of patients. All of the other lymphomas mentioned in the answers are high-grade lymphomas. *(Cotran, 6th ed., pp. 658–659)*

34. **(B)**

35. **(A)**

36. **(B)**

Explanations 34 through 36

The incidence of adenocarcinoma of the lung has increased significantly in the last two decades and is now the most common form of lung cancer in women and, in some studies, also in men. There may be mixtures of histologic patterns in the same cancers and, therefore, the finding of squamous cell carcinoma is not infrequent. A recent classification that is more common for clinical use has been developed in response to the necessity for the different therapies. These two large groups are divided into small cell versus nonsmall cell carcinomas. On histologic examination, the adenocarcinomas can be divided into bronchial-derived adenocarcinoma and bronchioloalveolar carcinoma. This classification is based on histologic findings alone. The lesions, in general, are peripherally located and tend to be smaller. Adenocarcinoma, including the bronchioloalveolar variant, is the least frequently associated with a history of cigarette smoking. Special stains for mucin are frequently positive. (Cotran, 6th ed., pp. 743–744)

37. **(A)** Malignant melanoma is a malignant neoplasm of the melanocyte. Most melanomas arise in the basal layer of the epidermis and remain confined to the epidermis in a radial growth phase for sometime. Later in the tumor development, it will grow down into the dermis (vertical growth phase) and gain access to the lymphatics. Clinically, most melanomas display a variegated brown, tan, pink, or black appearance. Irregular edges, enlargement and central nodular ulceration may be noted. The microscopic appearance is characterized by nests of cells and single cells with eccentrically located nuclei and prominent eosinophilic macronucleoli. Melanin is present in the cytoplasm. Squamous cell carcinomas are not pigmented and they are rare on the back. Basal cell carcinomas can sometimes be confused with the melanomas when they are the pigmented variety. (This was not a selection given.) Generally, those happen in the sun-exposed areas. The prognosis of melanoma is related to the depth of invasion measured by either the Clark's level or Breslow's thickness. Deeply invading tumor and thicker tumors are associated with poor prognosis. (Cotran, 6th ed., pp. 1177–1179)

38. **(C)**

39. **(E)**

40. **(E)**

Explanations 38 through 40

Adenocarcinoma of the colon is the most common type of malignancy arising in the large intestine. Iron deficiency and microcytic anemia may be the presenting symptoms due to the bleeding from the tumor's ulceration. Alternatively, the tumor may be suspected by detention of occult fecal blood test, bowel obstruction, or through the development of hepatic enlargement secondary to metastasis. The gross appearance of this tumor is usually polypoid and ulcerated. Many ulcerating tumors involve the full circumference of the bowel and appear radiologically as an "apple core" lesion. The microscopic appearance is that of gland-forming malignant cells and usually mucin production is present. The prognosis is related to the stage of the disease.

Ulcerative colitis is an inflammatory disease of uncertain etiology that has a relapsing course. Patients with ulcerative colitis have a higher than normal incidence of developing colon carcinoma, approximately 10%.

Carcinoid tumors originate in the neuroendocrine cells throughout the intestinal tract. The appendix is most frequently involved, followed by the terminal ileum. On histologic examination, carcinoids are composed of uniform, round cells forming small nests or cords without encapsulation. Special stains performed show neurosecretory granules in the cytoplasm, which are positive for chromogranin, neuron-specific enolase and other staining. (Cotran, 6th ed., pp. 833–836)

41. **(C)** Serous cystadenocarcinoma of the ovary is the most common malignant ovarian tumor and is frequently bilateral. Microscopically, they show a variegated appearance with papillary pattern. Different degrees of anaplasia of the cuboidal to columnar cells cover the papilla and occasional calcified concretions (Psammoma bodies) are present. These tumors almost never metastasize to the brain and they are not seen in children or young adults. (Cotran, 6th ed., pp. 1069–1070)

42. **(B)** Polycystic ovary syndrome is characterized by clinical manifestations related to the secretions of excess of androgen hormones. There is usually

a persistent anovulation, resulting clinically in irregular or absent menstruation. The ovaries are moderately enlarged and contain many small cysts located in the cortex. *(Cotran, 6th ed., p. 1066)*

43. **(E)** IgA nephropathy was described in 1968 and is primarily characterized by mesangial proliferative changes, seen on light microscopy as diffuse mesangial deposits of IgA by immunofluorescence. It is the most common type of glomerulonephritis worldwide. On electron microscopy, it is possible to demonstrate mesangial deposits on all of the glomeruli, indicating that this lesion is diffuse, not focal. Occasionally, small subendothelial deposits may be found. The pattern of immunofluorescence parallels to the distribution of the deposits seen by electron microscopy. *(Cotran, 6th ed., pp. 961–962)*

44. **(E)** The most important and frequent cause of painless hematuria is renal cell carcinoma. This symptom is usually associated with a palpable mass on the flank, as well as costovertebral pain. Occasionally, renal cell carcinomas are associated with a paraneoplastic syndrome, which includes polycythemia, hypercalcemia, hypertension, feminization or masculinization, Cushing's syndrome, and so on. The other answers listed are mostly seen in children. Transitional cell carcinoma is rarer than renal cell carcinoma and medullary fibroma is a benign tumor. *(Cotran, 6th ed., pp. 991–994)*

45. **(D)** Choriocarcinoma is a rare tumor of the testicles, but it is characterized by hemorrhage and necrosis. This tumor comprises only 1% of the malignant germ cell tumors and is rarely seen in a pure form. In general, they are small (no larger than 5 cm in diameter) and HCG can be readily demonstrated in the blood. The cells seen in the hemorrhagic areas are cytotrophoblastic, as well as syncytiotrophoblastic, cells. *(Cotran, 6th ed., pp. 1021–1022)*

46. **(A)** Because we suspect that this patient has suppurative arthritis, the test to be ordered would be a culture of the joint fluid from the affected knee to ascertain which organism is involved and, with further identification and sensitivity, to determine which would be the

antibiotic of choice. It would also be important to determine whether this is a hematogenous spread, secondary to osteomyelitis or contamination of the joint by a wound. *(Cotran, 6th ed., p. 1253)*

47. **(D)**

48. **(B)**

Explanations 47 and 48

Osteosarcoma most commonly occurs in the age group of 10–20 years (75% are under the age of 20), with a male predominance. The second most common age group is in the elderly population, but it is generally associated with other diseases such as Paget, bone infarcts, or previous radiation. Almost 50% of the osteosarcomas occur above the knee in the distal femur. *(Cotran, 6th ed., pp. 1236–1237)*

49. **(E)** Ewing sarcoma is a malignant neoplasm of the bone that originates in the medullary canal and is composed of small uniform round cells. This tumor belongs to the primitive neuroectodermal tumors (PNET) of childhood. Approximately, 85% of these tumors show the C-MYC oncogene expression and there is a reciprocal transformation of chromosomes 11 and 22. *(Cotran, 6th ed., pp. 1244–1245)*

50. **(B)** Giant cell tumors contain abundant multinucleated giant cells of the osteoclastic type. Another name for the tumor is osteoclastoma. It is a benign, locally aggressive neoplasm that is postulated to have a monocyte macrophage lineage. Grossly they are red-brown in color and undergo cystic degeneration. These lesions do not produce bone. It was thought that these tumors are always benign; recently a more aggressive type has been described in which up to 4% of these tumors metastasize to the lung. The other lesions mentioned, such as chondrosarcoma may contain areas of bone formation with calcification. Osteochondroma has a base formed by bone. In addition, osteosarcoma, particularly the well-differentiated variety, contains extensive areas of bone formation and mineralization. The osteoid osteoma also produces bony spicules. *(Cotran, 6th ed., pp. 1244–1245)*

51. (D)

52. (E)

53. (E)

Explanations 51 through 53

AIDS is caused by nontransforming human retrovirus. Two types of this virus have been found, HIV-1 and HIV-2. The HIV-1 is the most common type associated with AIDS in the United States, Europe, and central Africa. The virus infects the helper/inducer T lymphocytes, markedly impairing the function of the T cells and producing immunosuppression, affecting the cell-mediated immunity.

In addition to the loss of T cells, the monocytes and macrophages are also infected by the AIDS virus. These macrophages are not found in the peripheral blood, but rather in the tissues. More likely the macrophages are the reservoir for the human immunodeficiency virus. In the first stages of this disease, many patients present with peripheral lymphadenopathy. A biopsy of these enlarged nodes shows marked follicular hyperplasia. These follicles contain a pleomorphic amount of cells that are enlarged, irregular, and mitotically active. An attenuation of the mantle zone is seen. These enlarged germinal centers, which are composed of B cells, are showing hyperplasia of polyclonal type that is activated in patients infected with HIV particles. (*Cotran, 6th ed., pp. 238–239, 242–244*)

54. (C)

55. (E)

56. (B)

Explanations 54 through 56

Natural killer cells are a subset of T cells that can kill other cells whether neoplastic, transplanted tissue, or virus-infected cells. The lysis of cells (cytolytic action) is produced by producing holes in the surface membrane of an antigen-positive cell, particularly if it is coated with IgG. Interleukin-2 causes autocrine and paracrine proliferation of T cells. The T cells activated by interleukin-2 tend to accumulate on the sites of delayed hypersensitivity. A macrophage activation is obtained by secretion of cytokines (lymphokines) secreted by T cells, fibroblasts, and macrophages. The activation of the macrophages stimulates lysis of either organisms or neoplastic cells. Gamma interferon does not produce any activity. (*Cotran, 6th ed., p. 191*)

57. (B) In this case, the patient most likely has rheumatoid arthritis, an autoimmune chronic relapsing disorder that mostly affects the joints. The disease is usually seen in Western European and North American White females between the ages of 30 and 50. The clinical hallmark of the disease is symmetric swelling of the small joints of the hands and feet, particularly the proximal and interphalangeal joints. Swelling, pain, and stiffness are most severe in the morning. Pathologically, a pannus, or hypertrophic inflamed synovium, is produced that may eventually erode into the articular cartilage, with subsequent fibrosis, restriction of movements, and deformity. (*Cotran, 6th ed., pp. 1248–1251*)

58. (B) Goodpasture's syndrome is characterized by antibasement antibodies, with the lungs and kidneys bearing the brunt of the damage. Antibodies against platelet surface antigens, parietal cells, antigens, receptors, and colonic mucosal cells are seen in autoimmune thrombocytopenia, pernicious anemia, myasthenia gravis, and ulcerative colitis, respectively. (*Cotran, 6th ed., pp. 943–945*)

59. (E) Hemorrhagic infarcts, also called red infarcts, are usually encountered with venous occlusions. This is more likely in loose tissues, in tissues with double circulation, and in previously congested tissues. The other type of infarct, white or ischemic, is usually seen with arterial occlusion, single and arterial blood supply, and in solid tissues. The lungs characteristically have hemorrhagic infarcts. (*Cotran, 6th ed., pp. 132–133*)

BIBLIOGRAPHY

Cotran RS, Kumar V, Robbins SL. *Robbins Pathologic Basis of Disease*, 5th ed. Philadelphia, PA: W.B. Saunders, 1994.

Cotran RS, Kumar V, Collins T. *Robbins Pathologic Basis of Disease*, 6th ed. Philadelphia, PA: W.B. Saunders, 1999.

CHAPTER 8

Practice Test 1
Questions

Read each question carefully and in the order in which it is presented. Then select the one best response option of the choices offered. More than one option may be partially correct. You must select ONE BEST answer. You have 60 min to complete this test.

Setting I: Office/Health Center

You see patients in two locations: at your office suite, which is adjacent to a hospital, and at a community-based health center. Your office practice is a primary care generalist group. Most of the patients you see are from your own practice and are appearing for regularly scheduled return visits. Occasionally you will encounter a patient whose primary care is managed by one of your associates. Reference may be made to the patient's medical records. Known patients may be managed by the telephone. You may have to respond to questions about information appearing in the public media, which will require interpretation of the medical literature. The laboratory and radiology departments have a full range of services available.

1. On a routine school physical you note that an 11-year-old female has some freckles in her axillae. This is new since last year and there are no other new skin marks noted. She is doing well in school. The only other change is that there has been some increase in her scoliosis. Which condition does she likely have?

(A) Sturge Weber syndrome
(B) neurofibromatosis, type 1 ([NF-1], von Recklinghausen's disease)

(C) tuberous sclerosis
(D) CHARGE Association
(E) Beckwith-Wiedemann syndrome

Questions 2 and 3

2. A 38-year-old male is noted to have an elevated serum calcium level on yearly physical examination. A complete panel of laboratories is obtained which reveals an elevated ionized calcium, elevated serum parathyroid hormone, and a low serum phosphate level. Urine studies include a creatinine of 1.2 and a normal 24-h urine calcium excretion. Which of the following is the most likely diagnosis?

(A) metastatic prostate cancer
(B) acute renal failure
(C) sarcoidosis
(D) multiple myeloma
(E) primary hyperparathyroidism

3. Which of the following symptoms or signs would be an indication for surgical treatment in this patient?

(A) recurrent renal calculi
(B) low urinary calcium level
(C) high parathyroid hormone level
(D) high serum phosphate level
(E) lymphadenopathy found on a chest x-ray

Questions 4 through 6

A 62-year-old woman presents to the office with diarrhea. She is well-known to you, as you recently discharged her from the hospital after a 4-day admission for pneumonia. She has completed a course of a macrolide antibiotic. She is now having about 10 watery bowel movements a day. She has mild abdominal cramps and fever, but denies vomiting or blood in her stool. On examination, she is mildly ill appearing. Her temperature is 101°F and otherwise normal vital signs. Her abdominal examination is notable for hyperactive bowel sounds and diffuse, mild tenderness without rebound or guarding. A stool occult blood test is negative.

4. Which of the following tests is most likely to yield a diagnosis?

    (A) fecal leukocytes
    (B) stool culture
    (C) stool for ova and parasites
    (D) Gram stain of fresh stool specimen
    (E) stool for *Clostridium difficile* toxin

5. What would be the most appropriate management at this time?

    (A) oral rehydration only
    (B) antidiarrheal agent only
    (C) oral ciprofloxacin
    (D) oral metronidazole
    (E) oral vancomycin

6. The patient calls you on the phone 3 days later stating that she continues to have 10 watery stools a day and is still running a low-grade fever. Since you saw her in the office, the diagnostic test that you ordered initially came back with a positive result, confirming your suspicion. Which of the following would be the best intervention at this time?

    (A) increase the dose of the oral antibiotic you initially started
    (B) start oral vancomycin
    (C) start intravenous metronidazole
    (D) start intravenous vancomycin
    (E) perform a colonoscopy to confirm diagnosis

Questions 7 and 8

A 33-year-old married male is seen in the office for a routine visit. He comes to the appointment with his wife but enters the examination room alone. He quickly becomes tearful and, with further questioning, admits that he has been feeling "down" for the past several months. He feels fatigued and has lost 10 lbs. He casually mentions that "my life is not worth living." Consideration is given to hospitalizing this individual.

7. What is the most appropriate approach for this patient?

    (A) ask him directly if he has thoughts of suicide
    (B) immediately call in his wife and ask about suicide
    (C) inform him that his wife will not be told if he is suicidal
    (D) reassure him that his life is worth living
    (E) wait for him to bring up the subject of suicide

8. Which statement regarding his risk of suicide is most accurate?

    (A) If he has a family history of suicide, he will be more likely to attempt suicide.
    (B) If he has concurrent anxiety symptoms, he will be less likely to attempt suicide.
    (C) If he has prior suicide attempts, he will be less likely to make a lethal attempt.
    (D) If he is asked about a plan for suicide, he will be more likely to attempt suicide.
    (E) If he is severely suicidal, he will be less likely to respond to treatment.

9. A better control of cervical carcinoma has been attributed to which of the following?

    (A) early radical hysterectomy
    (B) external beam radiation therapy
    (C) treatment of precursor lesion after detection by cytology screening
    (D) development of multiagent chemotherapeutic regimes
    (E) public awareness of the risk factors for cervical cancer

Questions 10 and 11

A 64-year-old male has been suffering from lower back pain for over 10 years. You have been following him for this period. You have prescribed stretching exercises and, occasionally, an anti-inflammatory medication to alleviate his pain. Although he has had no neurologic deficits in the past, today he has shown up in your office unexpectedly, complaining of bilateral lower back pain with numbness and tingling over the dorsal aspect of both feet. His symptoms have become progressively worse over the past 2 weeks and he is now unable to stand for more than 5 min without developing extreme pain and numbness. His symptoms are much improved by sitting down or kneeling over a chair. Climbing stairs seems to be tolerated well, but walking greatly exacerbates the pain. He denies bladder or bowel incontinence or retention, point tenderness or anesthesia in the lower back along the spinal cord or in the saddle area.

10. What is the likely diagnosis?

    (A) spondyloathropathy of the sacro-illiac joint
    (B) age-related early degenerative joint disease (DJD) of the hips
    (C) spinal stenosis of the lumbo-sacral area
    (D) muscle spasm of the lower back
    (E) cauda equina syndrome

11. Which of the following imaging studies would be most helpful to confirm the diagnosis?

    (A) an MRI of the lumbo-sacral spine
    (B) an x-ray of the lumbo-sacral spine
    (C) a indium-tagged white blood cell (WBC) scan
    (D) a bone scan of the sacrum
    (E) nerve conduction study of the legs bilaterally

12. Which of the following statements regarding gastric lymphoma is true?

    (A) It is the second most common site of primary intestinal lymphoma (small bowel is first).
    (B) Chemotherapy is the treatment of choice.
    (C) Gastrointestinal bleeding is the most common presenting symptom.
    (D) Stage III disease is usually cured after resection alone.
    (E) In most cases, radiation therapy provides a long-standing remission that may be equal to that of resection.

Questions 13 through 16

A 36-year-old Black male presents to your clinic for a well adult examination. He has no significant medical history. His only medication is prn loratadine (Claritin) for occasional allergic rhinitis symptoms. His family history is positive for hypertension and coronary artery disease in his father, who died of a heart attack at age 81. His brother was diagnosed with prostate cancer at age 62 but is cancer free now. Mother is alive at age 80 with Alzheimer's disease and osteoarthritis. He has two healthy children aged 15 and 12. He denies tobacco or recreational drug use. He drinks a "couple of beers" on weekends. His vital signs in the clinic showed BP 134/80, HR 76, RR 18, temperature 97.9°F, and a body mass index (BMI) of 30.

13. Which of the following tests would be recommended at this visit?

    (A) a "baseline" electrocardiogram (ECG)
    (B) colonoscopy for colon cancer screening
    (C) rectal examination and prostate-specific antigen level for prostate cancer screening
    (D) complete blood count (CBC)
    (E) total cholesterol and high-density lipoprotein (HDL) cholesterol

14. He asks you if he needs any vaccinations at this time. You recommend

    (A) hepatitis A vaccine (HAV)
    (B) hepatitis B vaccine (HBV)
    (C) measles, mumps, rubella (MMR) booster every 10 years
    (D) diphtheria-tetanus (dT) booster every 10 years
    (E) pneumococcal vaccine

15. Two weeks later, the patient returns with the following results of a fasting lipid panel from a health fair at work: total cholesterol 234 mg/dL, triglyceride 158 mg/dL, LDL 153 mg/dL, HDL 38 mg/dL.

This patient's recommended low-density lipoprotein (LDL) goal is less than

(A) 160 mg/dL
(B) 130 mg/dL
(C) 120 mg/dL
(D) 100 mg/dL
(E) 90 mg/dL

16. To achieve this goal, you recommend

(A) continuation of his current diet and activity level as he is at his goal
(B) a prescription for cholestyramine
(C) therapeutic lifestyle changes in diet and exercise
(D) a prescription for a hydroxymethylglutaryl-coenzyme A (HMG-CoA) reductase inhibitor (statin)
(E) supplementation with over-the-counter niacin

Questions 17 and 18

A 26-year-old woman is a new referral to the primary care clinic. Review of her medical chart reveals numerous outpatient and urgent care visits over the past 12 months for different complaints relating to her concerns about having cancer. She has had extensive past workups, which were unrevealing of any significant major illness. On this visit she presents with "gas pains" and is focused on obtaining an abdominal computed tomography (CT) to diagnose her presumed stomach cancer. When educated about the low likelihood and her prior negative findings she states, "I know it's unlikely, but I can't stop feeling that I probably have stomach cancer." On further interview, she denies any past history of depression or substantial anxiety, except relating to her fears of developing a malignancy.

17. Which of the following is her most likely diagnosis?

(A) body dysmorphic disorder
(B) conversion disorder
(C) delusional disorder, somatic type
(D) hypochondriasis
(E) somatization disorder

18. Which of the following would be the most beneficial approach in treating this patient?

(A) confrontation regarding the lack of basis for her concerns
(B) extensive evaluation to provide reassurance
(C) initiation of a serotonin-specific reuptake inhibitor (SSRI)
(D) referral to a psychiatrist for management
(E) regularly scheduled medical appointments

19. A 54-year-old man with hypertension, 30 pack-year history of smoking, and a family history of premature coronary artery disease has a fasting lipid profile with total cholesterol 247 mg/dL, triglycerides 210 mg/dL, HDL cholesterol 35 mg/dL, and LDL cholesterol 177 mg/dL. The patient has been maintaining a low fat, low cholesterol diet. His physician decides to place him on a statin. What is the most appropriate next step?

(A) The physician should write a prescription for a statin stating that it will lower the patient's cholesterol but with no further explanation.
(B) If the physician is of the opinion that the statin is the best therapy for the patient, there is no need to suggest any other options.
(C) The physician should explain that blood tests may need to be checked periodically to be sure the patient is tolerating the medication.

(D) The physician should not inform the patient of potential liver or muscle toxicity so as not to unduly alarm the patient.

(E) Since statins are commonly advertised and used, it is not necessary for the physician to determine if the patient has any questions about taking the new medication.

20. At what age should an evaluation for primary amenorrhea be initiated if a female adolescent has had normal linear growth (height) and normal breast and pubic hair development?

(A) 13
(B) 14
(C) 15
(D) 16
(E) 18

Questions 21 and 22

You are asked by the health department to evaluate the prevalence of lung cancer in your hometown.

21. What would be the most appropriate study design to accomplish this?

(A) randomized-controlled study
(B) case-control study
(C) cross-sectional study
(D) prospective cohort study
(E) case series

Your study reveals the following:

The prevalence of lung cancer in the eastern half of the city is 5/1000 adults.
The prevalence of lung cancer in the western half of the city is 2/1000 adults.

Further investigations reveal that the prevalence of smoking is the same throughout the city, but that the eastern part of the city has several chemical factories.

22. Which of the following statements is true?

(A) This study proves that the chemical factories increase risk of lung cancer.

(B) If the population of the two halves of town is equal then more people have lung cancer in the eastern part of the city than the western part.

(C) More people will die from lung cancer in the eastern half of the city.

(D) If the prevalence of cigarette smoking is the same in both sides of town, then the chemical factories are responsible for the development of the lung cancer.

(E) A person could reduce his risk of getting lung cancer by moving from the eastern side of town to the western.

Questions 23 and 24

A 30-year-old gravida 2 para 2 female uses an intra-uterine device (IUD) for contraception. Over the last 6 months, she complains of feeling extremely irritable around the time of her menstrual period.

23. In order to meet diagnostic criteria for premenstrual syndrome (PMS), which of the following must be true?

(A) A patient must report being irritable and bloated in the follicular phase of her menstrual cycle.

(B) A patient must admit to feeling hopeless and suicidal before her menses.

(C) A patient must complain of constipation and hot flashes with the onset of her menstrual cycle.

(D) A patient must report at least one affective symptom (e.g., irritability, anxiety, social withdrawal) and one somatic symptom (e.g., mastalgia, bloating, headache) during the 5 days before menses for at least three prior consecutive menstrual cycles as documented on a symptom calendar.

(E) A patient must admit to feeling increasingly fatigued 1 week before her menstrual period.

24. Which of the following recommendations are based on consistent scientific evidence for the treatment of premenstrual syndrome?

(A) primrose oil
(B) vitamin B_6
(C) SSRIs
(D) natural progesterone
(E) avoidance of caffeine

25. A 74-year-old White female presents to your office with a 4-month history of abdominal distention, bloating, satiety, and associated shortness of breath. She reports an involuntary weight loss of 15 lbs, with associated lethargy and malaise. Her physical examination suggests mild cachexia, fluid wave, and a palpable abdominal mass. Her pelvic examination is unremarkable with the exception of thickened nodularity appreciated within the posterior cul de sac.

What is the appropriate diagnostic test to order at this point?

(A) pelvic ultrasound
(B) endoscopic retrograde cholangiopancreatography (ERCP)
(C) pelvic MRI
(D) abdominal/pelvic CT scan
(E) abdominal plain films

Setting II: Inpatient Facilities

You have general admitting privileges to the hospital, including the children's and women's services. On occasion you will see patients in the critical care unit. Postoperative patients are usually seen in their rooms, unless the recovery room is specified. You may also be called to see patients in the psychiatric unit. There is a short-stay unit where you may see patients undergoing same-day operations or being held for observation. Also, you may visit patients in the adjacent nursing home/extended care facility and the detoxification unit.

26. A 41-year-old patient with a 20 pack-year history of smoking is admitted with weight loss, nausea, fatigue, and hypertension. There is no history of diabetes, drugs, medications, arthritis, or travel. The patient reports noticing foamy urine. On physical examination, the patient is afebrile and her blood pressure is 194/106. The patient is thin. The fundi are normal. The remainder of the examination was unremarkable. Laboratory examination reveals the WBC to be 3000, Hgb 7.0 mg/dL, platelet count 110,000. The blood urea nitrogen (BUN) is 84, Cr 5.8, albumin 2.1. The urinalysis has no red blood cells (RBCs) or WBCs but has 4+ protein. Twenty-four hour urine protein is 5.4 g/24 h.

Which of the following is the most appropriate next step to diagnose this patient's illness?

(A) a bone marrow examination to evaluate the leukopenia and anemia
(B) a chest x-ray to rule out lung cancer
(C) complement levels to evaluate for systemic lupus erythematosis
(D) an antibody to human immunodeficiency virus (HIV) by enzyme-linked immunosorbent assay (ELISA)
(E) a monospot test

27. During prolonged starvation, the central nervous system will use which of the following as its primary fuel source?

(A) glucose
(B) fatty acids
(C) protein
(D) glycogen
(E) ketones

28. A 32-year-old woman presents at 18 weeks estimated gestational age for a prenatal assessment. The fundal height measures 14 cm. A sonogram is obtained that reveals a nonviable intrauterine pregnancy. A D&C is performed that reveals a small fetus and associated hydropic swelling in some of the placental tissue. The appropriate diagnosis to explain these findings is

(A) spontaneous miscarriage

(B) cervical incompetence

(C) partial mole

(D) luteal phase defect

(E) intrauterine growth retardation

29. A 44-year-old male patient presents with frequent regurgitation of undigested food particles and dysphagia. A thorough workup including a barium esophagogram reveals a pharyngoesophageal or Zenker's diverticulum. Which of the following is true regarding the management?

(A) Upper endoscopy is the best initial diagnostic study.

(B) Proper surgical treatment has a high risk of recurrence.

(C) When an operation is performed, a diverticulectomy is required.

(D) Division of the cricopharyngeal muscle is essential.

(E) Surgical correction carries a prohibitive risk of postoperative morbidity.

30. You are assisting in the nursery and are the first to examine a newborn. On your examination you find a palpable abdominal mass. What is the most common abdominal mass in a newborn infant?

(A) hydronephrosis

(B) neuroblastoma

(C) Wilms tumor

(D) hepatoma

(E) diaphragmatic hernia

Questions 31 and 32

A 22-year-old presents with a 2-week history of fever. The patient initially had sore throat and rash, then headache and nausea. On physical examination, the patient's oral temperature is 100°F, respiratory rate is 16, BP is 110/70, and pulse is 84. There is nuchal rigidity, the throat is red, there is cervical lymphadenopathy, and a faint macular rash (see Fig. 8-1). You perform a lumbar puncture (LP) with the following results: opening pressure 8 cm of water, glucose 78, protein 30, WBC 25 with 76% lymphocytes, RBC 2, CSF VDRL is negative.

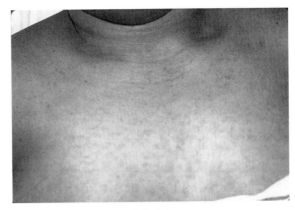

FIG. 8-1

31. What is the next most appropriate step?

(A) perform a monospot

(B) perform a rapid strep screen

(C) perform an HIV antibody test

(D) perform cultures for *Neisseria gonorrhea*

(E) perform an HIV RNA qualitative viral load

32. After getting the results of the LP, what is the next most appropriate step?

(A) treat with empiric therapy for tuberculosis

(B) treat for *Hemophilus influenza* meningitis

(C) perform an MRI scan of the head to rule out a brain tumor or lymphoma

(D) send serum antibody tests for West Nile virus

(E) consider repeating the LP in 2 days to see if there has been a change

33. Two days following a repair of an abdominal aortic aneurysm, a 57-year-old male develops episodes of bloody diarrhea. Which of the following is the most important intervention?

(A) immediate operative exploration

(B) serial hemoglobin evaluation and blood transfusion as indicated

(C) proctosigmoidoscopy

(D) arteriogram

(E) CT scan

Questions 34 and 35

A 6-year-old child with Down syndrome is noted to have a recent onset of bleeding gums and petechia on the upper torso. On CBC, the white count was found to be markedly elevated due to a monomorphic population of immature lymphoid cells (100,000).

34. What would be the most likely diagnosis in this case?

    (A) infectious mononucleosis
    (B) acute bacterial infection
    (C) septicemia
    (D) lymphoblastic leukemia
    (E) reactive lymphocytosis

35. Down syndrome is produced by the genotype

    (A) trisomy 13
    (B) trisomy 18
    (C) trisomy 21
    (D) XO
    (E) XXY

Setting III: Emergency Department

Most patients in this setting are new to you, but occasionally you arrange to meet there with a known patient who has telephoned you. Generally, patients encountered here are seeking urgent care. Also available to you are a full range of social services, including rape crisis intervention, family support, and security assistance backed up by local police.

36. A 6-month-old female infant is brought to the emergency room with vomiting and fever of 2 days duration. On examination, the infant is lethargic and appears dehydrated but has no other focal findings. Her WBC is elevated, a chest x-ray is clear, and a cath urine specimen shows WBCs and bacteria. What organism is most likely to be responsible for this infection?

    (A) group B *Streptococcus* (GBS)
    (B) herpes simplex virus

    (C) *Chlamydia trachomatis*
    (D) *Pseudomonas aerogenosa*
    (E) *Escherichia coli*

Questions 37 through 41

A 23-year-old White male, with a history of insulin-dependent diabetes mellitus and medical noncompliance, is brought into the emergency room by his girlfriend for decreased responsiveness. The girlfriend states that he ran out of his insulin 1 week ago. Moreover, he has been urinating frequently and recently started complaining of nausea, vomiting, and abdominal pain. His physical examination shows an oral temperature of 99.5°F, blood pressure of 95/40, heart rate of 125 bpm, and respiratory rate of 28. In general, he is tachypneic, lethargic, and unable to follow any commands. His mucus membranes are dry with very poor skin turgor. Cardiac examination reveals a tachycardic rate with a regular rhythm and no gallop. His lungs are clear. His abdominal examination is significant for mild diffuse tenderness but normoactive bowel sounds. His extremities are negative for edema. The laboratory results are as follows:

	Blood	Urine
Sodium	128	Specific gravity: 1.012
Potassium	6.5	Protein: trace
Chloride	92	RBCs: 1–3
CO_2	12	WBCs: 0–3
BUN	65	Ketones: 2+
Creatinine	2.0	No cellular casts
Glucose	900	

Glycosylated Hgb: 9.5
ECG: Sinus tachycardia, no ST/T wave abnormalities
Serum ketones: 3+
Arterial blood gas: pH: 7.38/pCO_2: 21/pO_2: 95
WBC: 11,300
Hgb: 16.5
HCT: 49.2
PLT: 400

37. What is this patient's "corrected" serum sodium level?

    (A) 120
    (B) 115
    (C) 141
    (D) 152
    (E) 156

38. What is this patient's acid-base status?

    (A) primary anion-gap metabolic acidosis
    (B) anion-gap and nonanion-gap metabolic acidosis
    (C) anion-gap metabolic acidosis and respiratory acidosis
    (D) anion-gap metabolic acidosis and respiratory alkalosis
    (E) anion-gap metabolic acidosis, nonanion-gap metabolic acidosis, respiratory alkalosis

39. In addition to volume replacement, which of the following statements is correct with regard to managing this patient?

    (A) His acidosis should be treated with IV sodium bicarbonate.
    (B) He should be started on subcutaneous 70/30 insulin until his blood glucose is below 200.
    (C) You should stop the intravenous insulin drip when his blood glucose is normalized.
    (D) You should start a dextrose-containing IV fluid when his blood glucose approaches 280.
    (E) You should immediately administer 60 g of kayexalate orally.

40. Four hours after the initiation of therapy, the patient complains of severe muscle weakness. Which electrolyte disturbance is most likely responsible for these symptoms?

    (A) hyperkalemia
    (B) hypocalcemia
    (C) hypophosphatemia
    (D) hypomagnesemia
    (E) hyponatremia

41. Toxic ingestion of which of the following could cause a similar acid-base disturbance?

    (A) isopropyl (rubbing) alcohol
    (B) lithium
    (C) ethylene glycol (antifreeze)
    (D) methanol
    (E) salicylate

42. Which of the following is the most likely cause of hypotension and tachycardia in an unconscious patient with an apparent isolated head injury following a high-speed motor vehicle collision?

    (A) neurogenic in origin
    (B) low plasma volume
    (C) cardiogenic in origin
    (D) herniation of the brain stem
    (E) subdural hematoma

Questions 43 and 44

A 20-year-old male is brought into the emergency room by the police after a disruption at the local college campus. According to his medical chart, he has been treated for a depressive episode in the past. He describes his mood as "great" but claims to have been awake for 4 days due to working on several inventions. He admits to rapid thoughts and believes that God has chosen him to be the next Messiah. In fact, angels have commanded him to steal from the student union in order to begin a new church.

43. Urine toxicology performed in order to rule out a substance of abuse as a cause of his symptoms would most likely reveal which substance?

    (A) alcohol
    (B) benzodiazepines
    (C) cannabis
    (D) cocaine
    (E) opiates

44. The toxicology screen is negative. The diagnosis of bipolar disorder is considered. Which of the patient's symptoms/signs is the most specific for a manic episode?

    (A) command hallucinations
    (B) decreased need for sleep
    (C) disruptive behavior
    (D) grandiose delusions
    (E) history of depression

45. A 45-year-old male sustains a stab wound to the left upper chest. In the emergency department he develops hypotension along with elevated jugular venous distention. His vital signs include a blood pressure of 90/65 and a heart rate of 135 bpm. A chest x-ray is obtained and shown in Fig. 8-2. The most appropriate intervention is

(A) bedside echocardiogram
(B) placement of a left chest tube
(C) placement of a three quarter occlusive dressing over the stab wound entrance site.
(D) needle pericardiocentesis
(E) emergency room thoracotomy

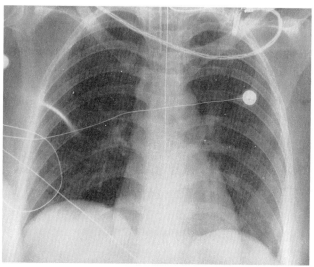

FIG. 8-2 (Reproduced, with permission, from Schwartz DT, Reisdorff EJ. Emergency Radiology. New York, NY: McGraw-Hill, 2000, p. 558.)

Questions 46 and 47

46. A 12-year-old boy is rushed to the emergency room after ingesting a caustic material. Following initial resuscitation and stabilization, the next most important intervention is

(A) induction of emesis
(B) oral ingestion of activated charcoal
(C) steroid therapy
(D) barium swallow
(E) esophagoscopy

47. Which of the following is a potential delayed complication that he may develop?

(A) diffuse esophageal spasm
(B) esophageal carcinoma
(C) Barrett esophagus
(D) achalasia
(E) Zenker diverticulum

Questions 48 through 50

A 48-year-old male presents to the emergency room with fever, chest pain, and cough for the past 2 days. His symptoms started abruptly. He describes the pain as a "sharp" pain in his left chest when he takes a deep breath or coughs. His coughs is productive of rusty-appearing sputum. He has a medical history of hypertension, for which he takes an angiotensin-converting enzyme (ACE) inhibitor. He does not smoke cigarettes. On examination, he is ill, but not toxic appearing. His temperature is 38.5°C, pulse is 115, respiratory rate is 26, and blood pressure is 110/70. His oxygen saturation is 93% on room air. His pulmonary examination reveals rhonchi and rales in the left hemithorax. His heart is tachycardic but regular. He has no physical examination signs of hypoxia. His chest x-ray is shown in Fig. 8-3(A) and (B).

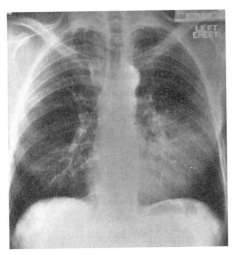 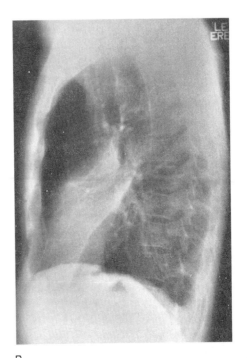

A   B

FIG. 8-3 (*Reproduced, with permission, from Chen MYM, Pope TL Jr, OH DJ.* Basic Radiology. *New York, NY: McGraw-Hill, 2004, p. 83.*)

48. Which of the following is the best description of the x-ray shown?

    (A) left lower lobe infiltrate
    (B) left upper lobe infiltrate
    (C) left lower lobe abscess
    (D) diffuse, bilateral, interstitial infiltrate
    (E) normal chest-x-ray

49. His history, examination, and radiographs are most consistent with which of the following?

    (A) aspiration pneumonia caused by enteric anaerobic organisms
    (B) pulmonary tuberculosis
    (C) *Pneumocystis carinii* pneumonia
    (D) community-acquired pneumonia caused by *Streptococcus pneumoniae*
    (E) pulmonary embolism

50. Which of the following is the most appropriate management of this patient?

    (A) hospitalization on the general medical floor for IV antibiotics
    (B) hospitalization in the intensive care unit for antibiotics, oxygen, and close monitoring
    (C) 23-h observation in the hospital with oral antibiotics; admission to the general medical floor for IV antibiotics if not improved at the end of the observation time
    (D) outpatient management with oral antibiotics and close follow-up
    (E) inpatient admission to the general medical floor for oxygen, IV heparin, and institution of oral warfarin

Answers and Explanations

1. **(B)** Axillary freckling (also called the Crowe sign) is highly associated with NF-1. Café-au-lait spots and hypermelanotic macules in the axillae make up two major criteria in the diagnosis of NF-1. Having both of these would fulfill the NIH consensus criteria for the diagnosis of NF-1. Children with NF-1 may develop Lisch nodules, which are hamartomas on the iris. Lisch nodules do not affect vision and do not have any malignant potential. They are usually not present in early childhood, but appear during adolescence. *(Smith's, pp. 508–509)*

2. **(E)**

3. **(A)**

Explanations 2 and 3

The diagnosis of primary hyperparathyroidism is readily established when a patient presents with an elevated serum calcium and parathyroid hormone with a concomitant low serum phosphate level. Other conditions associated with hypercalcemia include metastatic bone disease, myeloma, sarcoidosis, milk-alkali syndrome, hypervitaminosis, thyrotoxicosis, Addison's disease, and the overuse of thiazide diuretics. These conditions are associated with suppressed levels of parathyroid hormone.

Most patients with primary hyperparathyroidism present with nonspecific symptoms including weakness, fatigue, depression, musculoskeletal, and gastrointestinal complaints. Advanced or long-standing disease is associated with recurrent nephrolithiasis and osteitis fibrosa cystica, in which bone becomes softened, deformed, and may develop cysts. It is generally recommended that all symptomatic patients should undergo surgical treatment because of the high success rate and low morbidity rate. It is important to evaluate the 24-h urine excretion of calcium to rule out familial hypocalciuric hypercalcemia (FHH) before contemplation of surgery since patients with FHH do not benefit from surgery. Urinary calcium excretion will be low in FHH and high in primary hyperparathyroidism. *(Cameron, pp. 602–603)*

4. **(E)**

5. **(D)**

6. **(B)**

Explanations 4 through 6

Toxin-producing strains of *C. difficile* are the only identified cause of colitis induced by antibiotic use. The diagnosis of this type of colitis requires that the onset of symptoms occur during or within 4 weeks of administration of the antibiotic and that there be no other identifiable cause of the symptoms. The diagnosis is confirmed most often by an ELISA assay for *C. difficile* toxin A. The ELISA has comparable specificity and only slightly less sensitivity than a tissue culture assay, which requires more time, specialized facilities, trained technicians, and higher costs. Fecal leukocyte testing is likely to be positive, but is not specific for the cause of this patient's diarrhea. Neither stool ova and parasites nor Gram stain would play a role in the diagnosis of antibiotic-induced colitis.

The preferred initial treatment for *C. difficile* colitis is oral metronidazole. It is preferred to vancomycin because they have similar efficacy, while metronidazole is significantly less expensive and has not been associated with the development of vancomycin-resistant enterococci. When a patient continues to have diarrhea and signs of systemic toxicity after 48 h of treatment with metronidazole, changing to oral vancomycin would be a reasonable intervention. IV metronidazole could be used for a hospitalized patient or someone who could not take oral medication, but vancomycin must be given orally to be effective. (*Harrison's Principles of Internal Medicine, pp. 922–927*)

7. **(A)**

8. **(A)**

Explanations 7 and 8

This individual is likely suffering from a major depressive disorder. He is expressing thoughts of death and may be having active suicidal ideation. Calling in his wife prior to notifying the patient or asking him further about suicidal ideation may frighten and anger him, damaging feelings of trust. Assuring him about confidentiality, when a voluntary or involuntary hospitalization may be necessary, might be inaccurate and may also hurt the therapeutic alliance in the future. Reassuring an individual who is in the midst of a depressive illness and who may be contemplating suicide is not beneficial and may inadvertently promote further guilty feelings, conversely increasing suicidal intent. Often, patients who are having thoughts of committing suicide do feel guilty or embarrassed and, if not directly questioned, may not bring up the subject. Indeed, directly inquiring about suicidal ideation in a nonjudgmental way may help to comfort the patient and enable further discussion about the subject.

The rate of completed suicide is approximately 12 out of 100,000 persons in the United States. There are numerous factors that increase the risk of suicide. The presence of concurrent anxiety symptoms is one factor that increases the risk. Previous suicide attempts are actually the best indicator that a patient is at an increased risk to commit suicide. Asking about a specific plan for suicide is essential in a thorough risk assessment. It can demonstrate concern for patient and enhance the therapeutic alliance. Seriously suicidal individuals are often suffering from a severe depressive illness and can respond significantly to antidepressant therapy. A family history of suicide is another factor that increases the risk of attempted suicide. (*Synopsis, pp. 913, 917*)

9. **(C)** With the introduction of screening tests for cytologic evaluation of cervical cells, a dramatic decrease in mortality from invasive cervical carcinoma has occurred. This has been accomplished because of early detection of intraepithelial neoplasia of different degrees that may lead, if untreated, to carcinoma. Mild, moderate, and severe dysplasia can be diagnosed with regular pap smears and, more recently, with a different technique (ThinPrep). In cases of high-grade dysplasia, further adequate early treatment can be achieved before progressing into an invasive carcinoma. (*Cotran, 6th ed., pp. 1048–1052*)

10. **(C)**

11. **(A)**

Explanations 10 and 11

Although all of the given diagnoses could produce similar symptoms, there are distinct findings which suggest a diagnosis of spinal stenosis. Spinal stenosis is a degenerative disorder of the spine which normally presents after the age of 50. Neurologic symptoms, including dysesthesias and paraesthesias, and pain are often bilateral and not localized, since it commonly affects multiple vertebrae. The symptoms are improved with flexion of the spine (sitting or climbing stairs) and worsened by straightening the spine (standing). There is no localized pain in the sacrum and no bowel or bladder incontinence, so a diagnosis of cauda equina syndrome or spondyloarthopathy is less likely. Muscle spasms and early DJD should not produce such neurologic findings.

The most sensitive and specific imaging study in the diagnosis of spinal stenosis, among those given above, is an MRI of the spine at the affected area. Although x-rays of the spine have been frequently used in the past in the evaluation of lower back pain, they have been shown to be of limited value in diagnosing pathology. Bone scans may detect malignancy or infection before radiography does, but are of no value in spinal stenosis. Indium scans would be useful in occult inflammatory pathology and nerve conduction studies would suggest a neuropathic deficit, but would not help in localizing the defect. (*Harrison's Principles of Internal Medicine, p. 83*)

12. **(E)** Gastric lymphoma can occur as an isolated neoplasm confined to the stomach or it may be the manifestation of widespread infiltrative disease involving lymphatic and other organ systems. The stomach is the most common site of primary intestinal lymphoma. Anorexia and weight loss are the most common presenting complaints, whereas bleeding is relatively uncommon. Early satiety is a prominent symptom, as the gastric wall becomes thickened and the lumen is progressively compromised by the neoplastic infiltrate. Definitive diagnosis is made by endoscopy and biopsy. Radiation therapy provides a long-standing remission that may be equal to that of resection alone and has emerged as the treatment of choice. Patients who present with gastric outlet obstruction, however, are best treated by subtotal gastric resection and postoperative irradiation. A combined approach is associated with a 5-year survival rate of 85% when the malignant process is limited to the stomach. (*Schwartz, p. 1205*)

13. **(E)**

14. **(D)**

15. **(B)**

16. **(C)**

Explanations 13 through 16

The United States Preventative Services Task Force (USPSTF) has an A recommendation (strongly recommend) that clinicians routinely screen men aged ≥35 years and women aged ≥45 years for lipid disorders. The USPSTF has a D recommendation (against) routine screening with resting ECG. Colon cancer screening is recommended starting at the age of 50 for low-risk adults. The USPSTF has an I recommendation (insufficient evidence to recommend for or against routine screening) for prostate cancer using prostate-specific antigen (PSA) testing or digital rectal examination (DRE). Most major

U.S. medical organizations agree that the most appropriate candidates for prostate cancer screening include men older than 50 years and younger men at increased risk of prostate cancer, but that screening is unlikely to benefit men who have a life expectancy of less than 10 years. There is no recommendation for routine CBC screening of adults. (*USPSTF: www.preventiveservices.ahrq.gov*)

dT boosters are recommended every 10 years. HAV would be recommended for certain medical indications such as persons with clotting-factor disorders or chronic liver disease. It is also recommended for men who have sex with men, users of recreational drugs, persons working with hepatitis A-infected primates, or with HAV in a research laboratory setting. It should be considered by persons traveling to or working in countries that have high or intermediate endemicity of hepatitis A. (*MMWR 1999;48(RR-12):1–37; www.cdc.gov/travel/diseases/hav.htm*)

HBV is recommended for adults with certain indications. These include hemodialysis patients, patients who receive clotting-factor concentrates, health-care and public-safety workers who have exposure to blood in the workplace, persons in training for health professions. Behavioral indications for the HBV would include injecting drug users, persons with more than one sex partner in the previous 6 months, persons with a recently acquired sexually-transmitted disease (STD), all clients in STD clinics, and men who have sex with men. Household contacts and sex partners of persons with chronic HBV infection, clients and staff of institutions for the developmentally disabled, international travelers who will be in countries with high or intermediate prevalence of chronic HBV infection for more than 6 months, and inmates of correctional facilities should also be immunized. (*MMWR 1991; 40(RR-13):1–19*)

The CDC recommends that persons born after 1956 (like the patient in question) should have two doses of measles vaccine; additional doses should be given as MMR, but there is no need for MMR booster every 10 years. Pneumococcal vaccine should be given to patients with high-risk conditions, such as chronic obstructive pulmonary disease (COPD), chronic liver diseases, chronic renal failure, immunosuppressive conditions, and splenectomy.

This patient's LDL goal is less than 130 mg/dL as he has two coronary artery disease risk factors, a BMI of 30 and a low HDL. To achieve this goal you should recommend therapeutic lifestyle modification, including a low fat diet and regular exercises (30 min/day, most days of the week) to promote weight loss if overweight and stress management. He has normal triglycerides, so niacin is not indicated at this time. Lipid lowering medication would not be indicated at this time. However, if he continues to have high LDL readings after trying the recommended lifestyle modifications, one could then consider the addition of lipid lowering agents. *(National Heart, Lung and Blood Institute of the National Institutes of Health. The third report of the national cholesterol education program expert panel on the detection, evaluation and treatment of high blood cholesterol in adults (ATP III), 2001)*

17. (D)

18. (E)

Explanations 17 and 18

Body dysmorphic disorder involves the preoccupation with an imagined or exaggerated defect in appearance. Unlike the above case, the individual focuses on a perceived flaw rather than an internal symptom. Patients with conversion disorder display a neurologic deficit as a result of an unconscious conflict. The patient in the above case is anxious about having cancer, but she is not delusional regarding absolutely having the disease, as would be seen in delusional disorder. Somatization disorder requires the presence of multiple physical complaints covering several different body systems. The focus is on the somatic symptoms rather than having a specific disease. This individual displays features of hypochondriasis, a condition characterized by a preoccupation with fears of having a serious disease based on the misinterpretation of bodily sensations. In her case, it is her fearing having stomach cancer because of her gas pains (DSM IV).

Confrontation is only necessary in cases of malingering. Confronting a patient with hypochondriasis would likely increase the individual's anxiety and anger, as well as damage the therapeutic alliance. An extensive evaluation in this case will not likely reassure the patient, will increase costs, and expose the person to possible side effects or complications from tests and procedures. Beginning an SSRI is indicated if there is a comorbid mental illness that will respond to the medication, such as major depressive disorder or panic disorder, neither of which appear to be present in this case. While referring the above patient to a psychiatrist may be useful for the same reasons, individuals with hypochondriasis are often resistant to psychiatric interventions. The best approach is to have regularly scheduled visits. These can both help provide the needed reassurance and enable time for limited physical examinations if indicated. *(Synopsis, p. 653)*

19. (C) Informed consent is a means by which the physician demonstrates respect for the patient's autonomy, so that the patient can make up his own mind to accept or refuse a proposed treatment or diagnostic test. The process of informed decision-making involves two preconditions: that the patient is making the decision voluntarily (free of undue influence or coercion) and that the patient has the capacity to make the decision. Once these preconditions are met, the process of informed consent involves the disclosure of information, followed by the actual decision (either consent or refusal) made by the patient.

Disclosure of information must provide enough information on the patient's condition, the risks and benefits of the proposed treatment and the alternatives available, so that the patient can make a rational decision. The standard that is used today for the amount of information to disclose is based on what would be expected by a reasonable person in order to make a decision. The subjective standard would be the amount of information that a particular individual requires, based on the physician's knowledge of that patient's characteristics and/or circumstances. The clinician should be aware of the possibility of framing effects when giving information, since framing (e.g., presenting only one side of pertinent statistics) may influence the patient's voluntariness.

In the case presented, it is important for the physician to explain why she is prescribing the statin, especially in light of the patient's cardiac risk factors. The physician should explain that there are other options for managing the patient's hypercholesterolemia, including other classes of medications or further lifestyle modification. Relevant side effects of the medication, including the need to monitor for liver toxicity with periodic blood tests, should be mentioned and the patient should be alerted as to what symptoms to report to the physician in this regard. Once the physician has disclosed the information, she should determine if the patient has any questions, both to check for comprehension and to fill in any gaps of knowledge, before the patient makes a decision about the medication.

20. (D) The average age of menarche is dependent on race but averages 12.8 years. For an adolescent female who has made no pubertal progression, an evaluation for primary amenorrhea (and delayed puberty) should be initiated by age 14. In the adolescent female who has met all of her other normal pubertal milestones (linear growth, breast development, and pubic and axillary hair growth) it is appropriate to delay the evaluation for primary amenorrhea until age 16. *(Beckmann, p. 463)*

21. (C)

22. (B)

Explanations 21 and 22

A cross-sectional study is the best study design to determine the prevalence of an event or characteristic at a single point in time. It is not useful in determining the etiology of the event in question. A randomized-controlled study is a prospective study design used to assess differences between two or more groups receiving different intervention or treatment. It is most often used to compare outcomes between different treatments or used in clinical decision analysis to compare outcomes. A case-control study is an observational study in which affected and unaffected subjects are identified after the fact and then compared regarding specific characteristics to determine possible associations or risks for the disease in question. A prospective cohort study is an observational study in which exposed and unexposed populations are identified and followed prospectively over time to determine the rate of a specific clinical event. A case-series study design is an objective report of clinical characteristic or outcomes from a group of clinical subjects. A case series report can address almost any clinical issue, including screening test results, treatment outcomes, and natural history findings. It is most commonly used to describe clinical characteristics, such as signs and symptoms of disease or disease outcomes. *(Preventive Medicine and Public Health, NMS, 1992)*

23. (D)

24. (C)

Explanations 23 and 24

Documentation of both affective and somatic symptoms by a menstrual calendar is critical to establish the diagnosis of PMS. The University of California at San Diego criteria for the diagnosis of PMS includes at least one of the following affective and somatic symptoms during the 5 days before menses in each of the three previous cycles:

Affective symptoms: depression, angry outbursts, irritability, anxiety, confusion, social withdrawal
Somatic symptoms: breast tenderness, abdominal bloating, headache, swelling of extremities
Symptoms relieved from days 4 through 13 of the menstrual cycle.

The National Institute of Mental Health diagnostic criteria include a 30% increase in the intensity of symptoms of PMS (measured by a standard instrument) from days 5 to 10 of the menstrual cycle as compared with the 6-day interval before the onset of menses and documentation of these changes in a daily symptom diary for at least two consecutive cycles. *(Dickerson LM, Mazyck PJ, Hunter MH. Premenstrual syndrome. Am Fam Physician 2003;67:1743–1752)*

In clinical trials, SSRI therapy, particularly fluoxetine and sertraline, have been shown to be effective in treating PMS. While the other options listed, along with many others, are frequently tried, well-designed scientific studies have not consistently shown them to be helpful. *(Davis AJ and Johnson SR. Premenstrual syndrome. ACOG Pract Bull2000;(15))*

25. **(D)** This patient presents with the characteristic findings associated with undiagnosed ovarian cancer. The signs and symptoms in the early stages of the disease tend to be nonspecific, often gastrointestinal in nature. Patients with more advanced stage disease present with the classic constellation of abdominal distention, bloating, satiety, anorexia, dyspnea, and involuntary weight loss. The most appropriate diagnostic test to order in this situation would be a CT scan of the abdomen and pelvis to evaluate for extent of disease and potential respectability of disease. A CT scan can help to determine the presence or absence of liver metastases, hydronephrosis, and bowel obstruction.

Ultrasound is best reserved for the evaluation of the pelvic viscera, specifically the morphology and subtle detail associated with the uterus, ovaries, and fallopian tubes when abnormalities are suspected. It is not a good test to evaluate for abdominal extent of disease. Pelvic MRI, like ultrasound, does not provide any information relative to the abdominal extent of disease. Abdominal plain films are used primarily to assess bowel perforation or obstruction; it provides no fine detail about possible tumor burden or extent/location of disease. ERCP is used to evaluate the duct drainage of the gallbladder and pancreas. *(Togashi K. Ovarian cancer: the clinical role of US, CT, and MRI. Eur Radiol 2003;13(Suppl 4):L87–L104)*

26. **(D)** The patient has nephrotic syndrome. The patient is also noted to have anemia and leukopenia. HIV is one of the most common causes of nephrotic syndrome. While there are certainly many other conditions that can cause nephrotic syndrome, HIV is the most likely. A bone marrow examination would give important information to evaluate leukopenia and anemia but would be unlikely to yield a specific diagnosis. A chest x-ray is a poor way to rule out lung cancer. Other tests for systemic lupus erythematosus would be more useful than complement levels. The clinical history does not suggest mononucleosis. *(Mandell, pp. 1409–1410)*

27. **(E)** There is a fundamental difference between human body metabolism in normal physiology and during starvation. A healthy 70-kg individual expends an average of 1800 kcal/day of energy obtained from lipid, carbohydrate, and protein sources. Obligate glycolytic cells include neurons, leukocytes, and erythrocytes. These cells require 180 g of glucose per day for basal energy needs.

During acute starvation, glucose is initially derived from the breakdown of hepatic glycogen. However, within 24 h, hepatic glycogen storage is depleted. Thereafter, initiation of gluconeogenesis results in the production of glucose, mainly from the breakdown of amino acids and fatty acids. Ketones are derived from fatty acids during prolonged starvation. After 4 or 5 days, the rate of whole-body proteolysis diminishes significantly as the nervous system and other previous glucose-utilizing tissue begin to utilize ketones as the predominant energy source. Thus, ketones serve as the primary source of energy during prolonged starvation and have a protein sparing effect. *(Schwartz, pp. 26–28)*

28. **(C)** Hydropic swelling among the placental tissues suggests the presence of a molar gestation. There are two types of molar pregnancies, each with distinctive clinical and cytogenetic features.

The partial mole has a triploid karyotype that results from dispermic fertilization of an egg with retention of the maternal haploid set. The placental tissue of the partial mole is characterized by focal, variable hydropic villi and usually by focal, slight trophoblastic hyperplasia. The embryo associated with partial molar pregnancies survives much longer than with complete moles, with embryonic deaths typically occurring at approximately 8 weeks estimated gestational age. Frequently, at the time of evacuation, there is macroscopic or microscopic evidence of a fetus. Fetal blood vessels are identified and usually contain nucleated fetal erythrocytes.

The complete mole has a diploid karyotype, resulting from paternal fertilization of an "empty egg" and subsequent replication of the paternal haploid karyotype within the empty egg, to produce 46 chromosomes, all paternal in origin. The placental tissue of the complete mole is remarkable for generalized edema of the chorionic villi, including central cistern formation, which results in a macroscopic appearance similar to a "bunch of grapes." The embryo associated with the complete mole undergoes resorption before the development of the cardiovascular system, when the embryo is less than 1 cm in length. Thus, fetal vessels generally degenerate soon after formation and no nucleated fetal erythrocytes are seen in the villous capillaries.

Partial moles account for 25–40% of all molar pregnancies and are typically diagnosed in the second trimester, when they present most commonly as a missed abortion. In contrast to the extremely high serum human chorionic gonadotropin (hCG) levels found in association with complete moles, partial moles typically have hCG levels in the low to normal range. The risk of subsequent gestational trophoblastic neoplasia associated with partial moles is 5–10%, compared to the increased risk of 10–30% associated with complete moles.

Complete moles typically present with vaginal bleeding in the first trimester. They can also be associated with hyperemesis gravidarum, toxemia, and hyperthyroidism in the first or second trimester. Complete moles are associated with an extremely high hCG value and a characteristic ultrasound "snowstorm" appearance.

Spontaneous miscarriage involves the loss of a nonmolar gestation, typically in the first trimester. The causes can include genetic defects, uterine anomalies, poorly controlled diabetes, or luteal phase defect. Cervical incompetence generally presents with pain-

less cervical dilatation and spontaneous miscarriage at 18–22 weeks estimated gestational age. Intrauterine growth retardation generally refers to a viable intrauterine pregnancy in which fetal growth is inadequate for the gestational age. The causes range from uteroplacental insufficiency to genetic abnormalities to in utero infection. *(Altieri A. Epidemiology and etiology of gestational trophoblastic diseases. Lancet Oncol 2003; 4(11):670–678)*

29. **(D)** The diagnosis of pharyngoesophageal diverticula (Zenker's) is established by a barium esophagogram. Upper endoscopy carries a risk of perforation through the diverticula, especially if performed before the diagnosis is seen on esophagogram. The diverticulum arises over the cricopharyngeus muscle resulting from increased pharyngeal pressure. Therefore, a cricopharyngeal myotomy (division of the muscle) with or without diverticulectomy is the treatment of choice. Most diverticula less than 2 cm simply blend into the mucosa once the cricopharyngeal muscle is divided and do not require excision. The procedure carries a very low risk of recurrence or morbidity. *(Greenfield, pp. 726–728)*

30. **(A)** The most common abdominal mass in a newborn infant is hydronephrosis. It is a common finding in prenatal ultrasounds. It will usually resolve without therapy. Neuroblastoma is the most common abdominal tumor of infancy. It is much less common than the relatively common hydronephrosis. Hepatomas and Wilms tumors are even rarer than neuroblastoma. Diaphragmatic hernia will usually present with respiratory embarrassment and feeding difficulties, not an abdominal mass. *(Rudolph, pp. 1375–1376)*

31. **(E)**

32. **(E)**

Explanations 31 and 32

This case is a typical description of a person with acute HIV infection. The duration of this patient's illness is against strep pharyngitis.

The patient could have mononucleosis but a monospot would not be specific for this diagnosis. There is no history of oral sexual exposure, which would be necessary for *N. gonorrhea* pharyngitis. *N. gonorrhea* also does not cause meningitis in this setting. An HIV antibody test by ELISA is negative in a majority of cases of early acute HIV infection. The more sensitive polymerase chain reaction (PCR) test would be a better test to use.

After getting the results of the LP, the most appropriate next step is repeating LP in 2 days to see if there has been a change. The acute history is not indicative of tuberculosis. *Hemophilus influenza* meningitis usually affects children less than 5 years of age. The only time opportunistic infections or lymphoma occur in HIV is in the chronic setting of AIDS. Serum antibody tests for West Nile virus are indicated in patients with aseptic meningitis, but the clinical picture does not present with rash. Repeating an LP in 2 days to see if there is a change helps to exclude other infections that might cause a rash by identifying a change in the number and composition of cells. (*Mandell, pp. 1404–1405, 1432*)

33. **(C)** Any patient who develops bloody diarrhea following abdominal aortic surgery should be suspected of having ischemic colitis. It results from injury or ligation of the inferior mesenteric artery during the procedure. The estimated incidence is 1–6%. Patients may also present with abdominal distention, leukocytosis, and peritonitis as early as 24–48 h following surgery. Immediate sigmoidoscopy is the diagnostic modality of choice, since it facilitates direct visualization of the colonic mucosa. In most instances the injury is mucosal, which appears as edematous, friable, and hemorrhagic mucosa with patchy ulceration. In these patients, the process is self-limited and treated with supportive measures including hydration, transfusion, and serial examination. In cases of full-thickness involvement, the mucosa will appear black or grey, indicating transmural ischemia and impending gangrene of the bowel. Surgical resection of the ischemic segment with proximal colostomy is indicated in these patients or patients with signs of sepsis or

peritonitis. Arteriography and CT scan usually do not demonstrate specific vascular abnormalities. (*Schwartz, pp. 948, 1284, 1285*)

34. **(D)**

35. **(C)**

Explanations 34 and 35

Down syndrome is caused by a trisomy of chromosome 21. Prominent epicanthic folds, mental retardation, congenital cardiovascular abnormalities, increased susceptibility to infections, hyperflexibility, muscle hypotonia, dysplastic ears, and infertility characterize the syndrome. Individuals with Down syndrome have a 20-fold risk of developing lymphoblastic leukemia during childhood. Infectious mononucleosis, although it can show lymphocytosis, would not be monomorphic of such high proportion. Infectious diseases will give an increase in the myeloid series and leukemoid reaction. Reactive lymphocytosis is seen in viral infections and should not be considered in this case.

Down syndrome is the most common chromosome abnormality, occurring in 1 out of 800 live births. It is characterized by a trisomy 21 karyotype with an extra G group chromosome (chromosome 21), making 47 total chromosomes. The parents are phenotypically and genetically normal in the majority of cases and Down syndrome is secondary to a meiotic error in the ovum. The risk of having a Down syndrome child is proportional to increasing maternal age. The clinical features of Down syndrome include fat facies, epicanthic folds, oblique palpebral fissures, and mental retardation. The majority of affected individuals die early from cardiac or infectious complications. Thirty percent have a ventricular septal defect. Trisomy 13, also called Patau syndrome, causes microcephaly and severe mental retardation with absence of a portion of the forebrain. These children die soon after birth. Trisomy 18, or Edwards syndrome, is also a very severe genetic defect, and the average life-span is 10 weeks. Affected children have severe mental retardation and cardiac anomalies, including ventricular septal defect.

Persons with an XO karyotype have Turner syndrome and are phenotypically females. Only 3% of affected fetuses survive to birth; fetuses that do survive have severe edema of the hands, feet, and neck. Affected persons have a webbed neck, short stature, and congenital heart disease. At puberty, there is failure to develop normal secondary sex characteristics, so their genitals remain immature. Klinefelter syndrome, or testicular dysgenesis, is characterized by an XXY karyotype. It occurs in 1 out of 600 live births. Affected individuals usually are diagnosed after puberty and have eunuchoid habitus, long legs, small atrophic testes and penis and, often, low IQ. *(Cotran, 5th ed., pp. 170–173)*

36. **(E)** After the first 4–6 weeks of life, GBS begins to diminish as a cause of urinary tract infections (UTIs). The most common cause of UTIs then becomes *E. coli*. UTIs are more common in females. If infants develop fever and some degree of toxicity (vomiting, poor feeding, lethargy), they are commonly diagnosed clinically with pyelonephritis. The best clinical way to document pyelonephritis without any imaging would be seeing the presence of WBC casts in a urinary microscopic examination. *(Rudolph, pp. 1667–1673)*

37. **(C)**

38. **(D)**

39. **(D)**

40. **(C)**

41. **(E)**

Explanations 37 through 41

Hyperglycemia results in "translocational hyponatremia." Increases in glucose concentration of 100 mg/dL will decrease the serum sodium by approximately 1.7 mmol/L. In this case, the sodium will correct to approximately 141.

This patient has an anion-gap metabolic acidosis from diabetic ketoacidosis, with an anion gap of 24. Using the formula to determine appropriate respiratory compensation [expected $pCO_2 = 1.5 \times (HCO_3) + 8 \pm 2$], we would expect the pCO_2 to be 26 ± 2. However, the pCO_2 here is less, indicating a concurrent respiratory alkalosis. The anion gap and bicarbonate levels show that the acidosis stems completely from the presence of unmeasured anions. Therefore, a concurrent nonanion-gap metabolic acidosis is not present.

Volume resuscitation is necessary, as patients with diabetic ketoacidosis are frequently volume depleted. Treatment of the ketosis with insulin is also necessary. This is typically done with a continuous infusion of intravenous insulin. The drip is maintained based on the presence of persistent ketoacidosis and should not be discontinued based on blood glucose values. Furthermore, dextrose should be added to the intravenous fluids when the blood glucose decreases, in order to avoid hypoglycemia from the insulin infusion. The administration of kayexalate is unnecessary, as the etiology of the hyperkalemia is due to the relative deficiency in insulin and will correct with the insulin drip.

Serum phosphate must be monitored closely during the treatment of diabetic ketoacidosis. The insulin drip can lead to intracellular uptake of phosphate, creating hypophosphatemia. This can result in muscle weakness and even respiratory paralysis. Hypokalemia is also a potential complication of the treatment of diabetic ketoacidosis, as insulin will increase the cellular uptake of potassium.

This patient has a combined anion-gap metabolic acidosis and respiratory alkalosis, which also can be seen in salicylate toxicity. Lithium toxicity can lead to diabetes insipidus and may create a low anion-gap picture. Ingestion of methanol and ethylene glycol can lead to an anion-gap metabolic acidosis but not necessarily a respiratory alkalosis. Isopropyl alcohol ingestions can lead to an osmolar gap, but usually will not lead to an anion-gap acidosis. *(Brenner and Rector, pp. 966–968)*

42. **(B)** Shock is defined as a state of inadequate supply of essential nutrients to the tissues. In the trauma setting, hypotension should be

assumed to be secondary to hypovolemic shock resulting from an acute loss of plasma volume, regardless of the patient presentation. Massive external or internal hemorrhage is the most common cause. Hypovolemic shock may also result from the loss of plasma into burned or injured tissues. Initial resuscitative efforts are therefore directed toward hypovolemic shock with a rapid intravenous infusion of crystalloid. (*Cameron, p. 909*)

43.   (D)

44.   (B)

Explanations 43 and 44

This patient displays criteria for bipolar disorder, manic with psychotic features. While alcohol can present with psychotic symptoms, it more commonly creates a depressed picture. Benzodiazepine intoxication rarely causes manic or psychotic symptoms. Although cannabis use is not infrequently associated with paranoia, it rarely displays frank psychosis. Opiate intoxication will appear more as a depressed syndrome. Individuals intoxicated with cocaine classically show signs similar to mania. Frank psychotic symptoms can occur in up to 50% of individuals. (*Synopsis, p. 433*)

While psychotic symptoms such as hallucinations and delusions are common in patients with bipolar disorder, they are also seen in other illnesses, including depression, substance intoxication, and psychotic disorders such as schizophrenia. Disruptive behavior is not specific for bipolar disorder, as it is seen in the above illnesses, and other conditions such as deliriums, dementias, personality disorders, and so on. Although a history (or future episodes) of depression is frequent in bipolar disorder, it is not actually needed in order to diagnose bipolar disorder, manic episode. In fact, individuals who have bipolar disorder may have several manic episodes prior to developing a depressive episode. The only criterion specific for mania is decreased need for sleep (DSM IV).

45.   (D) The triad of hypotension, elevated jugular venous pressure, and decreased or absent heart sounds in a patient with history of penetrating chest trauma should immediately raise the suspicion of either pericardial tamponade or tension pneumothorax. The distinction can readily be made by chest x-ray, which will be normal in a patient with cardiac tamponade.

Cardiac tamponade develops when an injury causes blood to accumulate in the pericardial space between the heart and pericardium. Because the pericardium does not stretch, the heart is compressed and venous blood cannot enter the heart. The decreased diastolic filling results in a life-threatening decreased cardiac output.

Once the diagnosis of cardiac tamponade is established, immediate pericardiocentesis should be performed. Pericardiocentesis is successful in approximately 80% of cases and evacuation of as little as 15 cc may result in a dramatic response. Only if unsuccessful, and if the patient remains in severe hypotension, should an emergency room thoracotomy be performed. While the pericardiocentesis is being performed, the operating room should be prepared for emergent thoracotomy and definitive surgical repair. (*Schwartz, p. 150*)

46.   (E)

47.   (B)

Explanations 46 and 47

The initial management goals of caustic injuries are airway assessment, stabilization, and fluid resuscitation. The airway should be directly visualized with a fiberoptic nasopharyngoscope and, if edema or airway compromise is found, intubation is required. Induction of emesis reexposes the upper esophagus to the corrosive agent. Well-intended measures to neutralize the corrosive agent with water, milk, or activated charcoal are contraindicated as they may elicit vomiting or obscure endoscopic visualization. Early endoscopy is essential to evaluate the extent and severity of injury and should be performed within 12–24 h after injury. Recent controlled trials have shown no proven benefit of steroids.

The risk of developing a stricture is related to the degree of corrosive injury. Superficial mucosal injuries usually heal without complications, whereas deep or circumferential injuries usually result in a delayed stricture. The risk of malignant degeneration in the strictured segment is 100–1000 times higher than the incidence in the general population. The other listed choices are not related to caustic injuries. (*Cameron, pp. 47–50*)

48.   (B)

49.   (D)

50.   (D)

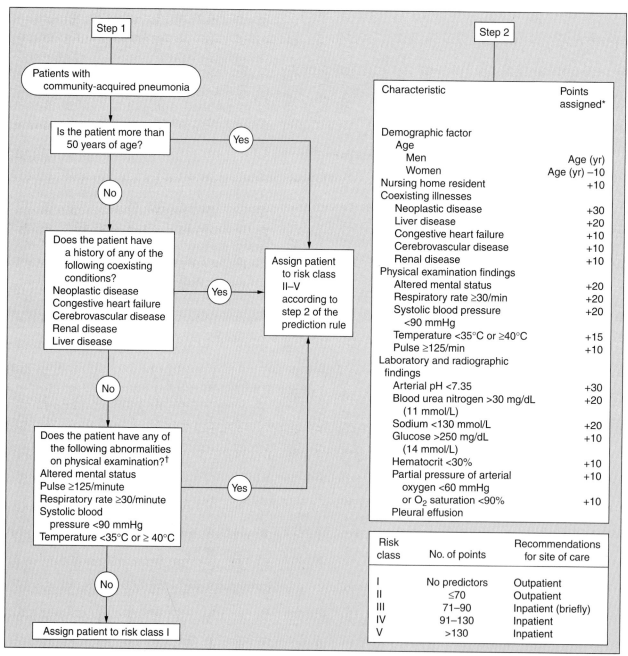

FIG. 8-4 Criteria for hospitalization of patients with pneumonia: the PORT score. *A risk score (total point score) for a given patient is obtained by summing the patient's age in years (age minus 10 for females) and the points for each applicable patient characteristic. †Oxygen saturation of <90% is also considered abnormal. (*Adapted from Fine et al., Bartlett et al., and Braunwald et al.*)

Explanations 48 through 50

The chest x-ray provided shows an infiltrate in the lingua of the left upper lobe. This is often confused with a left lower lobe infiltrate, but can be most readily distinguished by looking at the lateral image. On the lateral film, the left lower lobe—located posterior and inferior—is clear, documenting that the infiltrate is not in the lower lobe of the lung. The right lung is clear as well, ruling out bilateral interstitial infiltrates. Pulmonary abscesses, often associated with anaerobic infections, characteristically have air-fluid levels and are often located in dependent, poorly ventilated areas of the lung.

The most common cause of community-acquired pneumonia in adults is *S. pneumoniae.* Typical presentations would include a fairly sudden onset of a fever, productive cough, dyspnea, and pleuritic chest pain. *Pneumocystis carinii* pneumonia is almost always associated with AIDS or other profound immunocompromised states. It is often seen as a diffuse, "ground-glass" appearing, interstitial infiltrate but may occur in the presence of a relatively normal chest x-ray. A pulmonary embolus can cause the sudden onset of pleuritic chest pain, hypoxia, dyspnea, and cough but is less likely to cause a fever or a typical appearing infiltrate on chest x-ray. While aspiration pneumonias cannot be definitively ruled out based on the presentation, they tend to be more common in lower lung fields and are overall much less common than pneumococcal pneumonia.

Approximately 20% of patients with community-acquired pneumonia are hospitalized. One frequently used scoring system for the determination of risk class, and need for hospitalization, comes from the Pneumonia Patient Outcomes Research Team (PORT). They have created a system of assigning points based on the patient's age, comorbidities, symptoms and signs, from which a risk class can be determined (see Fig. 8-4). By applying this patient's age, lack of comorbidities, vital signs, and oxygen saturation, this patient falls into a risk class I and would be treated as an outpatient with oral antibiotics and close follow-up. *(Harrison's Principles of Internal Medicine, pp. 1475–1480)*

BIBLIOGRAPHY

American Psychiatric Association. *Diagnostic and Statistical Manual of Mental Disorders*, 4th ed., Text Revision. Washington, DC: American Psychiatric Association, 2000.

Beckmann CRB, Ling FW, Laube DW, et al., *Obstetrics and Gynecology*, 4th ed. Baltimore, MD: Lippincot Williams & Wilkins, 2002.

Braunwald E, et al. *Harrison's Principles of Internal Medicine*, 15th ed. New York, NY: McGraw-Hill, 2001.

Brenner BM. *Brenner & Rectors's The Kidney*, 7th ed. Philadelphia, PA: W.B. Saunders, 2004.

Cameron JL (ed.). *Current Surgical Therapy*, 8th ed. St. Louis, MO: C.V. Mosby, 2004.

Cotran RS, Kumar V, Collins T. *Robbins Pathologic Basis of Disease*, 6th ed. Philadelphia, PA: W.B. Saunders, 1999.

Cotran RS, Kumar V, Robbins SL. *Robbins Pathologic Basis of Disease*, 5th ed. Philadelphia, PA: W.B. Saunders, 1994.

Greenfield LJ, Mulholland MW, Oldham KT, et al. (eds.). *Surgery: Scientific Principles and Practice*, 3rd ed. Philadelphia, PA: Lippincott Williams & Wilkins, 2001.

Jones KL (ed.). *Smith's Recognizable Pattern of Human Malformations*, 5th ed. Philadelphia, PA: W.B. Saunders, 1997.

Last JM, Wallace RB, et al. *Maxcy-Rosenau-Last Public Health and Prventive Medicine,* 13th ed. Norwalk, CT: Appleton and Lange, 1992.

Mandell GL, Bennett JE, Mandell DR. *Mandell, Douglas and Bennett's Principles and Practice of Infectious Diseases*, 5th ed. Philadelphia, PA: Churchill Livingstone, 2000.

Rudolph CD, Rudolph AM, Hostetter MK, Lister GE, Siegel NJ, et al. (eds.). *Rudolph's Pediatrics*, 21st ed. New York, NY: McGraw-Hill, 2003.

Sadock BJ, Sadock VA. *Kaplan and Sadock's Synopsis of Psychiatry*, 9th ed. Philadelphia, PA: Lippincott Williams & Wilkins, 2003.

Schwartz SI, Shires GT, Spencer FC, et al. (eds.). *Principles of Surgery*, 7th ed. New York, NY: McGraw-Hill, 1999.

CHAPTER 9

Practice Test 2
Questions

Read each question carefully and in the order in which it is presented. Then select the one best response option of the choices offered. More than one option may be partially correct. You must select ONE BEST answer. You have 60 min to complete this test.

Setting I: Office/Health Center

You see patients in two locations: at your office suite, which is adjacent to a hospital, and at a community-based health center. Your office practice is a primary care generalist group. Most of the patients you see are from your own practice and are appearing for regularly scheduled return visits. Occasionally you will encounter a patient whose primary care is managed by one of your associates. Reference may be made to the patient's medical records. Known patients may be managed by the telephone. You may have to respond to questions about information appearing in the public media, which will require interpretation of the medical literature. The laboratory and radiology departments have a full range of services available.

Questions 1 through 4

A 43-year-old Black female presents to your office for elevated blood pressure (BP). She has been having headaches for the last 3 weeks. She is a pharmacist and she checks her BP at her pharmacy. She presents with readings ranging between 160/104 and 155/95. After some research she did on her own, she has been exercising and following the "DASH" diet for the past 3 months. Her BP in the office after more than 10 min of resting was 153/89 in her left arm and 145/90 in her right. She tells you that both her mother and father have hypertension. She denies chest pain, shortness of breath, dizziness, or blurred vision. She denies tobacco use, drinks 2–4 beers on weekends, and uses no recreational drugs.

1. At this point you diagnose the patient with

    (A) elevated BP without the diagnosis of hypertension
    (B) prehypertension
    (C) stage 1 hypertension
    (D) stage 2 hypertension
    (E) stage 3 hypertension

2. Your physical examination should include documentation of

    (A) cranial nerve examination
    (B) peripheral nerve examinations
    (C) auscultation for carotid, abdominal, and femoral bruits
    (D) palpation of the abdomen for hepatosplenomegaly
    (E) mental status examination

3. Which of the following tests would be recommended at this visit?

    (A) liver function tests
    (B) urine microalbumin
    (C) hemoglobin A1c
    (D) hematocrit
    (E) exercise stress test

4. Which of the following would be the most appropriate management recommendation at this time?

   (A) No intervention at this time, but bring the patient back in 2 weeks for BP check.
   (B) No pharmacologic treatment at this time, but advise her to continue life style modifications such as the "DASH" diet plan and increase her physical activity.
   (C) Continue life style modifications and add a thiazide diuretic.
   (D) Continue life style modifications and add a beta-blocker.
   (E) Continue life style modifications and add an angiotensin-converting enzyme (ACE) inhibitor.

5. A 6-year-old is brought in by his mother. The mother noticed a cold sore on his lip 3 days ago. The mother now notices some spots on the upper lid of the left eye. The child seems comfortable but the eye is mildly inflamed with conjunctival hyperemia.

   Which of the following is the most appropriate at this time?

   (A) prescribe tears for the redness and irritation
   (B) fluorescein stain of the cornea
   (C) give ointment to prevent bacterial infection
   (D) reassure the mother and ask her to check for fever
   (E) give Benadryl for itching

6. A 32-year-old man was diagnosed with diabetes 2 years ago. The diagnosis was made at the time of an insurance examination, when he was incidentally found to have a fasting glucose of 150 mg/dL. He had no symptoms at that time. He has no family history of diabetes. At the time of diagnosis, his weight was 175 lbs and he is 5 ft 10 in. tall. He had no end-organ damage from diabetes detectable at the time of diagnosis. He was started on glyburide 5 mg daily, which controlled his glucose initially. One year ago, his average home blood glucose read-ings were 120 mg/dL and his glycohemoglobin was 6.5% (normal 4–6%). However, over the past 2 months, he has become symptomatic with polyuria, polydypsia, and a 25 lb weight loss. His glyburide was increased to 10 mg twice daily without any improvement in his glucose readings. His current glycohemoglobin is 11%. Which of the following would be the most appropriate next step in his management?

   (A) initiate a strict diet of 1000 cal/day
   (B) switch glyburide to glipizide
   (C) switch to insulin therapy
   (D) add metformin 500 mg bid to his glyburide
   (E) add rosiglitazone 8 mg daily to his glyburide

7. The histologic changes seen in the connective tissue from the joint space of the great toe shown in the Fig. 9-1 are pathognomonic for

   (A) rheumatoid arthritis
   (B) suppurative arthritis
   (C) gout
   (D) osteoarthritis
   (E) ankylosing spondylitis

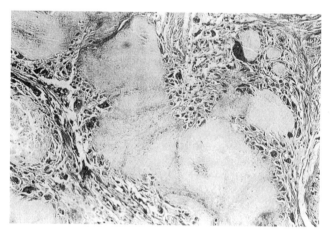

FIG. 9-1

Questions 8 and 9

A 21-year-old male is referred to the student health center because of unusual behavior in class for the past month. While discussing the reasons for the evaluation, the patient is noted to be glancing around the room nervously. When asked about this, he inquires whether there are any miniature-listening devices present. He further explains that he is being followed by the CIA, which is tapping the phone line in his dormitory room. He claims to be an "inactive operative," but that he has nonetheless been receiving instructions from a transmitter implanted in his skull. These experiences have been occurring for the past 8 weeks. He is greatly distressed by what he considers to be harassment by the government. He is sleeping poorly due to the transmitting device, but his energy and appetite have been unchanged. He has been distracted and unable to study as a result, but he denies any suicidal ideation.

8. Which of the following is his most likely diagnosis?

    (A) brief psychotic disorder
    (B) delusional disorder
    (C) schizoaffective disorder
    (D) schizophrenia
    (E) schizophreniform disorder

9. After a full history and physical examination, medical conditions and substances are ruled out as causes of his symptoms. Treatment is initiated with olanzapine (Zyprexa) rather than haloperidol (Haldol). When compared with older neuroleptics, the second generation or atypical antipsychotics are preferred as first-line medications due to

    (A) better treatment of delusions
    (B) fewer extrapyramidal symptoms
    (C) less weight gain
    (D) lower cost of medications
    (E) stronger potency

10. A 16-year-old female complains of worsening cyclic dysmenorrhea, lower back pain, and central pelvic pain. The pain with menses is no longer controlled with nonsteroidal anti-inflammatory agents. Her mother reports that she is missing 1 or 2 days of school each month due to the discomfort prior to her menstrual bleeding. Oral contraceptives are prescribed but do not relieve the symptoms significantly.

Which diagnostic test would be most likely to confirm the diagnosis?

(A) laparoscopy
(B) computed tomography (CT) of the abdomen and pelvis
(C) pelvic ultrasound
(D) hysteroscopy
(E) colonoscopy

Questions 11 through 14

A 24-year-old female presents to your office for the evaluation of 1 year of intermittent abdominal pain and diarrhea. The pain is most severe in the right lower quadrant, spastic, and often associated with fever. The patient intermittently manifests low-grade fevers, but often has asymptomatic periods as well. The pain does not seem to be related to her menses. The diarrhea is watery, nonbloody, and the patient states that she sometimes sees mucous in her stool. The patient smokes cigarettes but denies drug or alcohol use. Physical examination reveals a thin White female with unremarkable vital signs. She has one shallow oral ulcer that is mildly painful to her. Cardiopulmonary examination is normal. Her abdomen is flat, with normal bowel sounds and focal tenderness to palpation over the right lower quadrant. On rectal examination a perianal scar is noted. On questioning, the patient states that she once had an anal fissure that healed spontaneously.

11. An upper gastrointestinal (GI) series with small bowel follow through is performed. Which of the following would be the most likely finding?

    (A) gastric ulceration
    (B) duodenal ulceration
    (C) small bowel ulceration
    (D) small bowel volvulus
    (E) normal examination

12. A right upper quadrant ultrasound is obtained as part of the work up and gallstones are seen in the gallbladder, but the gallbladder wall is of normal thickness and there is no pericholecystic fluid. What is the likely cause of the gallstones in this patient?

    (A) hypocholesterolemia
    (B) failure of enterohepatic bile salt circulation
    (C) chronic cholecystitis
    (D) primary sclerosing cholangitis (PSC)
    (E) tobacco use

13. This patient is at increased risk for developing which of the following malignancies?

    (A) esophageal cancer
    (B) gastric cancer
    (C) small bowel cancer
    (D) ovarian cancer
    (E) uterine cancer

14. Which of the following is the most likely diagnosis for this patient?

    (A) Crohn's disease
    (B) chronic pancreatitis
    (C) irritable bowel syndrome
    (D) endometriosis
    (E) ulcerative colitis

15. One of the first pediatric manifestations of sickle cell disease is

    (A) cerebral infarcts
    (B) infections with *Streptococcus pneumoniae*
    (C) acute dactylitis
    (D) chest syndrome
    (E) papillary necrosis

Questions 16 through 18

A woman brings her 15-year-old son to the office for an evaluation. She became concerned after she heard on the news that a student in the same school died suddenly while he was playing basketball. Her son is a talented and competitive basketball player who is being recruited by several Division 1 colleges.

16. You tell them that the most common cause of sudden death in athletic adolescents is

    (A) coronary artery abnormalities
    (B) Marfan syndrome
    (C) mitral vale prolapse
    (D) aortic stenosis
    (E) hypertrophic cardiomyopathy

17. What is the most appropriate cardiovascular screening method for average risk student-athletes?

    (A) history and physical examination
    (B) history, physical examination, and screening echocardiogram
    (C) history, physical examination, and screening electrocardiogram
    (D) history, physical examination, and screening exercise stress test
    (E) history, physical examination, complete blood count (CBC), and lipid panel

18. While examining this patient you hear a heart murmur. Which one of the following characteristics should prompt a referral to a cardiologist for further evaluation?

    (A) any systolic murmur
    (B) any diastolic murmur
    (C) any murmur that gets softer with Valsalva maneuver
    (D) any murmur that gets softer when the patient stands
    (E) a late systolic murmur that is preceded by a midsystolic click

Questions 19 through 21

A 10-day-old infant is brought to your clinic for a check up. The infant was born after an uncomplicated term gestation via an uncomplicated vaginal delivery. The mother's labs were negative. Both the mother and the baby have type O+ blood. The infant is breast-fed and has normal stool and urinary patterns. The mother noted that the child became jaundiced on day of life (DOL) 4 and that it peaked around DOL 6. She says that the jaundice seems to be slowly getting better. The infant is afebrile and, on initial examination, you note an otherwise healthy infant with moderate jaundice. The mother brings a discharge note from the newborn nursery that indicates that on DOL 3 the total bilirubin was 8.7 with a conjugated bilirubin of 0.5.

19. What is the most likely diagnosis in this newborn?

   (A) biliary atresia
   (B) physiologic jaundice
   (C) breast milk jaundice
   (D) jaundice from isoimmune hemolysis
   (E) jaundice from late onset group B streptococcal sepsis

20. What is the most appropriate next step in management of this infant?

   (A) follow the clinical examination closely
   (B) admit to the hospital for a sepsis work-up and phototherapy
   (C) draw total and direct serum bilirubin levels
   (D) interrupt the breast feeding for 24 h and supplement with formula during that time
   (E) draw a hematocrit and Coombs test on the infant

21. On closer examination you notice a crop of 5 clear vesicles with a mildly erythematous base on the infant's left shoulder. The mother denies seeing these in the past. She also denies having a history of herpes or having any symptoms. What should you do next?

   (A) Begin the infant on topical mupirocin and oral cephalexin.
   (B) Un-roof one of the vesicles, send a swab from the base of the lesion for bacterial culture and herpes simplex virus (HSV) polymerase chain reaction (PCR), and treat only if positive.
   (C) Follow the clinical examination closely for any changes.

   (D) Admit to the hospital for a complete "sepsis work-up" and empiric parenteral acyclovir.
   (E) Un-roof a vesicle, send for bacterial culture and HSV PCR, and begin oral acyclovir and cephalexin.

22. A 42-year-old male with a history of ulcerative colitis has been to the emergency room three times over the past 6 months complaining of right upper quadrant pain, fever, and jaundice. His total bilirubin has fluctuated from 0.5 to 4.2 over this time. Work up has included an endoscopic retrograde cholangiopancreatography (ERCP) with the findings as shown in Fig. 9-2. The patient should be informed that

   (A) The symptoms will resolve if he undergoes a total colectomy.
   (B) The only definitive treatment is liver transplantation.
   (C) Hepatic ultrasound is the best modality to diagnose his condition.
   (D) His disease is more commonly associated with irritable bowel syndrome.
   (E) A bacterial pathogen is the responsible agent.

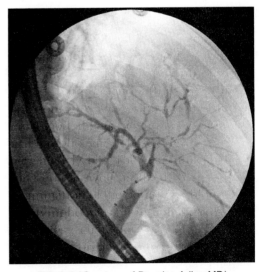

FIG. 9-2 (*Courtesy of Douglas Adler, MD.*)

Questions 23 through 25

A 33-year-old nulligravid female presents to her internist complaining of vaginal and pelvic pain of 8 months duration. The pain is diffuse, intermittent, 3/10 in severity, noncyclic, and does not radiate. It is exacerbated by bending and lifting and is not related to the timing of her menstrual cycle. She has internal vaginal pain with intercourse. The pain does not seem to be affected by urination or defecation. She has not noted any change in her vaginal discharge and is in a stable monogamous relationship. She has tried numerous over-the-counter medications, including acetaminophen and herbal remedies, without success. She has seen several other physicians for this problem, including a gynecologist, urologist, and gastroenterologist, none of whom "can find anything wrong with me."

23. An additional key element of her history today would include

    (A) whether or not she has had a work-up for systemic lupus erythematosus (SLE)
    (B) if she has had a history of recent travel outside the country
    (C) screening questions for depression, anxiety, and physical/sexual abuse
    (D) whether or not she has had a pelvic MRI
    (E) if she has a family history of colorectal cancer

24. On physical examination, the patient is afebrile with normal vital signs. Her urinalysis is unremarkable, she had a normal pap smear last month, her gonorrhea/chlamydia screen is negative, and her pregnancy test is negative. Her abdominal examination is normal with the exception of mild tenderness along the lower portion of her right abdomen which is exacerbated by raising her head from the table. Her cervix is normal appearing on speculum examination. On bimanual examination, she is tender along both lateral sidewalls of her vagina, and this tenderness increases with external rotation of her right hip. She had a pelvic ultrasound 1 week ago, which showed a 2-cm right ovarian cyst, normal uterus, and normal left adnexae.

Your most plausible diagnosis is

    (A) ovarian cancer
    (B) endometriosis
    (C) musculoskeletal pain
    (D) somatization disorder
    (E) irritable bowel syndrome

25. The most appropriate management at this time is

    (A) pelvic CT scan
    (B) laparoscopy
    (C) nonsteroidal anti-inflammatory drug (NSAID) and physical therapy
    (D) selective serotonin reuptake inhibitor (SSRI)
    (E) a high fiber diet and a prescription for dicyclomine (Bentyl)

26. A 42-year-old female patient with a history of diabetes develops necrolytic migratory erythema of her lower extremity. She most likely has

    (A) gastrinoma
    (B) glucagonoma
    (C) insulinoma
    (D) VIPoma
    (E) somatostatinoma

Setting II: Inpatient Facilities

You have general admitting privileges to the hospital, including the children's and women's services. On occasion you will see patients in the critical care unit. Postoperative patients are usually seen in their rooms, unless the recovery room is specified. You may also be called to see patients in the psychiatric unit. There is a short-stay unit where you may see patients undergoing same-day operations or being held for observation. Also, you may visit patients in the adjacent nursing home/extended care facility and the detoxification unit.

27. Tuboovarian abscess is one of the complications of acute pelvic inflammatory disease (PID), and occurs in up to 15–30% of women hospitalized with PID. The most cost-effective antibiotic regimen for treating inpatient women with tuboovarian abscess is:

(A) ampicillin IV plus gentamycin IV plus clindamycin IV
(B) cefotetan IV plus oral doxycycline
(C) gentamycin IV
(D) penicillin IM
(E) ancef IV

Questions 28 and 29

28. A 45-year-old female is undergoing radiation therapy for throat cancer. The patient develops slightly tender erythema of the face, chest, and hands as illustrated in Fig. 9-3. The most likely diagnosis is

(A) Sweet syndrome
(B) SLE
(C) radiation dermatitis
(D) drug reaction
(E) dermatomyositis

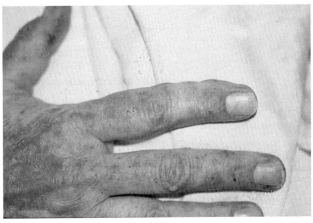

A

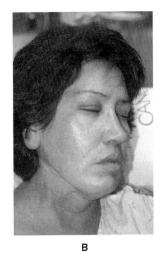

B

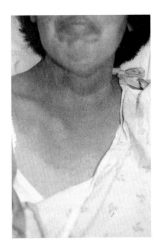

C

FIG. 9-3 Also see color plate. (*Courtesy of Steven Mays, MD.*)

29. Which of the following is the most appropriate initial treatment for this patient?

(A) IV immunoglobulin
(B) nonsteroidal anti-inflammatory drug
(C) topical midpotency steroid as needed for symptomatic relief
(D) oral prednisone
(E) oral diphenhydramine

30. A 62-year-old male smoker gradually develops dizziness, facial edema, and venous distention of the neck. An extensive workup including biopsy reveals the presence of a small cell carcinoma of the lung. Which of the following is the most appropriate management?

(A) loop diuretics
(B) radiation therapy
(C) angioplasty
(D) jugular vein bypass
(E) thoracotomy with operative resection

Questions 31 and 32

31. You are examining a male infant in the newborn nursery. He was born 6 h ago by spontaneous vaginal delivery to a 16-year-old primagravida mother. The prenatal course was unremarkable and the delivery was uncomplicated. Which of the following vaccines is recommended to be given to all newborn infants?

(A) DTaP
(B) BCG
(C) varicella
(D) hepatitis B
(E) Rhogam

32. Prophylaxis for which infectious agent is routinely given to all newborns?

(A) group B *Streptococcus*
(B) HSV
(C) *Chlamydia trachomatis*
(D) *Neisseria gonorrhea*
(E) *Escherichia coli*

33. A 42-year-old male, who has been on long-term oral steroid therapy, undergoes a partial small bowel resection for a near-obstructing Crohn's stricture. Which of the following vitamins is known to help counteract the ill effects of steroids on wound healing?

(A) vitamin A
(B) vitamin B_{12}
(C) vitamin C
(D) vitamin D
(E) vitamin E

34. A 19-year-old nulliparous patient is being evaluated for a palpable abdominal mass and complaints of pelvic pain and pressure. A CT scan is obtained and suggests the presence of bilateral solid adnexal masses, each approximately 6 cm in diameter. As part of your preoperative assessment, you order appropriate tumor markers to assess the malignant potential of this pelvic mass. In this setting, what tumor markers would you order?

(A) ovarian cancer antigen 125 (CA-125)
(B) carcinoembryonic antigen (CEA), CA-125
(C) CA 19-9
(D) inhibin
(E) alpha-fetoprotein (AFP), lactic dehydrogenase (LDH), beta hCG

35. A 45-year-old female, with a history of oral contraceptive use and right upper quadrant abdominal pain, has a 4 cm lesion in the right lobe of the liver seen on ultrasound. A CT scan reveals a hypodense lesion consistent with a hepatic adenoma. Which of the following is the most feared complication of the lesion?

(A) malignant transformation
(B) rupture and bleeding
(C) obstructive cholangitis
(D) anaphylactic shock
(E) peritoneal sepsis

36. A biopsy of a lateral neck mass in a 55-year-old man reveals normal thyroid tissue. Which of the following is the most appropriate management?

(A) suppression therapy with thioamides
(B) local excision of the neck mass
(C) excision of the neck mass and ipsilateral thyroid lobectomy
(D) excision of the neck mass and total thyroidectomy
(E) radioactive iodine ablation therapy

Setting III: Emergency Department

Most patients in this setting are new to you, but occasionally you arrange to meet there with a known patient who has telephoned you. Generally, patients encountered here are seeking urgent care. Also available to you are a full range of social services, including rape crisis intervention, family support, and security assistance backed up by local police.

37. A 2-year-old female developed generalized edema and, on urine examination, revealed a heavy proteinuria of 5 g over the 24-h period. Which of the following would be the diagnosis?

    (A) acute diffuse proliferative glomerulonephritis
    (B) membranoproliferative glomerulonephritis
    (C) membranous glomerulonephritis
    (D) minimal-change disease (lipoid nephrosis)
    (E) rapidly progressive glomerulonephritis

Questions 38 and 39

A 58-year-old incoherent and agitated man wanders into the emergency room. He has no specific complaints, but he appears confused and mumbles about being homeless for a long time. His vitals are unremarkable except for a pulse of 110. His physical examination is remarkable for poor hygiene, body odor, a diffusely tender abdomen, nystagmus, and an unsteady gait.

38. Intravenous administration of what substance would be the most appropriate next step in the management of this patient?

    (A) benzodiazepines
    (B) naloxone (Narcan)
    (C) thiamine
    (D) glucose
    (E) insulin

39. He is subsequently admitted to the medicine service for hepatitis. On day 3 of his admission, the nurses are concerned because he has mental status changes. On evaluation, he complains of extreme anxiety. He appears diaphoretic and tremulous. His vital signs demonstrate a temperature of 101.5°F, BP of 167/98, pulse of 120, and respirations of 24. Oral administration of which of the following benzodiazepines would be the most appropriate in the management of this patient?

    (A) alprazolam (Xanax)
    (B) clonazepam (Klonopin)
    (C) diazepam (Valium)
    (D) lorazepam (Ativan)
    (E) triazolam (Halcion)

40. A 32-year-old female with anorexia nervosa complains of chronic epigastric pain, nausea, and bilious vomiting. Her symptoms are relieved when she assumes a knee to chest position. The etiology of the disorder is most likely

    (A) compression of the bowel by the inferior mesenteric artery
    (B) kinking and obstruction of an afferent loop
    (C) obstruction of the third portion of the duodenum
    (D) obstruction from a cholangiocarcinoma
    (E) obstructing gastric ulcer

Questions 41 through 43

While working in the emergency room, you see a patient with a cough, mild pleuritic chest pain, and a reduced oxygen saturation. Your differential diagnosis includes pulmonary embolus (PE). You order a D-dimer titer as a screening test, with a subsequent result of 6.2 (normal range 0–5.0). Your lab reports to you that this test has a sensitivity of 90% and a specificity of 50% for the diagnosis of pulmonary embolism.

41. If the occurrence of pulmonary embolism in persons with these symptoms and signs is 1 in 3, what is the predictive value of a positive test for the diagnosis of pulmonary embolism?

    (A) 33%
    (B) 47%
    (C) 53%
    (D) 67%
    (E) 91%

42. What would be the predictive value of a negative D-dimer test?

    (A) 99%
    (B) 91%
    (C) 85%
    (D) 77%
    (E) 67%

43. After a reanalysis of the test is performed, it is decided by the hospital laboratory director to change the reference range for the D-dimer test. Now, a normal D-dimer result will be 0–3.5. The lab director states that the new sensitivity will be 95% and the new specificity will be 30%. Based on this change, which of the following statements is true?

    (A) The test now has a higher positive predictive value (PPV).
    (B) The test now has a higher negative predictive value (NPV).
    (C) Both the PPV and NPVs are now higher.
    (D) The test will now have more false negative results.
    (E) The test will now have more true negative results.

44. A 14-month-old develops a fever in the middle of summer. His parents state that he has had mild upper respiratory symptoms. On examination, he is febrile and fussy, but otherwise is well appearing. A CBC reveals an elevated white blood cell count. A urinalysis is normal. A lumbar puncture is performed and the following cerebrospinal fluid (CSF) results are found: WBC 50/hpf (60% lymph, 40% PMN), RBC 3/hpf, protein 75, glucose 88. What is the most likely infectious agent?

    (A) group B *Streptococcus*
    (B) HSV
    (C) *Neisseria meningitidis*
    (D) nonpolio enterovirus
    (E) *Streptococcus pneumoniae*

Questions 45 through 49

A 48-year-old Black woman, with a history of hypertension, cocaine abuse, and medical noncompliance, arrives at the emergency room complaining of progressive dyspnea on exertion, fatigue, nausea, vomiting, and generalized malaise. She also has had generalized pruritis for the past 4 weeks. She was last seen by her primary care physician approximately 2-$\frac{1}{2}$ years ago but never followed-up. On questioning, she has not been taking her antihypertensive medication for the last 1 year because she "ran out of them." On physical examination, she has a BP of 185/98, with a heart rate of 85 bpm. She is somnolent but oriented and follows commands. Her examination is significant for pale conjunctiva and nail beds. The cardiac examination shows a regular heart rate and rhythm with a S4 gallop. Her lungs have few bibasilar crackles and the abdominal examination is unremarkable. There is no audible abdominal bruit. Her extremities are significant for 1+ bilateral ankle edema and the neurologic examination was unremarkable. Rectal examination was negative for occult blood.

The laboratory values are:

Blood, serum value	Urinalysis:
Sodium 138	Specific gravity: 1.010
Potassium 5.8	Proteinuria: trace
Chloride 107	Leukocytes (per HPF): 0–2
CO_2 15	RBCs (per HPF): 1–3
BUN 75	Casts: 3–5 hyaline casts
Creatinine 8.4	
Glucose 80	
Phosphate 9.5	Urine electrolytes
Calcium 7.7	Na^+: 80
LDH 235	K^+: 30
Total bilirubin 0.2	Cl^-: 50
WBC 10.5	
Hemoglobin 7.7	Toxicology: positive for cocaine
Hematocrit 22.3	
Platelets 194	

An ECG shows sinus rhythm at a rate of 75 with left ventricular hypertrophy. The chest x-ray (CXR) shows clear lung fields with an enlarged cardiac silhouette.

A kidney ultrasound shows bilateral 7.5 cm kidneys (normal >11–12 cm) with increased echogenicity.

45. Which statement regarding the etiology of this patient's kidney failure is correct?

    (A) This patient has chronic kidney disease most likely from renal artery stenosis.

    (B) She has chronic kidney disease most likely secondary to hypertensive nephrosclerosis.

    (C) Her ultrasound findings are suggestive of HIV-associated nephropathy.

    (D) This patient has acute renal failure resulting from hypertensive emergency due to cocaine.

    (E) She has chronic kidney disease most likely from chronic glomerulonephritis.

46. What diagnostic test would be necessary to perform next?

    (A) cardiac catheterization to evaluate patient for coronary artery disease

    (B) a renal artery angiogram to evaluate for renal artery stenosis

    (C) a kidney biopsy

    (D) HIV serology to evaluate for HIV-associated nephropathy

    (E) no further diagnostic testing is indicated

47. Which statement best describes the mechanism explaining this patient's anemia?

    (A) development of polyclonal antibodies against erythropoietin

    (B) diminished production of erythropoietin by bone marrow

    (C) decreased production of erythropoietin by kidney cells

    (D) increased erythropoietin production by red blood cells

    (E) decreased production of bone marrow erythropoietin receptors due to uremic toxins

48. Which of the following would be the next best step?

    (A) placement of an arterio-venous fistula and initiation of hemodialysis

    (B) intravenous infusion of sodium bicarbonate and furosemide

    (C) placement of a temporary hemodialysis catheter and initiate hemodialysis immediately

    (D) intravenous infusion of calcium gluconate, insulin, and dextrose to treat hyperkalemia

    (E) placement of an arterio-venous graft and initiate hemodialysis as soon as possible

49. Which of the following is an indication for emergent hemodialysis?

    (A) BUN of 110 and creatinine of 10.0

    (B) urine output of <5 cc/h for the past 24-h

    (C) pericardial friction rub on physical examination

    (D) ingestion of toxic levels of acetaminophen

    (E) asymptomatic, but profound, hyponatremia (Na 115)

50. A 33-year-old male is brought to the ER by paramedics because of a severe asthma attack. He is intubated and placed on a mechanical ventilator on an assist control (AC) mode with a rate of 18, FiO_2 of 70%, and an appropriate tidal volume for his size. Appropriate treatment of his asthma is instituted and a CXR confirms appropriate endotracheal tube placement. One hour after intubation, an arterial blood gas is drawn with the following results: pH 7.47/pCO_2 30/pO_2 280/O_2 saturation of 100%.

    Which of the following ventilator setting changes would be most appropriate?

    (A) Increase the ventilator rate to 20 and keep the FiO_2 at 70%.

    (B) Increase the ventilator rate to 20 and reduce the FiO_2 to 50%.

    (C) Reduce the ventilator rate to 16 and keep the FiO_2 at 70%.

    (D) Reduce the ventilator rate to 16 and reduce the FiO_2 to 50%.

    (E) Keep the ventilator rate at 18 and the FiO_2 at 70%.

Answers and Explanations

1. **(C)**

2. **(C)**

3. **(D)**

4. **(C)**

Explanations 1 through 4

The seventh report of the Joint National Committee on the prevention, detection, evaluation, and treatment of high blood pressure (JNC VII) key recommendations classify this patient in hypertension stage 1, as most of her BP readings are systolic blood pressure (SBP) in the 140–159 range and diastolic blood pressure (DBP) between 90 and 99.

Category	SBP and/or DBP
Normal	<120 and <80
Prehypertension	120–139 or 80–90
Hypertension stage 1	140–159 or 90–99
Hypertension stage 2	≥160 or ≥100

The primary purpose of the initial physical examination is to look for causes of secondary hypertension and for early organ damage due to untreated hypertension. In your physical examination for a newly diagnosed patient with hypertension, you should include BP measurement in both arms, examination of the optic fundi, BMI calculation, auscultation for carotid, abdominal and femoral bruits, palpation of the thyroid gland, examination of the heart and lungs, and examination of the abdomen for enlarged kidneys, masses, and abnormal aortic pulsation. Cranial/peripheral nerve examination, mental status examination, and palpation of the abdomen for hepatosplenomegaly are not an essential part of this physical examination.

Initial laboratory tests should include urinalysis (not urine microalbumin), blood glucose (not hemoglobin A1c), hematocrit, lipid panel and serum potassium, creatinine and calcium, which is part of a basic metabolic panel (not liver function tests). There is no indication for exercise stress testing at this time.

The JNC VII recommends that the most appropriate initial management for this patient is lifestyle modification and a thiazide-type diuretic. Lifestyle modification includes weight reduction (goal BMI 18.5–24.9), adopting the DASH diet plan, dietary sodium reduction, regular aerobic physical activity such as brisk walking at least 30 min/day most days of the week, and no more than 2 alcoholic drinks per day in most men and no more than 1 alcoholic drink per day in women.

Beta-blockers should be the initial pharmacologic agents in postmyocardial infarction patients. ACE inhibitors should be the initial pharmacologic agents in patients with chronic kidney diseases. (*National Heart, Lung and Blood Institute. The 7th report of the joint national committee on prevention, detection, evaluation and treatment of high blood pressure, 2003*)

5. **(B)** The presence of a red eye in a patient with signs of a herpes viral infection (cold sore) raises the possibility of herpetic infection of the eye. This can be in the form of eyelid involvement only, conjunctivitis or corneal disease, with corneal disease being the most serious and potentially vision threatening. The most appropriate and important intervention at this time would be flourescein staining of the cornea with a slit-lamp examination to look for the presence of corneal epithelial ulcers, particularly dendritic ulcers characteristic of HSV, or abnormalities of the deeper corneal stroma. Most cases of herpes simplex can be diagnosed clinically, but corneal scrapings or viral

cultures may be taken. Patients with corneal herpes infections require antiviral therapy—either topical or systemic—and frequent ophthalmologic follow up. *(Wills, Section 4.14)*

6. **(C)** The patient appears to be insulin deficient with uncontrolled hyperglycemia and weight loss. He now weighs 150 lbs, which is about 15 lbs below his ideal body weight. Type 1 diabetes can occur at any age. Although there is a genetic component to type-1 diabetes, it is less consistent than type 2 diabetes, so his negative family history tends to favor this entity. Each of the oral medications, even if effective, would only reduce glycohemoglobin by 1–2%. Therefore, there is no single agent that will correct his glucose level into a target range. As he is underweight and losing weight, it is unlikely that insulin resistance is playing a major role. Thus, rosiglitazone or metformin would not be advisable. Glyburide and glipizide are similar sulfonylureas, so there is no advantage in switching from one to another. Only insulin will immediately correct the hyperglycemia and the weight loss. *(Larsen, pp. 1460–1466)*

7. **(C)** The pathognomonic lesion of gout is the tophus, a collection of crystalline or amorphous urates surrounded by an inflammatory response consisting of macrophages, lymphocytes, fibroblasts, and foreign body giant cells. In the photomicrograph that accompanies the question, the darker stellate deposits denote the center of the tophus. These urate deposits would appear golden brown, in contrast to the pink-staining tissue about them on hematoxylin-eosin staining. Gout is a systemic disorder of uric acid metabolism resulting in hyperuricemia. Urates precipitate out of the supersaturated blood and deposit in the joints and soft tissue. Rheumatoid arthritis and ankylosing spondylitis are characterized by a diffuse proliferative synovitis; suppurative arthritis, by a prominent neutrophilic inflammation; and osteoarthritis, by cartilaginous and subchondral bone changes. *(Cotran, 5th ed., pp. 1253–1257)*

8. **(E)**

9. **(B)**

Explanations 8 and 9

This individual is experiencing a psychotic illness, manifested by paranoia, delusions and hallucinations, lasting for several months. Brief psychotic disorder is characterized by psychotic symptoms similar to those above but only lasting for 1 day up to 1 month, with a subsequent return to premorbid functioning. Delusional disorder typically affects patients in midlife and involves the presence of a non-bizarre delusion without prominent hallucinations or significant impairment in functioning, as seen in the above case. A diagnosis of schizoaffective disorder requires both 1 month of psychotic symptoms and an additional mood disorder; this patient does not display evidence of a significant affective component. The diagnosis of schizophrenia similarly necessitates at least 1 month of active psychosis, but some indication of the disorder must be present for at least 6 months. While this patient may actually have and be eventually diagnosed with schizophrenia, his above presentation is consistent with schizophreniform disorder, the criteria of which require prominent psychotic symptoms to be present for at least 1 month but less than 6 months (DSM IV).

The introduction of second generation, so called atypical, antipsychotics have markedly improved the armamentarium in the treatment of psychotic disorders such as schizophrenia. They are at least as effective as older medications in decreasing the positive symptoms, such as delusions, hallucinations, or disorganized speech/behavior. Their advantage over neuroleptics such as haloperidol comes with the superior management of negative symptoms, including apathy, anhedonia, and poor attention. As a class, second-generation antipsychotics do have disadvantages. They can cause a significant amount of weight gain and are substantially more expensive when compared directly to the cost of older agents. Potency of a drug is the amount needed to obtain efficacy. While the efficacy of the second-generation medications is similar across the board, their potency varies significantly and is not necessarily greater when compared to the older neuroleptics. One of the greatest improvements is that, as a group, the atypical antipsychotics cause substantially fewer extrapyramidal side effects and, therefore, may be better tolerated overall. (*Synopsis, p. 498*)

10. **(A)** Direct visualization of the pelvic organs during laparoscopy is required to definitively diagnose endometriosis. In some cases, a biopsy of one or more of the lesions for pathologic confirmation may also be useful. Cystic collections of endometriosis in the ovaries, termed endometriomas, can often be visualized by CT, MRI, or ultrasonography. However, intraoperative confirmation is still required to exclude other common causes of cystic ovarian masses. (*Stenchever, p. 532*)

11. **(C)**

12. **(B)**

13. **(C)**

14. **(A)**

Explanations 11 through 14

The history and physical examination are all highly suspicious for Crohn's disease, an inflammatory bowel disorder that can affect the entire gut from the mouth to the anus. Gastric and duodenal ulcers would likely present with bleeding and not diarrhea. A small bowel volvulus would be more acute and would have signs of an obstruction. A normal examination would be unlikely.

Patients with Crohn's disease often have ileal inflammation, which leads to the loss of bile acid receptors in the terminal ileum. This results in net bile salt loss with a decreased overall bile acid pool and, thus, bile in the biliary tree that is more lithogenic. Hypercholesterolemia, not hypocholesterolemia, is associated with gallstones. PSC is associated with ulcerative colitis, not Crohn's disease. The ultrasound findings are not compatible with chronic cholecystitis, as the gallbladder wall is normal and there is not pericholecystic fluid. Tobacco use is not associated with gallstones.

Patients with Crohn's disease are at increased risk of developing cancer in areas of chronic inflammation. In this patient, as she has primarily small bowel disease, she is at risk for small bowel adenocarcinoma. Adenocarcinoma of the ileum, where this patient likely has the most inflammation, can be seen 100 times more frequently in Crohn's patients than in age and sex matched controls. The other malignancies listed are not strongly associated with Crohn's disease, although patients with Crohn's disease are also at increased risk for squamous cell cancers of the anus and vulva, as well as certain hematologic malignancies such as lymphomas. Patients with Crohn's colitis are at increased risk for colorectal cancer.

The history and physical are most consistent with Crohn's disease. The patient is young, a smoker, and has right lower quadrant pain associated with diarrhea. The presence of oral ulcers and a history of an anal fissure are all strongly associated with Crohn's disease. Irritable bowel syndrome is not associated with fevers, but can produce diarrhea and abdominal pain. Ulcerative colitis would likely produce bloody diarrhea. Endometriosis would be expected to flare during menses. Chronic pancreatitis could present with diarrhea but would be very unusual in a young female who does not consume alcohol. (*Harrison's Principles of Internal Medicine, pp. 1683–1692*)

15. **(C)** Acute dactilitis (hand-foot syndrome) is one of the first manifestations of sickle cell disease. This entity is due to bone marrow necrosis of the hands and feet. The first attack usually occurs before the end of the first year of life, when the hemoglobin F level declines. Acute dactilitis becomes infrequent after age 6, when hematopoiesis shifts from the small bones to the axial skeleton. (*Hoffman, pp. 531–532*)

16. **(E)**

17. **(A)**

18. **(B)**

Explanations 16 through 18

Sudden cardiac death is defined as a nontraumatic, nonviolent, and unexpected event resulting from sudden cardiac arrest within 6 h of a previously witnessed state of normal health. It occurs in about 1 per 200,000 high school athletes per academic year. The most common cause of sudden death in athletic adolescents is hypertrophic cardiomyopathy (36%), followed by coronary artery abnormalities (19%). Marfan syndrome, aortic stenosis, and mitral valve prolapse are rare causes of sudden death in athletic adolescents.

Detection of cardiovascular abnormalities that may cause sudden death is difficult, as congenital cardiac abnormalities relevant to athletic screening account for a combined prevalence of only about 0.2% in athletic populations. Currently, there is no cost-effective battery of tests to identify all, or even most, dangerous cardiovascular conditions. A complete, careful, personal and family history, and physical examination is recommended to identify, or raise suspicion of, cardiovascular lesions known to cause sudden cardiac death or disease progression in young athletes.

During the physical examination, auscultation of the heart should be performed with the patient in standing and supine positions. The following murmurs should be referred to cardiologist for further evaluation: any systolic murmur grade 3/6 or higher, any diastolic murmur, and any murmur that gets louder with Valsalva maneuver. Murmurs that get softer when a patient stands include tricuspid stenosis (most commonly rheumatic in origin), and atrial or ventricular septal defects. A late systolic murmur that is preceded by a midsystolic click is characteristic of mitral valve prolapse. (*Lyznicki JM, Nielsen NH, Schneider JF. Cardiovascular screening of student athletes. Am Fam Physician 2000;62:765–784*)

19. **(B)**

20. **(A)**

21. **(D)**

Explanations 19 through 21

Approximately one-third of newborn infants will have some degree of recognizable jaundice. This is termed physiologic jaundice. This physiologic jaundice is usually present after the first 2 days of life and will usually peak by day 5. This jaundice usually lasts no longer than 10–14 days and has no conjugated portion. Breast milk jaundice is seen when the jaundice in a newborn is prolonged, typically longer than 2 weeks. Group B Streptococcus (GBS) infection is a cause of jaundice in the newborn infant, but it is very rare compared to physiologic jaundice. Biliary atresia causes a cholestatic (or conjugated) jaundice. Isoimmune hemolysis is the cause of a rapid increase in the bilirubin level and is usually seen in the first 1–3 days of life. Jaundice from hemolysis is much less common than physiologic jaundice.

Physiologic jaundice is usually a benign, self-limited condition. It usually does not require therapy once it begins to resolve. Breast milk jaundice may improve with interruption of breast feeding, but that is not recommended by the American Academy of Pediatrics. If this infant's bilirubin level were increasing, it could be anticipated that hemolysis were present. If that were the case, the amount of hemolysis could be judged by a hematocrit and reticulocyte count. (*Rudolph, pp. 164–169*)

What is described in the vignette is cutaneous herpes simplex infection (HSV). A negative maternal history for HSV is seen in approximately 50% of infants with perinatally acquired HSV disease. The absence of a maternal history of HSV should not dissuade one from entertaining the diagnosis. Neonatal HSV occurs in one of three common presentations: skin-eye-mucous membrane (SEM), disseminated, and CNS disease. What is described is the SEM manifestation. Approximately one-third of infants with SEM HSV will develop CNS or disseminated disease. All infants with SEM HSV in the newborn period should be treated aggressively with a full evaluation and parenteral acyclovir. Oral acyclovir has no role in the management of perinatal HSV disease. SEM manifestation of HSV needs to be distinguished from a simple impetigo, which may present with cloudy blisters, most commonly in the diaper region. This entity could potentially be treated with topical or oral antimicrobials. If HSV cannot be adequately ruled-out, aggressive intervention is warranted. *(Red Book, pp. 344–353)*

22. **(B)** Sclerosing cholangitis is a chronic progressive disease of the liver in which an inflammatory process results in intrahepatic and/or extrahepatic biliary strictures. The disease is progressive and may eventually result in biliary cirrhosis and portal hypertension. Sclerosing cholangitis is strongly associated with ulcerative colitis and to a lesser extent with Crohn's disease. The precise cause is unknown; however, it has been suggested that it may result from a local response to viral infection.

     The diagnosis should be considered in a patient with inflammatory bowel disease who presents with abnormal liver function tests and a clinical picture of jaundice, intermittent right upper quadrant pain, nausea, vomiting, and fever. The diagnosis is traditionally established by ERCP demonstrating characteristic biliary strictures alternating with areas of dilatation that has been referred to as a "string of beads." The appropriate management of sclerosing cholangitis is supportive, with no known medical cure. Definitive treatment of the underlying ulcerative colitis with total colectomy does not prevent progression of the disease. In patients with diffuse and advanced parenchymal disease, hepatic transplantation is the only known cure. *(Cameron, pp. 428–430)*

23. **(C)**

24. **(C)**

25. **(C)**

Explanations 23 through 25

Physical and sexual abuse are associated with various chronic pain disorders. Studies have found that up to 50% of women with chronic pelvic pain have a history of past or current abuse. *(Jamieson EF, Steege JF. The association of sexual abuse with pelvic pain complaints in a primary care population. Am J Obstet Gynecol 1997;177:1408–1412)*

Primary or secondary myofascial pelvic pain is an under-recognized and under-treated aspect of pelvic pain. Common findings include exacerbation of symptoms with movement, lifting, and/or vaginal penetration, along with localization to the abdominal wall and/or vaginal sidewalls. NSAIDs and physical therapy can be helpful for these patients. *(King PM, et al. Musculoskeletal factors in chronic pelvic pain. J Psychosom Obstet Gynaecol 1991;12(Suppl):87–98; Weiss JM. Pelvic floor myofascial trigger points: Manual therapy for interstitial cystitis and the urgency-frequency syndrome. J Urol 2001;166:2226–2231)*

26. **(B)** Glucagonoma is a tumor that arises from α_2 cells in the islets of Langerhans of the pancreas. They produce a distinctive syndrome consisting of migratory necrolytic dermatitis of the legs and perineum, weight loss, stomatitis, hypoaminoacidemia, anemia, and diabetes mellitus. Patients also have a risk of venous thrombosis and pulmonary emboli. The diagnosis is confirmed by demonstrating elevated plasma glucagon levels. Workup should include an abdominal CT scan and, if necessary, arteriography to localize the lesion. The majority of glucagonomas are malignant and have metastasized by the time of diagnosis. The most common sites of metastases include the liver, lymph nodes, adrenal gland, and vertebrae. Treatment includes surgical excision of the primary tumor and debulking of metastases. Oral zinc supplement may improve the dermatitis. Somatostatin has been reported to return serum glucagon and amino acid levels to normal, clear the rash, and promote weight gain. Streptozotocin and dacarbazine are the most effective chemotherapeutic agents. *(Schwartz, p. 1496)*

27. **(A)** A tuboovarian abscess is more likely to respond to triple antibiotic therapy. Lack of response within 48 h usually requires surgical intervention. *(McNeely S, et al. Medically sound, cost-effective treatment for pelvic inflammatory disease and tubo-ovarian abscess. Am J Obstet Gynecol 1998;178(6): 1272–1278)*

28. (E)

29. (D)

Explanations 28 and 29

This patient has the classic cutaneous manifestations of dermatomyositis: the purple discoloration and edema of the upper eyelids (heliotrope erythema); malar erythema; purple macules over the knuckles (Gottron's sign); and erythema of the sun-exposed upper chest (V sign). The skin lesions of dermatomyositis are photoexacerbated. Many patients also have nail fold telangiectasias, which are also seen in scleroderma and systemic lupus. The five diagnostic criteria for dermatomyositis are: (1) characteristic skin lesions; (2) symmetric proximal muscle weakness; (3) elevated skeletal muscle enzymes, especially creatinine phosphokinase; (4) characteristic electromyelogram findings; and (5) characteristic muscle biopsy findings.

Some patients may present with the cutaneous manifestations only. They may later develop the characteristic symmetric proximal weakness that particularly involves the neck flexors, shoulder abductors and adductors, and hip flexors. Patients may complain of having difficulty getting up from a chair, climbing steps, or combing their hair. Muscle involvement in dermatomyositis may be confirmed by electromyelogram or by muscle biopsy. Activity of muscle disease can be monitored by following serum levels of creatine phosphokinase (CPK (MM)). Approximately 20–30% of adult patients with dermatomyositis have an associated underlying malignancy, in particular ovarian, lung, pancreatic, colon, and non-Hodgkin's lymphoma. Patients with dermatomyositis may have involvement of other organ systems, such as GI (with dysphagia); cardiac (with arrhythmias, conduction defects, and cardiomyopathy); and pulmonary (with interstitial lung disease and respiratory failure from muscle weakness). Approximately 30% have arthralgias of the peripheral joints. Fifty percent of patients have high-titer antinuclear antibodies (ANA).

The initial treatment of choice for dermatomyositis is oral prednisone. After an initial period of high dose treatment, the prednisone will be tapered slowly until the lowest possible dose that controls the disease is reached. Immunosuppressive drugs may be required if the disease is not responsive to steroids. Approximately 75% of patients will eventually require immunosuppressive therapy. IVIG can improve symptoms in refractory cases, but the benefit is short lived and repeated treatments are required. NSAIDs and antihistamines do not play a role in the treatment of dermatomyositis. (*Harrison's Principles of Internal Medicine*, 15th ed., pp. 2524–2529)

30. (B) Superior vena cava (SVC) obstruction is caused by a bronchogenic carcinoma in over 85% of cases. The majority of these carcinomas are small cell tumors. Obstruction is caused by compression or direct invasion and results in impairment of the venous return from the head, neck, and upper extremities. Patients present with venous distention, facial edema, and plethora. Less common symptoms include headache, respiratory symptoms, and life-threatening laryngeal edema with airway compression.

The presence of SVC obstruction in a patient with a bronchogenic carcinoma portends a grave prognosis, with survival measured in weeks to months. Radical surgical resection in these patients is contraindicated and treatment is aimed at palliation. Palliative radiation, with or without chemotherapy, has proven effective to help downsize the tumor and ameliorate many of the accompanying symptoms. It is therefore the preferred treatment modality. (*Schwartz, p. 784*)

31. (D)

32. (C)

Explanations 31 and 32

The current recommendations are that all newborn infants receive the hepatitis B vaccine in the newborn period, specifically within the first 12 h of life. The vaccine should be administered in the newborn nursery. Rhogam is not a vaccine. It is pooled IgG used to prevent Rh-isoimmunization in Rh-negative mothers. BCG is a vaccine used in other countries to prevent tuberculous meningitis in the neonate. It is not used in the United States. Varicella vaccine is not administered until after the child is 12 months of age.

All newborn infants in the United States receive ophthalmia neonatorum prophylaxis in the immediate newborn period. This commonly is a topical dose of erythromycin or tetracycline. This is used to prevent trachoma, which is the leading infectious cause of blindness in the world. Trachoma is a manifestation of a *C. trachomatis* ocular infection. Historically, ophthalmia neonatorum prophylaxis was with topical silver nitrate but, as it caused a significant contact irritation, it is no longer routinely used. (*Red Book, pp. 24, 238–243*)

33. **(A)** Vitamin A plays an important role in wound healing. It is involved in the stimulation of fibroblasts, collagen cross-linking, and epithelialization. In addition, it has been shown to help reverse many of the inhibitory effects of glucocorticoids on the inflammatory phase of wound healing. Vitamin A may be indicated in steroid-dependent patients undergoing extensive surgery or for those with problematic wounds. (*Greenfield, p. 78*)

34. **(E)** Epithelial ovarian tumors arise from the surface epithelium of the ovary and comprise approximately 75–80% of all ovarian neoplasms; the mean age of onset is 60 years of age. Germ cell neoplasms arise from the germ cell, or eggs of the ovary, and comprise 10–15% of ovarian tumors; the mean age of onset is 19 years of age. Sex cord stromal neoplasms arise from the connective tissue of the ovary and comprise approximately 5% of ovarian neoplasms. Their occurrence is rather evenly spread over the childhood and adult years, with a minimal propensity toward bilateralism.

Ovarian tumors are capable of producing peptides that can be detected in the peripheral circulation and, if present, that can suggest the presence of these tumors preoperatively. For example, CA-125 will be elevated in the presence of epithelial ovarian cancers in approxi-

mately 80% of all cases. Unfortunately, elevations in CA-125 are found most commonly in association with advanced stage, incurable disease. CA-125 will be elevated in less than 50% of curable stage 1 disease. The usefulness of CA-125 as a screening tumor marker for epithelial ovarian cancer is also limited by the fact that CA-125 can be elevated in association with a number of benign gynecologic conditions including endometrioisis, PID, menstruation, adenomyosis, leiomyomata, and pregnancy.

Germ cell neoplasms comprise the second largest category of ovarian neoplasm. Characteristic germ cell neoplasms include dysgerminoma, immature teratoma, endodermal sinus tumor, embryonal tumor, gonadoblastoma, and mixed germ cell neoplasms. Dysgerminomas comprise 50% of all germ cell neoplasms and have a propensity toward bilateralism. Dysgerminomas are associated with elevated levels of LDH, endodermal sinus tumors with elevated levels of AFP, and embryonal tumors with elevated levels of AFP and beta hCG. Immature teratomas can be associated with elevated levels of LDH and AFP.

CEA is a nonspecific tumor antigen that can be elevated in the setting of GI tumors, breast cancer, and mucinous ovarian neoplasms. Inhibin is a tumor marker that can be elevated in association with granulosa cell tumors, a specific type of ovarian sex cord stromal neoplasms.

Given the age of the patient in this case, the most likely category of ovarian tumor present would be a germ cell tumor. Thus, the appropriate panel of tumor markers to order would be AFP, LDH, and beta hCG. (*Schwartz PE. Ovarian masses: serologic markers. Clin Obstet Gynecol 1991;34:423–432*)

35. **(B)** Hepatic adenoma is a benign tumor of the liver that is strongly associated with oral contraceptive use. Ninety percent of patients with hepatic adenomas have a history of oral contraceptive use. The diagnosis is typically made in women of childbearing age who present with right upper quadrant pain or mass effect. Liver function tests are usually normal. The hepatic lesion is identified on US, CT, and MRI. Characteristic findings include a hypodense

lesion on CT scan and early enhancement on MRI with contrast. Percutaneous biopsy is contraindicated because it is associated with a high risk of bleeding.

Hepatic adenomas are associated with up to a 30% risk of spontaneous rupture with life-threatening massive hemorrhage. Although much less common, malignant transformation has also been described.

Although regression and disappearance of hepatic adenomas have been reported after the discontinuation of contraceptives, the potential for bleeding and malignant transformation warrants routine surgical resection. They often can be removed by enucleation with a narrow rim of normal hepatic parenchyma. *(Cameron, p. 318)*

36. **(D)** The finding of normal thyroid tissue in the lateral side of the neck, previously known as lateral aberrant thyroid, is, in fact, a metastasis from an occult papillary type thyroid carcinoma. Therefore, definitive treatment mandates total thyroidectomy with excision of the metastatic neck lesion. Medical therapy and radioactive iodine ablation are treatment modalities for benign disease, such as a toxic goiter. *(Charles V. Mann, R.C.G. Russell, Norman S. Williams. Bailey & Love's Short Practice of Surgery, 22nd ed. London: Chapman & Hall, 1995)*

37. **(D)** In minimal-change disease (lipoid nephrosis) the classic clinical findings secondary to glomerular injury are massive proteinuria, hypoalbuminemia, peripheral edema, and hyperlipidemia. Lipoid nephrosis is of unknown etiology and pathogenesis. Epidemiologically it is seen in children, usually between the ages of 1 and 4. The clinical picture gives the pure nephrotic syndrome, which is selective proteinuria in over 90% of the cases (only albumin is lost in the urine). The BP generally remains normal and the urine sediment is free of RBCs or WBCs. Of the other selections listed, membranous glomerulonephritis occurs in adults, while rapidly progressive glomerulonephritis and acute diffuse proliferative glomerulonephritis have different symptomatology and clinical presentation. *(Cotran, 6th ed., pp. 954–956)*

38. **(C)**

39. **(D)**

Explanations 38 and 39

This case is demonstrative of Wernicke's encephalopathy, caused by acute thiamine deficiency. Intravenous benzodiazepines would be an appropriate treatment for delirium caused by either alcohol or benzodiazepine withdrawal, which might present with confusion and agitation. However, the patient would likely display an elevated BP, as well as flushing, diaphoresis, and tremor. Intravenous naloxone is the treatment of choice for acute opiate overdose. This would more likely present with a diminished level of consciousness, a decreased pulse, BP, and respirations, as well as constricted and unresponsive pupils. Intravenous insulin would be essential for treating diabetic ketoacidosis. The classic triad of Wernicke's encephalopathy includes confusion, oculomotor disturbances, and ataxia. The treatment of choice is parenteral thiamine given prior to glucose, as administering glucose prior to thiamine can cause a worsening of symptoms or even permanent damage. *(Synopsis, p. 908)*

This presentation is consistent with acute alcohol withdrawal. While the primary treatment for alcohol withdrawal is benzodiazepines, alprazolam is a shorter acting but high potency drug, which would require more frequent dosing and may potentially build up in the patient's system given his hepatic disease. Clonazepam is longer acting but also higher potency, and could cause over-sedation given its active metabolites. Diazepam can be an appropriate treatment for alcohol withdrawal; however caution should be used in patients with questionable hepatic function given the long half-life of the medication and its metabolite. It is also poorly absorbed when given intramuscularly. Triazolam is a very short-acting benzodiazepine, used only for insomnia, and as such can cause rebound anxiety in individuals. Lorazepam has the advantage of having an intermediate half-life and not being dependent on liver function for its breakdown. It is also well absorbed when given orally and parenterally. *(Synopsis, pp. 908, 404–405)*

40. (C) The superior mesenteric artery arises directly from the aorta and crosses in front of the third portion of the duodenum to enter the root of the mesentery. Superior mesenteric artery compression syndrome occurs when the acute angle between the aorta and superior mesenteric artery results in compression of the third portion of the duodenum. This syndrome usually occurs in young, thin women who have a loss of the retroperitoneal fat cushion. The syndrome is also known as "cast syndrome" because of its association with patients in body casts. Symptoms include bilious vomiting and postprandial pain. Medical treatment consists of eliminating all contributing factors (such as casts), lying in the supine position and increasing weight. Surgery is reserved for those who fail conservative measures. Surgical interventions include releasing the ligament of Treitz, which moves the duodenum out from beneath the superior mesenteric artery, or bypassing the obstruction. (*Schwartz, p. 1560*)

41. (B)

42. (B)

43. (B)

Explanations 41 through 43

In order to determine the answers to Questions 41 and 42, we must first take the information provided and place it into 2 × 2 table form. With the given prevalence of the disease being 1 in 3, we will assume a population of 300 people, as this makes the mathematical calculations as easy as possible—100 people will have a PE and 200 will be free of this disease.

With the sensitivity of the test being 90%, then the number of true positive test results is calculated as: $0.9 \times 100 = 90$. The number of false negative test results would then be: $100 - 90 = 10$.

With the specificity of the test being 50%, then the number of true negative test results is calculated as: $0.5 \times 200 = 100$. The number of false positive test results would then be: $200 - 100 = 100$.

A 2 × 2 table with this information would appear as follows:

Disease: Pulmonary Embolism

		+	−
D-dimer	+	True positives 90	False positives 100
	−	False negatives 10	True negatives 100

The calculation of predictive values is then:

$$PPV = \text{true positives}/(\text{true positive} + \text{false positive})$$
$$PPV = 90/(90 + 100) = 0.47 = 47\%$$
$$NPV = \text{true negatives}/(\text{true negative} + \text{false negative})$$
$$NPV = 100/(100 + 10) = 0.91 = 91\%$$

The answer to Question 43 requires the understanding of the concepts of sensitivity and specificity as characteristics of a test. By lowering the threshold for a test to be abnormal, in this case lowering the upper limit of the normal D-dimer range from 5.0 to 3.5, one can reasonably expect to have more test results that are abnormal (i.e., all of the test results from 3.6 to 4.9 that used to be considered normal will now be considered abnormal). Some of these results will be true positives and some of them will be false positives. The net effect of this will be to increase the sensitivity of the test and to lower its specificity. However, the prevalence of the disease in the population will remain the same, because changing a test characteristic does not change the occurrence of the disease. Putting the new numbers into a 2 × 2 table results in:

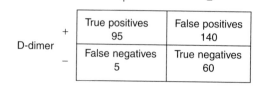

Disease: Pulmonary Embolism

		+	−
D-dimer	+	True positives 95	False positives 140
	−	False negatives 5	True negatives 60

The PPV now equals $95/(95 + 140) = 0.40 = 40\%$

The NPV now equals $60/(60 + 5) = 0.92 = 92\%$

Conceptually, this can be remembered by using the following mnemonics: SpPIn and SnNOut. In the first, when a test is highly **Sp**ecific, a **P**ositive test helps to rule **In** a disease (SpPIn). In the second, when a test is highly **Sen**sitive, a **N**egative helps to rule **Out** a disease. *(Slawson D, Shaughnessy A. Becoming an information master. Course materials, 2003)*

44. **(D)** The "summer flu" is commonly a nonpolio enterovirus infection. In children this may manifest itself in a range from simply fever to shock and encephalitis. Most infants and children with enteroviral infection have fever, fussiness, and a nominal amount of upper respiratory infection (URI) symptoms. The CSF findings described are most consistent with aseptic meningitis. The lymphocytic predominant CSF pleocytosis, with a normal glucose and protein level, would speak against this being bacterial meningitis. The CSF findings may also be consistent with HSV meningoencephalitis, but the child would not typically be well appearing clinically. Enterovirus infections usually warrant supportive care only. *(Red Book, pp. 269–270)*

45. **(B)**

46. **(E)**

47. **(C)**

48. **(C)**

49. **(C)**

Explanations 45 through 49

This patient most likely has hypertensive nephrosclerosis. Furthermore, the findings in her history suggest that she has chronic kidney disease. The presence of LVH and an S4 gallop suggest long-standing hypertension with end-organ damage. Small, echogenic kidneys are consistent with a chronic process; therefore, this is unlikely to be a presentation of acute renal failure. HIV-associated nephropathy is usually associated with large kidneys on ultrasound. There is no evidence, by urinalysis, of glomerulonephritis.

At this time, there is no indication for any invasive evaluation of coronary artery disease. Moreover, there is nothing on physical examination (such as abdominal bruit) to suggest renal artery stenosis. Given the small, echogenic kidneys, any intervention at this point would not likely make a difference in her kidney function. HIV-associated nephropathy usually is associated with significant proteinuria and large kidneys on ultrasound—neither of which is presented in this case. Lastly, a kidney biopsy would not likely yield any information that could improve the renal outcome in this case. Moreover, biopsy of small, scarred kidneys is not recommended, as this poses a significant risk of bleeding.

Erythropoietin is a glycoprotein that is synthesized in kidney cells adjacent to the proximal tubule. Erythropoietin then stimulates erythropoiesis in the bone marrow. In chronic kidney disease, the synthesis of erythropoietin is diminished, resulting in anemia. This anemia can be treated by administering recombinant human erythropoietin.

This patient requires urgent hemodialysis as she is presenting with uremic symptoms, i.e., nausea, vomiting, and malaise. An arteriovenous fistula is the best form of permanent hemodialysis access (owing to its less frequent rate of infections), followed by arterio-venous graft. However, an AV fistula takes weeks to mature. Similarly, an AV graft cannot be used immediately. As this patient has chronic kidney disease with symptoms of uremia, she will need dialysis much sooner. Placement of a temporary dialysis catheter, which can be used immediately, would be the best choice at the present time. An alternative access would be the placement of a tunneled permanent hemodialysis catheter, if this could be done in quick fashion. The acid-base and electrolyte abnormalities will be managed with hemodialysis and, at this time, there is no emergency stemming from the hyperkalemia and metabolic acidosis.

Emergent hemodialysis is indicated for hyperkalemia, metabolic acidosis, or pulmonary edema that are refractory to medical management. The presence of symptomatic uremia, including uremic encephalopathy or uremic pericarditis (characterized by the presence of a pericardial friction rub), would also be an indication for emergency dialysis. Ingestions or overdoses of certain toxic substances, such as ethylene glycol, lithium, or salicylates, are an indication for emergent hemodialysis. Acetaminophen overdose is treated with acetylcysteine, not dialysis. High levels of BUN and creatinine and low urine output are not strict indications for emergent hemodialysis. *(Brenner and Rector, pp. 1085–1095, 2567)*

50. **(D)** Most patients who are started on ventilator support are placed on either an AC or a synchronized intermittent mandatory ventilation (SIMV) mode. In the AC mode, an inspiratory cycle is initiated either by the patient's inspiratory effort or by a timer within the ventilator, if the patient does not make spontaneous respiratory efforts. In the SIMV mode, mandatory breaths are delivered in synchrony with the patient's inspiratory efforts, at a frequency set, by the operator, and spontaneous respiratory effort without ventilator assist is allowed between the delivered ventilator breaths. Once the patient's oxygenation has been stabilized, appropriate therapy for the cause of the respiratory failure must be initiated, and changes in the ventilator therapy provided as appropriate for the patient's clinical status.

This patient's blood gas reveals a respiratory alkalosis, secondary to hyperventilation. The most appropriate response to this, of the options given, is to reduce the ventilatory rate. One of the priorities of ventilator management is to reduce the fraction of inspired oxygen to reduce the risk of oxygen toxicity. Oxygen toxicity can occur in as little as 72 h with a FiO_2 ≥60%. As this patient has a high oxygen saturation and partial pressure of oxygen measured by blood gas, we can safely reduce his inspired oxygen to 50% (or less). Therefore, option D is correct. *(Harrison's Principles of Internal Medicine, pp. 1526–1530)*

BIBLIOGRAPHY

American Academy of Pediatrics. *The Red Book, 2003 Report of the Committee on infectious Diseases*, 26th ed. Elk Grove Village, IL: American Academy of Pediatrics, 2003.

American Psychiatric Association. *Diagnostic and Statistical Manual of Mental Disorders*, 4th ed., Text Revision. Washington, DC: American Psychiatric Association, 2000.

Braunwald E, et al. *Harrison's Principles of Internal Medicine*, 15th ed. New York, NY: McGraw-Hill, 2001.

Brenner BM. *Brenner & Rectors's The Kidney*, 7th ed. Philadelphia, PA: W.B. Saunders, 2004.

Cameron JL (ed.). *Current Surgical Therapy*, 8th ed. St. Louis, MO: C.V. Mosby, 2004.

Cotran RS, Kumar V, Collins T. *Robbins Pathologic Basis of Disease*, 6th ed. Philadelphia, PA: W.B. Saunders, 1999.

Cotran RS, Kumar V, Robbins SL. *Robbins Pathologic Basis of Disease*, 5th ed. Philadelphia, PA: W.B. Saunders, 1994.

Greenfield LJ, Mulholland MW, Oldham KT, et al. (eds.). *Surgery: Scientific Principles and Practice*, 3rd ed. Philadelphia, PA: Lippincott Williams & Wilkins, 2001.

Hoffman R, et al. *Hematology: Basic Principles and Practice*, 3rd ed. New York, NY: Churchill Livingstone, 2000.

Kunimoto DY, et al. *The Wills Eye Manual: Office and Emergency Room Diagnosis and Treatment of Eye Disease*, 4th ed. Philadelphia, PA: Lippincott Williams & Wilkins, 2004.

Larsen PR, et al. *Williams Textbook of Endocrinology*, 10th ed. Philadelphia, PA: W.B. Saunders, 2003.

Rudolph CD, Rudolph AM, Hostetter MK, Lister GE, Siegel NJ, et al. (eds.). *Rudolph's Pediatrics*, 21st ed. New York, NY: McGraw-Hill, 2003.

Sadock BJ, Sadock VA. *Kaplan and Sadock's Synopsis of Psychiatry*, 9th ed. Philadelphia, PA: Lippincott Williams & Wilkins, 2003.

Schwartz SI, Shires GT, Spencer FC, et al. (eds.). *Principles of Surgery*, 7th ed. New York, NY: McGraw-Hill, 1999.

Stenchever M, et al. *Comprehensive Gynecology*, 4th ed. St. Louis, MO: C.V. Mosby, 2001.

CHAPTER 10

Practice Test 3
Questions

Read each question carefully and in the order in which it is presented. Then select the one best response option of the choices offered. More than one option may be partially correct. You must select ONE BEST answer. You have 60 min to complete this test.

Setting I: Office/Health Center

You see patients in two locations: at your office suite, which is adjacent to a hospital, and at a community-based health center. Your office practice is a primary care generalist group. Most of the patients you see are from your own practice and are appearing for regularly scheduled return visits. Occasionally you will encounter a patient whose primary care is managed by one of your associates. Reference may be made to the patient's medical records. Known patients may be managed by the telephone. You may have to respond to questions about information appearing in the public media, which will require interpretation of the medical literature. The laboratory and radiology departments have a full range of services available.

Questions 1 and 2

You see a 6-year-old girl in your office for leg aches. The mother relates that she has been complaining that her knees and ankles have been bothering her for the past 3 months. The pain is worse in the morning. She has not noticed any swelling, redness, or warmth in her joints. The mother says that she seems to have a fever once a day. She has never taken her temperature, but she seems flushed and has a lacy rash in the evening. She has not lost any weight. Her examination is essentially normal, with the exception of mild fluid notable in both of her knees. The knees have full range of motion and do not seem to bother her when you move them. You perform some blood tests which reveal the following: white blood cell (WBC) 28,000 (polymorphonuclear [PMN] 88%, lymph 10%, and no blasts on the smear), hematocrit 10.2 mg/dL, platelets 765,000, and erythrocyte sedimentation rate (ESR) 112.

1. What is the most likely diagnosis?

   (A) juvenile rheumatoid arthritis (JRA) (Still's disease)
   (B) growing pains
   (C) osteogenic sarcoma
   (D) infectious arthritis
   (E) acute toxic synovitis

2. What is the most appropriate next step?

   (A) diagnostic arthrocentesis
   (B) bilateral hip, knee, and ankle x-rays
   (C) a trial of oral corticosteroids
   (D) a trial of nonsteroidal anti-inflammatory medication (NSAID)
   (E) MRI of both knees

3. A 74-year-old woman presents for routine physical examination. She is accompanied by her daughter, who reports that her mother has become increasingly forgetful. The patient has been misplacing objects and forgetting the names of her children and grandchildren. On examination, the patient demonstrates some paucity of speech, with frequent nodding and smiling in response to questions posed. A mini-mental status examination reveals her score to be 21/30. The physician suspects she has dementia and may benefit from initiation of donepazil. Before doing so, the physician wants to order some tests to rule out treatable causes of dementia. In getting the patient's consent for both the tests and the treatment, what statement is correct when determining whether the patient has the ability to make her own decisions?

(A) Since the patient has dementia, she automatically does not have decision-making capacity.

(B) If the patient's condition were life threatening, the physician would not have to worry about whether the patient had decision-making capacity.

(C) If the patient agrees with the recommendations of the physician, it does not matter whether she has decision-making capacity.

(D) The patient may have the capacity to make a decision about whether or not to have the tests but not have the capacity to accept or refuse the proposed treatment.

(E) The determination of capacity need not factor in whether there is any concomitant depression.

Questions 4 and 5

The patient is a 16-year-old girl attending a primary care clinic appointment with her mother. The mother is worried that her daughter is "too skinny." She apparently picks at her food, skips meals altogether, and exercises several hours per day. When asked about her behavior, she claims to be "fat" and expresses the need to lose more weight. She appears pale and cachectic, and her weight is markedly below that expected for her height.

4. Which of the following would be the most likely associated finding in this patient?

(A) absence of menstrual cycles

(B) abuse of diuretics or laxatives

(C) eating large amounts of food

(D) self-induced vomiting

(E) sense of loss of control over behavior

5. Which of the following laboratory results would most likely be present in this individual?

(A) decreased corticotropin-releasing hormone level

(B) elevated fasting glucose level

(C) high serum cholesterol level

(D) hyperthyroidism

(E) leukocytosis

Questions 6 and 7

A 38-year-old manager of a construction company presents to your office for the first time for evaluation of diffuse joint pain and swelling that has persisted for the past 4 weeks. His symptoms began with gradual pain and swelling in his knees which subsequently involved the joints of his hands and wrists. He reports some improvement with over-the-counter nonsteroidal anti-inflammatory agents but "the symptoms keep coming back." He denies any genitourinary symptoms. His physical examination demonstrates symmetrical swelling and warmth of his proximal interphalangeal joints (PIP), metacarpophalangeal joints (MCP), and knees bilaterally.

6. At this time, what would be the best test to order to confirm your diagnosis and affect the management of this patient?

(A) HLA-B27

(B) urinalysis

(C) plain radiographs of the sacroiliac joints

(D) antinuclear antibodies (ANA)

(E) plain radiographs of the hands and knees

7. You suspect that your patient may have rheumatoid arthritis. In addition to the test you ordered above, you also order rheumatoid factor (RF) testing. Imaging studies demonstrate bony decalcification that is most marked adjacent to the PIP, MCP, and knee joints. Laboratory testing demonstrates mild leukocytosis, an elevated ESR, and a negative RF test.

How will the result of RF testing affect your management of this patient?

(A) Since the RF test is negative, he does not have rheumatoid arthritis and should not be exposed to the side effects of medications such as methotrexate and prednisone, but instead should receive anti-inflammatory medications.

(B) Test the patient for ANA, as the negative RF suggests that your diagnosis of rheumatoid arthritis is incorrect.

(C) Make the diagnosis of "general" arthritis NOS (not otherwise specified) and treat the patient with 10 mg of daily prednisone as sole therapy, as this will control his inflammation and has relatively few side effects.

(D) Diagnose the patient with rheumatoid arthritis and refer the patient to a rheumatologist for management with methotrexate.

(E) Verify your suspicion that this is indeed rheumatoid arthritis by ordering a c-reactive protein (CRP).

Questions 8 through 10

A 67-year-old Hispanic female is seen in the clinic for a well woman examination. The patient has a history of type II diabetes mellitus (DM) and hypertension. Her medications include hydrochlothiazide 50 mg qd and metformin (Glucophage) 500 mg bid. She does not check her blood pressure (BP) at home and she told you that her fasting blood sugar is ranging 110–140 mg/dL. In reviewing some health maintenance issues, she tells you that her last dT was 5 years ago, she had a normal mammogram 1 year ago, she had an undilated eye examination at "a place in the mall" 1 year ago that was normal and she had a screening colonoscopy 8 years ago that was normal. She has had normal pap smears throughout her life, including annually for the last 5 years. She is widowed and not sexually active. Today she has no complaints. Her vital signs are: BP 140/85, heart rate 84, respiration rate 18, temperature 98.7°F.

8. At this office visit, you should order which of the following?

(A) CA-125 for ovarian cancer screening
(B) pap smear
(C) chest x-ray for lung cancer screening
(D) referral to an ophthalmologist
(E) colonoscopy for colon cancer screening

9. After the patient rested for more than 10 min, you rechecked her BP and it was 144/88. Her goal BP should be less than

(A) 120/80
(B) 130/80
(C) 135/85
(D) 140/85
(E) 140/90

10. At this time the most appropriate management would be to

(A) add low dose of atenolol
(B) increase the hydrochlothiazide dose
(C) add low dose amlodipine
(D) add low dose lisinopril
(E) add low dose clonidine

11. A 15-year-old male presented with fever, sore throat, generalized lymph node enlargement, and lymphocytosis with atypical lymphocytes on the peripheral smear. These findings are characteristic of which of the following?

(A) chronic lymphocytic leukemia
(B) infection with Epstein-Barr virus (EBV)
(C) streptococcal pharyngitis
(D) allergic drug reaction
(E) pulmonary tuberculosis

Questions 12 and 13

A 23-year-old mother brings her 5-month old child to your office for nasal congestion, runny nose, mild wheezing, red watery eyes, and vomiting that started suddenly 45 min ago. The mother took her child's temperature and it was 98.5°F. The child had not had a cough or diarrhea. There have been no known ill contacts. This is the first time that her baby has had these symptoms. Further history reveals that this happened after the child was breast fed and given a small part of a boiled egg. On examination, the infant's pulse is 140, respiratory rate is 24, and temperature is 98.6°F. The patient has nasal and conjunctival congestion, bilateral wheezing and flushing of the skin over the trunk.

12. At this time you should

   (A) Tell the mother that this is a self-limited viral illness and ask her to return to your office in 3 days if symptoms persist.

   (B) Give a prescription for Tylenol as needed and advise mother to give the child plenty of water.

   (C) Order a chest x-ray in your office to rule out pneumonia.

   (D) Ask the mother to take her child to the emergency room (ER), which is a 10-min drive from your office.

   (E) Call 911 and closely monitor the patient until they arrive to transport the patient to the ER.

13. One month later, the mother brings her child for a well child examination. Which of the following vaccinations would be contraindicated?

   (A) diphteria, tetanus, acellular pertussis (DTaP)

   (B) *Haemophilus influenzae*, type B (HIB)

   (C) hepatitis B

   (D) injectable polio (IPV)

   (E) influenza

14. The major method of action of combined oral contraceptives (containing both an estrogen and a progestin) is due to

   (A) cervical mucus thickening

   (B) decreased fallopian tube transport of the fertilized egg

   (C) suppression of endogenous follicle-stimulating hormone (FSH)

   (D) changes in the uterine endometrium

   (E) suppression of endogenous LH

15. A 22-year-old woman presents with depression, hypertension, 20 lb weight gain over 6 months, and amenorrhea. She is currently on fluoxetine and oral contraceptives. She admits to drinking 4–6 beers per day on weekends. On examination, she weights 160 lbs, her height is 5 ft, and she has supraclavicular fullness, abdominal striae, ecchymoses on her arms, and facial acne.

Which of the following would be the most appropriate next step?

   (A) morning adrenocortiotropic hormone (ACTH) level

   (B) morning cortisol level

   (C) MRI of pituitary

   (D) 24-h free urinary cortisol

   (E) 1 µg cosyntropin stimulation test

Questions 16 through 18

A 46-year-old man presents with a 2-year history of dysphagia. Initially the dysphagia was for solid foods only, especially meats, but has progressed over time to the point where he mostly consumes liquids or soft foods such as pudding and ice cream. He occasionally awakens with regurgitated food on his pillow in the morning. He has lost 10 lbs over the past year. His physical examination is unremarkable. He has no other medical problems. He drinks one to two alcoholic beverages per day and smoked 1 pack of cigarettes per day for 10 years, stopping 15 years ago.

16. The most appropriate test to evaluate the patient would be

   (A) upper endoscopic examination (esophagogastroduodenoscopy)

   (B) barium swallow

(C) computed tomography (CT) scan of the chest and abdomen

(D) esophageal pH testing

(E) esophageal manometry (motility testing)

17. Further studies reveal the following: the esophageal mucosa is normal, as is the proximal stomach. The esophagus is dilated and contains residual food despite an overnight fast. The lower esophageal sphincter (LES) is tight.

Which condition is the patient most likely to have?

(A) Barrett's esophagus

(B) diffuse esophageal spasm (DES)

(C) achalasia

(D) nutcracker esophagus

(E) scleroderma

18. The patient is at increased risk for which of the following disorders?

(A) eesophageal squamous cell carcinoma

(B) esophageal adenocarcinoma

(C) gastroesophageal reflux disease

(D) gastric adenocarcinoma of the proximal stomach

(E) Barrett esophagus

19. Gastrin secretion is enhanced by

(A) antral distention

(B) antral acidification

(C) presence of fat in the antrum

(D) sympathetic nerve stimulation

(E) duodenal acidification

Questions 20 and 21

20. A 19-year-old college student calls your answering service requesting a prescription for emergency contraception. During intercourse 6 hours ago her partner's condom broke. You call her in *Plan B*, which is comprised of

(A) misiprostol 300 µg

(B) gonadotropin releasing hormone (GnRH) agonist

(C) ethinyl estradiol and norgestimate

(D) levonorgestrel 0.75 mg

(E) conjugated equine estrogens (Premarin) 0.625 mg

21. The patient asks you how emergency contraception works and if it will work for her. You understand that

(A) It inhibits ovulation and works for up to 1 week after the last unprotected intercourse.

(B) It causes insufficient corpus luteum function, alters the histology of the endometrium, and must be taken within 72 h of unprotected intercourse.

(C) It interrupts an implanted pregnancy within 18 h of ingestion.

(D) It causes an imbalance between testosterone and estrogen if taken within 24 h.

(E) It evokes a surge in inhibin and decrease in FSH which diminishes ovarian follicular production if taken within 5 days of unprotected intercourse.

Questions 22 through 24

A 36-year-old White female comes to your office complaining of an unintentional 15 lb weight loss in the last 3 months. Her review of systems is notable for fatigue, a skin rash over her face and upper chest, hair loss, mild bilateral knee swelling, and shortness of breath with exertion. On physical examination, there is an erythematous macular rash on her face and upper chest. She has a pericardial friction rub and a normal pulmonary examination. She has mild bilateral knee swelling and tenderness.

22. Which of the following laboratory tests would be most likely to help in diagnosing this patient's condition?

(A) complete blood count

(B) comprehensive metabolic panel

(C) CRP

(D) antinuclear antibody

(E) RF

23. A chest x-ray would be most likely to show which of the following?

(A) cardiomegaly
(B) bilateral pulmonary congestion
(C) bilateral pleural effusion
(D) pulmonary fibrosis
(E) diffuse bilateral infiltrates

24. You institute appropriate therapy and 2 months later the patient returns for follow up. She is feeling much better, has regained some of her weight, her skin rash has resolved, and her knee pain has improved. She would like to get pregnant in the next few months.

You tell her that

(A) She can get pregnant at any time as she is much better now.
(B) She should wait until her symptoms resolve completely and she regains her initial weight.
(C) She can get pregnant, but she needs to stop her medications now.
(D) She should wait until the disease has been quiescent for at least 6 months.
(E) This is a life-long disease that needs chronic treatment; therefore, she should not attempt to become pregnant.

25. A 33-year-old female complains of a sore throat and general malaise over the past week after being treated for an upper respiratory infection. On examination, her thyroid gland is nodular and tender to palpation. Which of the following is the best treatment?

(A) penicillin G
(B) salicylates
(C) fluconazole (Diflucan)
(D) subtotal thyroidectomy
(E) total thyroidectomy

Setting II: Inpatient Facilities

You have general admitting privileges to the hospital, including the children's and women's services. On occasion you will see patients in the critical care unit. Postoperative patients are usually seen in their rooms, unless the recovery room is specified. You may also be called to see patients in the psychiatric unit. There is a short-stay unit where you may see patients undergoing same-day operations or being held for observation. Also, you may visit patients in the adjacent nursing home/extended care facility and the detoxification unit.

26. Eight hours following an uneventful kidney transplant, a 57-year-old patient develops fever and renal failure. The most likely cause is

(A) preformed antibodies
(B) immunosuppresive drug reaction
(C) T-cell-mediated immune response
(D) wound infection
(E) graft versus host disease

27. An 18-year-old G_1 White woman who has received no prenatal care is brought in to Labor and Delivery by rescue squad. She called for an ambulance when she noted the sudden onset of heavy vaginal bleeding. Earlier the same day she noted the onset of painful hardening of her abdomen every 5–7 min. She reports that she believes she is about "7 months" pregnant. She has no significant medical or surgical history. She denies use of alcohol, tobacco, or illicit drugs. You confirm fetal heart tones in the range of 140–150 beats per minute and place the patient on a fetal heart rate monitor and tocometer. You explain to the patient that she needs an ultrasound evaluation.

You opt to proceed with ultrasound as your first diagnostic test to rule out

(A) placenta accreta
(B) multiple gestation
(C) preterm labor
(D) placenta previa
(E) chorioamnionitis

Questions 28 and 29

A 60-year-old female is treated with trimethoprim/sulfamethoxazole (Bactrim) for a urinary tract infection. One week after completing the course, she develops blisters on her abdomen and thighs. After another 2 weeks, the patient presents for evaluation and has multiple flaccid bullae and superficial erosions on the chest, abdomen, back, and thighs. She also has painful erosions of the oral mucosa. A skin biopsy reveals an intraepidermal split.

28. The most likely diagnosis is

    (A) toxic epidermal necrolysis
    (B) bullous pemphigoid
    (C) primary varicella
    (D) pemphigus vulgaris (PV)
    (E) disseminated herpes simplex

29. The most appropriate initial therapy for this patient would be

    (A) oral valacyclovir
    (B) inpatient admission to the Burn Unit
    (C) oral prednisone
    (D) oral dicloxacillin
    (E) watchful observation

30. An 82-year-old female returns to the intensive care unit after a partial colectomy with a diverting colostomy for an acute large bowel obstruction. The following morning, the nurse records a total of 100 cc of urine over the past 6 h. Which of the following criteria suggest prerenal failure?

    (A) urine osmolarity of 300 mOsm/kg
    (B) urine sodium level of 50 meq/L
    (C) urine/plasma creatinine ratio of 15
    (D) fractional excretion of sodium <1
    (E) central venous pressure greater than 15 cm H_2O

31. A 69-year-old male with history of coronary artery disease and high lipids is admitted to the coronary care unit (CCU) with an acute inferior myocardial infarction. He is placed on a continuous infusion of unfractionated heparin and undergoes a cardiac catheterization with stent placement. On day 7, he complains of a swollen left leg. A Doppler ultrasound confirms a deep vein thrombosis of the femoral vein. The intern notices that his platelet count has dropped to 70,000 from 300,000 at admission.

What is the next step in the management of this patient?

    (A) continue heparin at the same dose
    (B) increase the dose of heparin since it seems not to be working
    (C) stop heparin
    (D) start warfarin and continue heparin
    (E) stop heparin and start a low molecular weight heparin

32. A 3 cm lesion in the right lobe of the liver is found in a 65-year-old male suspected of having cholethiasis. A CT scan is obtained which reveals that the lesion has an enhancing rim with centripetal filling. The most appropriate management is

    (A) observation
    (B) estrogen therapy
    (C) percutaneous CT guided biopsy
    (D) laparotomy with wide excision with 1 cm margins
    (E) laparotomy with right hepatic lobectomy

Questions 33 and 34

You are called to the newborn nursery to see a baby with a birthmark on his face. You note a port-wine stain on the right forehead and cheek. The port-wine stain is only on the right side.

33. What is the most likely condition?

    (A) Sturge Weber syndrome
    (B) neurofibromatosis, type 1 (von Recklinghausen's disease)
    (C) tuberous sclerosis
    (D) CHARGE association
    (E) Beckwith-Wiedemann syndrome

34. The most common complication of the above disorder is

    (A) cardiac abnormalities
    (B) seizures and mental retardation
    (C) polycystic kidney disease
    (D) cystic or fibrous pulmonary changes
    (E) hypoglycemia

35. A patient who sustained extensive burns developed shock and acute renal failure. Which would be the most accurate description of pathologic changes seen in the kidney?

    (A) crescents in the glomeruli
    (B) fibrinoid necrosis of the arterioles and hyperplastic atherosclerosis
    (C) patchy necrosis of the proximal tubular epithelium
    (D) multiple infarctions
    (E) pus within the tubules and abscess in the interstitium

36. Which of the following is the most appropriate treatment for a 32-year-old male with a toxic nodular goiter and compressive airway symptoms?

    (A) radioactive iodine therapy
    (B) propranolol
    (C) propylthiouracil
    (D) Lugol's solution
    (E) total lobectomy

37. Several days following an uneventful laparoscopic cholecystectomy, the pathology report reveals gallbladder cancer that is invasive into the submucosa of the specimen. The most appropriate management is

    (A) observation and close follow up
    (B) chemotherapy with a 5-fluorouracil (5-FU)-based regimen
    (C) laparotomy with 2–3 cm wedge resection of the gallbladder liver bed

    (D) laparotomy with 2–3 cm wedge resection of the gallbladder liver bed and regional lymphadenectomy including the portal and hepatic nodal basins
    (E) radiation to the gallbladder liver bed

Setting III: Emergency Department

Most patients in this setting are new to you, but occasionally you arrange to meet there with a known patient who has telephoned you. Generally, patients encountered here are seeking urgent care. Also available to you are a full range of social services, including rape crisis intervention, family support, and security assistance backed up by local police.

Questions 38 and 39

38. A 3-year-old child is seen in the ER with a history of a recent acute respiratory infection. The mother reports that the child has been complaining of bilateral knee pain and abdominal discomfort. On examination, you notice a palpable purpuric rash on the buttocks extending to both lower extremities. What is the most likely diagnosis?

    (A) immune thrombocytopenic purpura (ITP)
    (B) Henoch-Schonlein purpura (HSP)
    (C) Evans syndrome
    (D) meningococcemia
    (E) hemolytic uremic syndrome (HUS)

39. Treatment of the above condition should include

    (A) course of antibiotics
    (B) no specific treatment is required at this time
    (C) blood transfusion
    (D) corticosteroids
    (E) Intravenous immunoglobulin (IVIG)

Questions 40 through 42

A 23-year-old male checks into the ER with his girlfriend. His chief complaint is "I can't look to my side." The patient was released from a local community hospital 5 days prior, after a 3-week hospitalization. While there, he was diagnosed with schizophreniform disorder and treated with risperidone (Risperdal), which was just increased to 2 mg orally two times per day. His mental status examination is notable for significant anxiety without overt psychotic symptoms. He is afebrile and his vital signs are normal. His physical examination is remarkable for rotation of his head toward the left, with tender neck musculature in spasm.

40. What is the most likely etiology of his presentation?

(A) acute dystonic reaction
(B) akathisia
(C) conversion disorder
(D) parkinsonism
(E) tardive dyskinesia

41. What is the most appropriate next step in the management of his condition?

(A) discontinue the risperidone
(B) intramuscular injection of benztropine (Cogentin)
(C) intramuscular injection of haloperidol (Haldol)
(D) intramuscular injection of lorazepam (Ativan)
(E) reassurance and suggestion that it will improve

42. The patient returns to the ER 1 week later complaining of "feeling more agitated." He states he has felt "edgy" over the past several days. His girlfriend confirms that he has been pacing around the apartment both during the day and night. On mental status examination, he demonstrates good hygiene and is cooperative. He displays some psychomotor agitation with moving in his chair and standing up frequently. His thought processes are logical without looseness of association. His thought content is without suicidal or homicidal ideation. He

denies paranoia, ideas of reference, or delusions. He denies perceptual disturbances and does not appear to respond to internal stimuli.

What is the most appropriate next step in the management of this patient?

(A) add a mood stabilizer to the regimen
(B) add propranolol (Inderal) to the regimen
(C) decrease the dose of risperidone
(D) increase the dose of risperidone
(E) switch to another antipsychotic

Questions 43 through 46

A 68-year-old woman, with a history of hypertension, type 2 diabetes, and a previous myocardial infarction, presents to the ER with dyspnea. She gives a history of progressively worsening dyspnea on exertion and lower extremity edema. She sleeps on three pillows and will get short of breath if she tries to lay flat for any period of time. She came to the ER because she feels "like I'm not getting any air." On examination, her pulse is 110 bpm, BP is 160/100, and her respiratory rate is 28. Her oxygen saturation is 91% by pulse oximetry at room air.

43. Which of the following physical examination findings is she most likely to have?

(A) tracheal deviation
(B) pericardial rub
(C) diastolic murmur along the left sternal border
(D) perioral cyanosis
(E) S3 gallop

44. Which of the following should be administered first?

(A) furosemide 80 mg IV
(B) continuous infusion of IV nitroglycerin
(C) aspirin 650 mg po
(D) enalapril 1.25 mg IV
(E) oxygen

45. A subsequent echocardiogram reveals an ejection fraction of 35%. Which of the following medications has been shown to reduce mortality in this setting?

(A) angiotensin converting enzyme (ACE) inhibitors

(B) digoxin

(C) dihydropyridine calcium channel blockers

(D) alpha-adrenergic antagonists

(E) warfarin

46. Which of the following medications would be contraindicated in this patient?

(A) insulin

(B) metformin (Glucophage)

(C) glyburide (DiaBeta, Micronase)

(D) acarbose (Precose)

(E) glimepiride (Amaryl)

Questions 47 and 48

A 52-year-old male, with past medical history of gallbladder stones and hypertension, presents to the emergency department with midabdominal pain radiating to the back and nausea and vomiting for 2 days. Initial labs showed WBC count of 19,000, hemoglobin of 14 g, total bilirubin of 1.1, aspartate transaminase (AST) of 430 mg, alanine transaminase (ALT) of 420, amylase of 860, lipase of 620, lactate dehydrogenase (LDH) of 590, glucose of 364, creatinine of 0.8, and blood urea nitrogen (BUN) of 19. Abdominal x-ray was negative and CT scan is consistent with acute pancreatitis.

47. Which of the following is the most appropriate management of this patient?

(A) outpatient management with oral pain medications and antiemetics, with follow up in a week

(B) 23-h observation

(C) admission to the general medical floor, NPO, pain medications, and antiemetics

(D) ICU admission, NPO, nasogastric (NG) tube, IV fluid, antibiotics

(E) immediate surgery for debridement of pancreatic debris

48. The estimated mortality of this patient is

(A) 2%

(B) 15%

(C) 40%

(D) 80%

(E) 100%

49. A 65-year-old gentleman suddenly notices he cannot see from one eye but he is not having any pain or redness. Which of the following is the most likely diagnosis?

(A) cataract

(B) angle closure glaucoma

(C) corneal abrasion

(D) retinal detachment

(E) primary open angle glaucoma

50. A 32-year-old male is seen in the ER with a nondisplaced fracture of the ulna after a fall. Incidentally, you notice that the patient is jaundiced and has a palpable spleen. You order a CBC which shows hemoglobin of 10.2 g/dL. The patient reveals a history of having chronic anemia and that he has intermittently been prescribed iron pills to take. He says that at age 23 he had a cholecystectomy. He has several family members with similar symptoms. You review the peripheral smear and find spherocytes. The best way to confirm this man's diagnosis would be by

(A) splenectomy

(B) hemoglobin electrophoresis

(C) osmotic fragility

(D) glucose-6-phosphate dehydrogenase (G-6PD) level

(E) indirect Coombs test

Answers and Explanations

1. **(A)**

2. **(D)**

Explanations 1 and 2

Leg aches are a common complaint and are usually nonspecific in nature. The presence of a lacy rash with arthralgias and daily fever spikes, in an otherwise healthy child, is a common presentation of systemic onset JRA (Still's disease). "Growing Pains" is a term used for a common, yet nonspecific, constellation of complaints. The typical compliant associated with growing pains is in a 7–12-year-old who has vague pain in the midthigh or calf (but not the joints) which is at its worst in the evening time. The pain is usually symmetric and the therapy is usually massage and analgesia. Osteogenic sarcomas are rare bone tumors. Their most common location is around the knee, but the bilateral nature of this child's presentation makes a tumor unlikely. Infectious arthritis (or septic arthritis) is usually a single joint which is very tender and warm. A septic joint has an acute course with limp, fever, and some degree of toxicity. In septic arthritis, the ESR and WBC counts will usually be markedly elevated, but the 3-month history would exclude this diagnosis. Acute toxic synovitis (ATS) is a postinfectious arthralgia. The screening tests of a CBC and ESR are typically normal in ATS.

The best first-line therapy in the treatment of JRA is a trial of NSAIDs. If this trial fails then a course of prednisone is usually undertaken. Given the "classic" nature of this child's presentation, and the nominal fluid in the joint, an arthrocentesis is uncalled-for. Plain films of the entire lower extremity would be unrevealing and expose the child to excessive radiation. Close follow-up of this child is a necessity until the diagnosis is made and the disease under control. Some children with JRA can have other systemic findings, the most concerning of which is uveitis *(Rudolph, pp. 836–839)*.

3. **(D)** Decision-making capacity can be determined by the patient's attending physician and need not involve consultation with a psychiatrist, although this may provide helpful information when there is cognitive impairment or mental illness. Cognitive impairments, such as mental illness, mental retardation, or dementia, do not automatically entail decisional incapacity. Decision-making capacity is not to be confused with competency, which is a legal determination made by a court of law to decide whether the patient can handle her own affairs. Determination of decision-making capacity is dependent on the decision to be made, wherein complex or riskier decisions require a higher threshold in assessing capacity. This sliding scale notion of capacity may entail that a patient is capable of making some medical decisions but not others.

There are seven requirements for decision-making capacity: (1) ability to communicate a choice and preference; (2) ability to understand medical condition; (3) ability to understand risks and benefits of condition and treatment options; (4) intact judgment (e.g., not impaired through depression or substance abuse); (5) consistency with previously expressed wishes or values; (6) ability to reason through issues at hand; (7) some fixity in the decision made (although this does not exclude the possibility of a patient changing her mind for compelling reasons).

In the case presented, the patient may be able to weigh the risks, benefits, and options of testing but may not have this capacity for the proposed treatment. Just because the patient may agree with the recommendations made by the physician does not imply that she has capacity or that it is not necessary to assess decisional capacity. Were the patient found to lack decision-making capacity, the physician is obligated to obtain consent from the patient's appropriate surrogate decision-maker, whether it is an appointed health care agent or a decision-maker chosen from a hierarchy of relationships (spouse, adult child, parent, other relative, close personal friend).

4. **(A)**

5. **(C)**

Explanations 4 and 5

This patient likely has anorexia nervosa. Abuse of diuretics, laxatives or enemas, and self-induced emesis are all considered to be purging behaviors. While there is a purging subtype of anorexia, these symptoms are also commonly seen in bulimia nervosa. Eating excessively large amounts of food, or binging, can also be present during an episode of anorexia, but, like purging, binging is not specific for anorexia nervosa. Binging is necessary for the diagnosis of bulimia nervosa. Feeling a loss of control is part of the clinical picture of bulimia, but in anorexia the patients display a dramatic sense of denial regarding their weight loss and physical appearance. Amenorrhea, or the absence of three consecutive menstrual cycles, is not only characteristic of but also necessary for the diagnosis of anorexia nervosa (DSM IV).

Because of the recurrent vomiting, the purging type of anorexia nervosa can demonstrate electrolyte disturbances such as a hypokalemic, hypochloremic alkalosis and elevated serum amylase levels. The prolonged state of starvation seen in anorexia can also cause various laboratory abnormalities, including hypersecretion of corticotrophin-releasing hormone, low fasting glucose concentrations, mild hypothyroidism, leukopenia, and elevated serum cholesterol levels. These irregularities normalize with regaining sufficient weight. *(Synopsis, p. 743)*

6. **(E)**

7. **(D)**

Explanations 6 and 7

This patient presents with symptoms typical for rheumatoid arthritis but has not met diagnostic criteria. He has had arthritis of three different joint areas simultaneously, involvement (swelling) of the MCP and PIP joints and a symmetrical arthritis. These three symptoms plus one of the following would make the diagnosis of rheumatoid arthritis: morning stiffness greater than 1 h, rheumatoid nodules, serum RF or radiographs demonstrating erosions or unequivocal bony decalcification. In the event that the patient does have erosions on plain radiographs, your management of his rheumatoid arthritis would be more aggressive and referral to a rheumatologist would be indicated. HLA-B27 is associated with spondyloarthropathy but should never be ordered when there is no clinical suspicion for spondyloarthropathy (due to the presence of this antigen in the normal population). The diagnosis of spondyloarthropathy requires inflammatory spinal pain or asymmetric synovitis and either family history, psoriasis, inflammatory bowel disease, urethritis, buttock pain or sacroiliitis, which this patient does not have. A urinalysis would not confirm a diagnosis. Plain radiographs of the sacroiliac joints, in the absence of symptoms of spondyloarthropathy, are not indicated. Similar to HLA-B27 testing, ANA testing, in the absence of clinical history and examination suggesting a connective tissue disease, is not indicated, due to the false positive results occurring in the normal population.

This patient has clinical criteria suggestive of rheumatoid arthritis and the radiographic changes fulfill criteria for rheumatoid arthritis (as there can be erosions OR bony decalcification). The absence of RF does not contradict the diagnosis of rheumatoid arthritis. However, once rheumatoid arthritis has been diagnosed, patients who are RF-positive tend to have more severe disease. Joint inflammation is more severe and there is more joint destruction in RF-positive compared to RF-negative rheumatoid arthritis patients. However, RF-negative patients are still at risk for joint damage and warrant therapy with a disease modifying antirheumatic drugs (DMARD), such as methotrexate, under the supervision of a rheumatologist. ANA testing is a "fishing expedition" in the absence of clinical suspicion for a connective tissue disease and, therefore, should not be ordered. Arthritis NOS is a vague diagnosis, but the side effects of 10 mg of prednisone, as sole therapy, are very clear and very real. Although prednisone will control his inflammation, steroid-induced osteoporosis, avascular necrosis, or other steroid-associated morbidities may ensue. This is the reason that DMARD therapy is used in rheumatoid arthritis. DMARD therapy will enable the physician to either lower the dosage of or discontinue prednisone and effectively treat the rheumatoid arthritis. CRP is an acute-phase reactant produced by the liver. It can be elevated as early as 4 h after tissue injury and peaks within 1–3 days. It is elevated in many diseases associated with inflammation. Even if this test was positive in this patient, systemic inflammation was already indicated by the mild leukocytosis and the elevated ESR. *(Ruddy, pp. 970–980, 1001–1003)*

8. **(D)**

9. **(B)**

10. **(D)**

Explanations 8 through 10

The basic guidelines for diabetic care recommend that patients with type 2 DM should have a dilated eye examination by a trained expert shortly after diagnosis and then every year afterward. The U.S. Preventive Services Task Force (USPSTF) has a D recommendation (Against) checking CA-125 levels for ovarian cancer screening. They also have a D recommendation (Against) routinely screening women older than 65 for cervical cancer if they have had adequate recent screening with normal pap smear and are not otherwise at high risk for cervical cancer. The USPSTF has an I recommendation (insufficient evidence for recommending for or against screening asymptomatic persons) for lung cancer with chest x-ray, low dose CT, sputum cytology, or a combina-

tion of these tests. The USPSTF has an A recommendation (found fair to good evidence that several screening methods are effective in reducing mortality) for screening for colorectal cancer in men and women 50 years of age or older with colonoscopy every 10 years. There are other equally effective methods for screening for colorectal cancer, such as sigmoidoscopy every 5 years, double-contrast barium enema every 5 years, or fecal occult blood testing (FOBT) yearly, or the combination of sigmoidoscopy and FOBT every 5 years. There are insufficient data to determine which strategy is best in terms of the balance of benefits and potential harm or cost-effectiveness.

In this patient with a history of hypertension and DM, her BP goal is 130/80, as recommended by the JNC VII. To achieve this goal for patients with DM or chronic renal disease, the best management is to add a low dose of an ACE inhibitor, such as lisinopril. The American Diabetes Association (ADA) recommends an ACE inhibitor for all patients over the age of 55 years with hypertension or without hypertension but with another cardiovascular risk factor (history of cardiovascular disease, dyslipidemia, microalbuminuria, smoking). *(American Diabetes Association. Standards of medical care in diabetes. Diabetes Care 2004;27:S15–S35; USPSTF: www.preventiveservices.ahrq.gov)*

11. **(B)** Infection with EBV is transmitted by close human contact. The clinical picture of infectious mononucleosis is typically fever, generalized lymphadenopathy, sore throat, and splenomegaly. On examination of the peripheral blood, there is a lymphocytosis with atypical lymphocytes. These cells are proved to be activated T cells. The virus attacks the epithelial cells as well as the B lymphocytes. On examination of the peripheral blood, the atypical lymphocytes represent suppressor T lymphocytes characteristic of this disease. Lymphoid organs, such as spleen and lymph nodes, are enlarged, although the architecture is usually preserved. The final diagnosis of this disease includes specific findings such as lymphocytosis, atypical lymphoid cells previously described, a positive heterophile reaction

(monospot test), and specific antibodies for EBV antigens. *(Cotran, 6th ed., pp. 371–373)*

12. (E)

13. (E)

Explanations 12 and 13

This child is showing the symptoms of an anaphylactic reaction, most likely to egg protein. Cutaneous manifestations, with or without angioedema, are characteristic of systemic anaphylactic reactions. Upper or lower airway obstruction may occur, which can cause hoarseness, stridor, or wheezing. Gastrointestinal symptoms may include nausea, vomiting, diarrhea, or abdominal pain. Vascular collapse or shock may occur. In this patient, vascular collapse or respiratory compromise due to bronchospasm or laryngeal edema could occur quickly. Therefore, the child should be closely monitored while emergency medical technicians are called for safe transport. As the child's condition could quickly deteriorate, allowing the parent to drive the child to the ER would be unsafe.

Eggs, milk, seafood, and nuts are common food causes of anaphylaxis. The influenza vaccine is contraindicated in persons who have a history of anaphylaxis to egg proteins, as the virus is grown in chicken eggs and small amounts of egg protein may be present in the vaccine. Vaccines to measles, mumps, and yellow fever are also prepared in eggs and would be similarly contraindicated. *(Harrison's Principles of Internal Medicine, pp. 785, 1915–1916)*

14. (E) Combination oral contraceptives have both an estrogen and a progestin component. The overall effect of oral contraceptives is progestational. Although progestins can affect fallopian tube function, endometrial maturation, and cause thickened cervical mucus, the major contraceptive effect of progestins is to suppress luteinizing hormone (LH) release thereby preventing ovulation. Estrogen in the oral contraceptive primarily acts to suppress FSH release. *(Beckmann, pp. 331–333)*

15. (D) The patient has the clinical features of Cushing's syndrome. Initial screening tests for determining if she has hypercortisolism include dexamethasone suppression testing, midnight cortisol measurement, and urinary free cortisol. Of these tests, the urinary free cortisol is best in this patient as depression, obesity, and oral contraceptives all interfere with the 1 mg dexamethasone suppression test. Depression is known to be associated with abnormal glucocorticoid metabolism and oral contraceptives increase cortisol binding globulin, thus increasing total serum cortisol levels. The other tests listed are not useful in the initial evaluation of hypercortisolism. *(Larsen, pp. 509–511, 516)*

16. (A)

17. (C)

18. (A)

Explanations 16 through 18

The next best test would be an upper endoscopy. The patient has some alarm symptoms in his history, including progression of his dysphagia and weight loss. His history of smoking also puts him at increased risk for squamous cell esophageal cancer. Endoscopy would allow direct inspection of the esophagus, stomach, and duodenum. An obstructing malignancy, if present, could be identified and biopsies could be obtained. A barium swallow or a CT scan would be helpful, but would not allow tissue samples to be obtained were a mass identified. Esophageal pH testing and esophageal manometry are not yet indicated at this time.

The patient has achalasia, manifesting as failure of relaxation of the LES despite the initiation of a swallow. His esophagus has dilated over time in response to swallowing against a chronic obstruction, although the LES does still occasionally relax. DES and nutcracker esophagus would have a normal appearing esophagus endoscopically but would have manometric abnormalities on formal testing. Scleroderma esophagus is associated with chronic relaxation of the LES, esophagitis, and strictures. Barrett esophagus would not manifest as dysphagia, but represents a mucosal change seen at the gastroesophageal junction in patients with gastroesophageal reflux disease(GERD).

Patients with achalasia are at increased risk for esophageal squamous cell carcinoma, possibly secondary to chronic esophageal inflammation from retained food. The tumors often arise in the dilated portion of the esophagus. Other complications in patients with achalasia include aspiration pneumonia and chronic cough. GERD and its complication, Barrett's esophagus, are less common in patients with achalasia as gastric contents usually cannot reflux through the chronically closed LES. (*Harrison's Principles of Internal Medicine, pp. 233–236, 1644–1645*)

19. **(A)** Gastrin secretion is stimulated by vagal stimulation, antral distention, and the presence of protein in the antrum. Antral acidification decreases gastrin secretion by a feedback mechanism. Acid secretion ceases when antral pH reaches 1.5. The same is true with duodenal acidification. (*Sabiston, pp. 848–849*)

20. **(D)**

21. **(B)**

Explanations 20 and 21

Plan B is comprised of two tablets, each containing 0.75 mg of the progesterone agent levonorgestrel. The second pill is ingested 12 h after the first.

Although a single mechanism of action for emergency contraception has not been clearly established, it is generally thought to work by inhibiting ovulation, causing insufficient corpus luteum formation, and alteration of the histology and biochemistry of the endometrium. The method does not interrupt an implanted pregnancy. Effectiveness ranges from 75 to 90% and is more likely to be successful in preventing pregnancy if taken within 72 h of unprotected intercourse. (*Chez R. Emergency oral contraception. ACOG Pract Bull 2001;(25)*)

22. **(D)**

23. **(A)**

24. **(D)**

Explanations 22 through 24

Systemic lupus erythematosis (SLE) is diagnosed by the presence of 4 of the following 11 signs or symptoms: malar rash; discoid rash; photosensitivity; oral ulcers; arthritis; serositis; renal disorder; neurologic disorder; hematologic disorder; immunologic disorder; ANA. In this case, the patient has the presence of a characteristic rash, arthritis, and serositis (pericardial friction rub suggestive of a pericardial effusion). The presence of ANA on blood testing would, therefore, be diagnostic for SLE. The other tests listed may be helpful but are nonspecific.

All of the chest x-ray findings listed can occur in the presence of SLE. Pericarditis is the most common manifestation of cardiac lupus and effusions can occur. Pleurisy and pleural effusions are also common. Lupus pneumonitis can cause fleeting infiltrates on x-ray, but the most common cause of pulmonary infiltrates in patients with SLE is infection. (*Harrison's Principles of Internal Medicine, pp. 1924–1925*)

SLE can lead to recurrent pregnancy loss. Reports have indicated that during pregnancy, approximately one-third of women reported that their lupus improved, one-third stayed the same, and one-third worsened. In general, pregnancy outcomes are better if the disease has been quiescent for at least 6 months, there is no active renal involvement, superimposed preeclampsia does not develop, and there is no evidence of antiphospholipid antibody. (*Williams Obstetrics, pp. 1386–1387*)

25. **(B)** Subacute thyroiditis (giant cell, granulomatous, or de Quervain's thyroiditis) is an acute inflammatory disease of the thyroid gland. The cause is thought to be viral and it is often preceded by an upper respiratory tract infection. Patients may also experience a viral prodrome marked by muscle aches, fever, and general malaise. The thyroiditis is characterized by constant and often severe pain over the gland that is aggravated with swallowing. It

often presents as a sore throat. Physical examination reveals a firm, nodular, and tender thyroid gland with overlying erythema and warmth. Patients may have symptoms of hyperthyroidism due to the release of thyroid hormone from the gland, secondary to the inflammation.

The disorder is usually self-limited and treatment focuses on conservative measures for pain control. Salicylates and nonsteroidal anti-inflammatory agents are successfully used in mild to moderate cases. For severe pain and swelling, oral glucocorticoids such as prednisone may be required. If symptoms of hyperthyroidism are present, beta-adrenergic blockage may also be needed. Antithyroidal medications are ineffective because the hyperthyroidism is not caused by increased thyroid hormone synthesis. (Cameron, p. 599)

26. **(A)** Transplant rejection is classified as hyperacute, acute, and chronic. Hyperacute rejection is a B-cell-mediated process and occurs when the serum of the recipient has preformed antidonor antibodies. These antibodies adhere to and kill endothelium, which results in rapid graft infarction. The rejection characteristically occurs within the first 24 h. The presence of preformed antibodies can be predicted by a positive cross-match and is an absolute contraindication to transplant. The rejection does not respond to medical treatment and the transplanted organ must be removed.

Acute rejection is a cell-mediated immune response initiated by helper T cells. It occurs 1 week to 3 months following the transplant and rarely occurs after 1 year. The diagnosis is made by detection and work-up of graft dysfunction, culminating in a biopsy. It can be treated medically by a course of high-dose immunosuppressive drugs.

Chronic rejection usually occurs more than 1 year posttransplant. It has an insidious onset and is multifactorial, with both the cell-mediated and humoral arms of the immune system involved. Chronic rejection is usually not reversible.

Graft versus host disease occurs with transplant of tissues that contain immunocompetent cells, such as during a bone mar-

row transplant. Surgical wound infection typically takes place 3–5 days after surgery and does not result in organ failure. (Bruce E. Jarrell, R. Anthony Carabasi, III, John S. Radomski. National Medical Series For Independent Study, Surgery, 4th ed. Philadelphia, PA: Lippincott Williams & Wilkins, 2000, p. 464)

27. **(D)** In a patient with no prenatal care who presents with vaginal bleeding, ultrasound should be the first diagnostic test. It is needed to rule-out placenta previa or vasa previa. It would be dangerous to proceed with a digital or speculum examination when the placenta or its vessels might be located at or near the cervical os. (Marx J, Hockenberger R, Walls R. Rosen's Emergency Medicine: Concepts and Clinical Practice, 5th ed. St. Louis: Mosby, Chap. 172, 2002)

28. **(D)**

29. **(C)**

Explanations 28 and 29

PV is an autoimmune blistering skin disease that occurs mainly in elderly patients. Affected patients have circulating autoantibodies against keratinocyte adhesion molecules (desmogleins). The typical skin lesion of pemphigus is a flaccid blister that ruptures to leave large erosions, especially on the head, neck, axillae, and trunk. Mortality in untreated patients is often due to bacteremia (or fungemia) that occurs in the setting of a severely compromised cutaneous barrier. Most patients with PV have oral mucosal erosions; other mucosae may be affected as well.

Skin biopsy of a pemphigus blister shows an intraepidermal split. Biopsy for direct immunofluorescence reveals intercellular deposits of IgG in the epidermis. By contrast, the skin biopsy of a patient with Stevens-Johnson syndrome shows a subepidermal split. In addition, the cutaneous manifestations of Stevens-Johnson syndrome are unlikely to continue to progress 3 weeks after the causative drug has been discontinued.

Standard therapy for PV is oral prednisone at an initial dose of about 1 mg/kg/day. Patients may also be treated with a steroid-sparing agent such as azathioprine. *(Harrison's Principles of Internal Medicine, pp. 311–312)*

30. (D) Oliguria is defined as urine output less than 400 cc/day and results from prerenal, renal, or postrenal failure. Prerenal failure is the most common type following surgery and usually results from a relative state of hypovolemia. Renal causes include intrinsic renal pathology, such as acute tubular necrosis (ATN). Postrenal causes are obstructive in nature, as in those with benign prostate hyperplasia or ureteral stone. The distinction between prerenal and renal oliguria can be made based on laboratory data. In prerenal oliguria, the kidneys function to preserve water and sodium, which results in a highly concentrated urine with Na sparing. Fractional excretion of sodium (FeNa) is characteristically less than one in prerenal failure, as in the chart *(Schwartz et al., p. 503)*:

	Prerenal	Renal
Urine osmolarity	>500	<350
U/P osmolarity	>1.25	<1.1
U/P creatinine	>40	<20
Urine Na	<20	>40
FeNa	<1%	>1%

31. (C) This patient has heparin-induced thrombocytopenia with thrombosis (HITT). Heparin-induced thrombocytopenia (HIT) is estimated to occur in about 1% of individuals exposed to heparin. The diagnosis should be considered in any individual who develops thrombocytopenia (platelet count less than 100,000/μL) or a fall in platelet count greater than 50% after the initiation of heparin. Thromboembolic complications (arterial and/or venous) can occur in 10–70% of patient with HIT. HIT seem to be caused by the development of heparin-dependent antibodies that recognize platelet factor 4 and heparin complexes. The mainstay of treatment is the cessation of heparin. The use of low molecular heparin is not recommended because in vitro cross-reactivity surpasses 90%. *(Hoffman, p. 2052)*

32. (A) Hemangioma is the most common benign lesion of the liver. Unlike hepatic adenomas, malignant degeneration does not occur and spontaneous rupture is rare. Most patients are asymptomatic and the lesion is found incidentally. Large lesions, however, can result in a palpable right upper quadrant mass and abdominal pain. In addition, platelet trapping in giant hemangiomas may result in thrombocytopenia.

The diagnosis of hepatic hemangiomas can usually be made on CT scan with the classic findings of a rim-enhancing lesion with central filling. If needed, additional studies including a T2-weighted MRI, technetium-labeled red blood cell scan, and arteriogram can be helpful to confirm the diagnosis. Percutaneous biopsy often provides the histologic diagnosis but is rarely indicated and is associated with the complication of bleeding.

Most hepatic hemangiomas should not be excised. Even large lesions followed for long periods of time show no notable increase in size or clinical manifestations. The potential for rupture is minimal and should not constitute an indication for excision. Pain, mass effect, significant growth, platelets trapping, and early rupture are indications for surgical excision. In these patients, large lesions may necessitate anatomic resection, but enucleation is often feasible. *(Schwartz, pp. 1407–1409)*

33. (A)

34. (B)

Explanations 33 and 34

Sturge Weber syndrome is a neurocutaneous syndrome which involves port-wine stains, typically in V_1 or V_2 (trigeminal nerve) distribution. The port-wine stain usually is unilateral and respects the midline. There is a concomitant leptomeningeal vascular anomaly and underlying cerebral cortical atrophy. Seizures develop in most patients during the first year of life. Typically, they are tonic-clonic in nature and may involve the contralateral side of the facial nevus. In at least 50% of children, mental retardation or severe learning disabilities will be present. *(Smith, p. 495; Behrman, p. 2018).*

35. (C) ATN is a clinico-pathologic entity characterized pathologically by destruction of tubular epithelium and clinically by acute renal failure. ATN is the most common cause of acute renal failure. ATN can be divided into ischemic, in which the causes are shock, burns, and crush injury, and toxic tubular necrosis, caused by heavy metals, drugs, and organic solvents. The clinical course has an initial phase followed by a maintenance phase in which there is a decrease in urine output (oliguria), elevated BUN, hyperkalemia, and metabolic acidosis. All of this is followed by a recovery phase. *(Cotran, 6th ed., pp. 969–971)*

36. **(E)** Toxic nodular goiter, also know as Plummer's disease, is a consequence of one or more thyroid nodules secreting inappropriately high levels of thyroid hormone independently of thyroid-stimulating hormone (TSH) control. Hyperthyroidism in patients with toxic nodular goiter is milder than in those with Graves disease and the condition is not accompanied by extrathyroidal manifestations such as ophthalmopathy, pretibial myxedema, vitiligo, or thyroid acropathy.

   Patients with toxic multinodular goiter are older at presentation than those with Graves disease. The thyroid gland goiter characteristically has one or more nodules on palpation. Local symptoms of compression, such as dysphasia and dyspnea, may occur. The diagnosis is suggested by a thorough history and physical examination and confirmed by documenting suppressed serum TSH level and raised serum thyroid hormone level.

   Therapy with antithyroid medications or beta-blockers may help alleviate symptoms but is not definitive treatment, especially if the patient possesses local symptoms of compression. Radioiodine therapy is not as effective as in Graves disease because of lower uptake. I[131] ablation may be used in patients who are unsuitable for surgery but, because of the high failure rate, local resection is considered the treatment of choice. For solitary nodules, nodulectomy or thyroid lobectomy is the treatment of choice. *(Schwartz, p. 1674)*

37. **(A)** Carcinoma of the gallbladder accounts for 2–4% of gastrointestinal malignancies. Less than 1% of patients undergoing biliary tract operations have carcinoma either as an anticipated diagnosis or as an incidental finding. The calcified "porcelain" gallbladder is associated with a 20% incidence of gallbladder carcinoma.

   Signs and symptoms of carcinoma of the gallbladder are generally indistinguishable from those associated with cholecystitis and cholelithiasis. They include abdominal discomfort, right upper quadrant pain, nausea, and vomiting. Most long-term survivors are patients who underwent cholecystectomy for cholelithiasis and in whom the malignancy was an incidental finding on the pathology report. The management of these patients is based on the depth of tumor penetration into the wall of the gallbladder. No further surgical intervention is required if the tumor invades superficially into the mucosa and submucosa. These patients are placed on surveillance programs. However, if the lesion penetrates deeper into the muscularis or perimuscular connective tissue of the gall bladder wall, a radical second procedure is undertaken which includes radical lymphadenectomy and partial hepatic resection.

   If a malignancy is identified at the time of initial surgery, removal of the regional lymph nodes, partial liver resection and, in some cases, pancreaticoduodenectomy are indicated. *(Schwartz, p. 1457)*

38. **(B)**

39. **(B)**

Explanations 38 and 39

HSP is also commonly referred to as anaphyllactoid purpura. HSP is a small vessel vasculitis. The rash of HSP is very characteristic and is commonly located on the lower extremities and buttocks. Abdominal pain, joint pain, and nephritis are common features of the disease as well. These complaints are usually self-limiting. Symptomatic treatment including hydration and pain control with acetaminophen may be given. Avoidance of competitive activities and elevation of the lower extremities may help reduce any local edema. *(Rudolph, pp. 842–844; Behrman, p. 827)*

40. (A)

41. (B)

42. (B)

Explanations 40 through 42

This individual is being treated with an antipsychotic medication. The presumed mechanism of action involves the blockade of dopamine receptors in the mesolimbic and mesocortical regions of the brain. Dopamine blockade in other areas, such as the nigrostriatal pathways, accounts for many of the side effects seen with this class of medications. Akathisia is described as an inner feeling of restlessness, which usually appears after several weeks of treatment with antipsychotics. Conversion disorder is the unconscious production of neurologic deficits due to unconscious conflict. Antipsychotic-induced Parkinsonism also appears after several weeks of treatment and is characterized by the triad of a resting (*pill-rolling*) tremor, bradykinesia, and rigidity (either lead-pipe or cogwheel). Tardive dyskinesia is a long-term consequence of chronic antipsychotic use. It involves involuntary choreoathetoid movements, especially of the face, mouth, tongue, and hands. It occurs in up to 25% of patients medicated over 4 years and often progresses over time. Acute dystonic reactions, as in this case, occur within hours to days of initiating or increasing an antipsychotic medication and are categorized by the painful contraction of muscles.

Although consideration should always be given to either lowering the dose of or switching to another medication if intolerable side effects occur, discontinuing the risperidone will not immediately treat the dystonic reaction and will increase the risk for a relapse of psychotic symptoms. Injection of haloperidol or lorazepam may be indicated in the management of an acutely agitated patient. In this example, the individual is without current psychotic symptomatology and is anxious due to his painful muscle spasms. Injection of haloperidol may also worsen his dystonia. Reassurance and suggestion are often effective in managing conversion symptoms, but acute dystonia requires immediate treatment with an anticholinergic agent, such as benztropine, or an antihistaminic agent, such as diphenhydramine.

This patient is exhibiting symptoms and signs of akathisia. Adding a mood stabilizer or increasing the dose of antipsychotic might be appropriate if he were showing indications of manic excitement or psychotic agitation, but his psychotic symptoms appear to be in remission. Increasing the risperidone may actually worsen his akathisia. Decreasing the current dose or switching to another antipsychotic would be indicated if he were experiencing intolerable side effects. Both of these options could also result in a relapse of his psychosis. Given the apparent remission of his symptoms on risperidone, the most reasonable approach would be to add a B-adrenergic blocker, such as propranolol, which has been shown to be beneficial in treating akathisia. (*Synopsis, pp. 992–995, 1058*)

43. (E)

44. (E)

45. (A)

46. (B)

Explanations 43 through 46

This patient is presenting with symptoms and signs of congestive heart failure. She has evidence of both left and right ventricular failure, with orthopnea, hypoxia, and peripheral edema. Along with peripheral edema, signs that one would be expected to find on physical examination would include pulmonary rales, elevated jugular venous pressure, hepatojugular reflux, and an S3 gallop. This is a "protodiastolic" sound that would be expected to occur 0.13–0.16 s after the second heart sound. These sounds may occur in healthy children and young adults, but are rare in healthy adults over the age of 40 and are common in persons of any age in heart failure. Tracheal deviation may be expected to occur in a person with a tension pneumothorax. A pericardial friction rub, while possible in the setting of heart failure, is less likely to occur than an S3 gallop and may lead toward a consideration of the diagnosis of pericarditis. A diastolic murmur along the left sternal border may be associated with, among other valvular abnormalities, aortic insufficiency. This may be a specific cause of heart failure but, again, is much less likely to be heard than an S3 gallop in this setting. Perioral cyanosis is unlikely to occur at an oxygen saturation of 91%. In a hypoxic patient presenting with dyspnea, the first drug to be administered should be oxygen. In the primary survey of emergency patients, the mnemonic "ABC"—for airway, breathing, and circulation—should always come first. The other medications listed, all of which may play a role in the management of this patient in the acute or long-term settings, would be appropriate after assuring airway, breathing, and circulation.

Alpha-adrenergic antagonists have been shown to be no better than placebos in their reduction in mortality in heart failure. Dihydropyridine class calcium channel blockers have not been shown to produce improvement in congestive heart failure. Some agents in this class may worsen symptoms and actually increase mortality. Newer dihydropyridines—felodipine and amlodipine—do not appear to worsen mortality, so they may be safe to use in this setting. In patients with sinus rhythm and reduced ejection fraction, digoxin is often used. Study results have been conflicting; however mortality does not seem to be affected by the use of digoxin in this setting. The use of warfarin in systolic dysfunction is controversial. While many patients with moderate to severe left ventricular dysfunction are given warfarin in order to reduce the risk of thromboembolic events, evidence of improved outcomes is, at present, lacking. Warfarin would be indicated in those with atrial fibrillation, visualized thrombus, or previous thromboembolic disease. Multiple studies have consistently shown an improvement in the natural history of congestive heart failure, along with reductions in mortality, with the use of ACE inhibitors. Their use should be considered first-line in all patients with congestive heart

failure due to systolic dysfunction. (*Braunwald, pp. 503–543, 570–582, 645*)

The use of metformin is contraindicated in the setting of congestive heart failure that requires drug treatment. The thiazolidinediones are also contraindicated for NYHA class III and IV heart failure and must be used with caution in class I and II heart failure. The other diabetic medications listed may be used in the clinical setting of congestive heart failure. Caution may be required, however, in the setting of renal or hepatic insufficiencies that may be associated with congestive heart failure.

47. (D)

48. (B)

Explanations 47 and 48

Several scales and criteria have been devised to assess the prognosis of patients with pancreatitis. The most widely used is Ranson's criteria. Ranson's criteria are not diagnostic; however, they help estimate the severity of the disease, the prognosis, and serve as a guide to management decisions. Ranson's criteria are divided into two groups. The first group contains five criteria that are used to assess the severity in the first 24 h of admission. This group includes: age above 55 years, WBC count higher than $16,000/mm^3$, serum glucose higher than 200 mg/dL, serum AST higher than 250 IU/L, serum LDH higher than 350 IU/L. The second group is the 48-h criteria (the second day of admission) and includes: hematocrit decrease more than 10%, increase in blood urea nitrogen level of more than 5 mg/dL, serum calcium level lower than 8 mg/dL, partial pressure of oxygen in arterial blood lower than 60 mmHg, base deficit higher than 4 meq/L, and fluid sequestration of more than 6 L.

If a patient meets 0–2 of the criteria, the mortality rate is only 2%, whereas the presence of 3–4 criteria bears a mortality rate of 15%. If a patient meets 5–6 criteria, the mortality rate is 40%, and if patient meets 7 criteria, the mortality rate is nearly 100%. Patients presenting with three or more of the Ranson's criteria should be admitted to the intensive care unit for aggressive resuscitation, bowel rest, NG tube decompression, and serial laboratory and physical examination. Surgery is reserved for complications of pancreatitis, including pancreatic abscess formation, hemorrhagic pancreatitis, infected pancreatic necrosis, or recalcitrant disease with deterioration of the patient's general status. *(Schwartz, pp. 1476–1478)*

49. **(D)** Common causes of sudden, painless vision loss lasting more than 24 h would include retinal detachment, retinal artery or vein occlusion, and ischemic optic neuritis. Cataracts and open angle glaucoma would be among the most common causes of painless vision loss that is gradual over the course of months or years. Acute angle closure glaucoma is a cause of acute, painful vision loss. Corneal abrasions are usually painful and associated with eye redness. *(Wills Eye Manual, Chap. 1)*

50. **(C)** Hereditary spherocytosis (HS) is a hemolytic anemia characterized by abnormal flexibility and shape of red cells, due to a deficiency or dysfunction of multiple membrane proteins. Clinically, patients with HS can vary from having an asymptomatic condition with almost normal hemoglobin levels to severe hemolysis and anemia, leading to life-threatening jaundice and congestive heart failure in neonates. Patients that maintain mild anemia are usually diagnosed later in life during evaluation for unrelated conditions. Some patients may develop bilirubin gallstones at early age that require cholecystectomy. The hallmark for the diagnosis of HS is the presence of sphrerocytes in the peripheral smear. In addition to the indices of hemolysis (reticulocytosis, elevated LDH, and elevated unconjugated bilirubin), the red cell osmotic fragility is characteristically increased. Splenectomy in these individuals is the main treatment producing improvement in red cell survival and a rise in hemoglobin levels. *(Hoffman, pp. 584–585)*

BIBLIOGRAPHY

American Psychiatric Association. *Diagnostic and Statistical Manual of Mental Disorders*, 4th ed. Text Revision. Washington, DC: American Psychiatric Association, 2000.

Beckmann CRB, Ling FW, Laube DW, et al. *Obstetrics and Gynecology*, 4th ed. Baltimore, MD: Lippincot Williams & Wilkins, 2002.

Braunwald E, et al. *Harrison's Principles of Internal Medicine*, 15th ed. New York, NY: McGraw-Hill, 2001.

Braunwald E. *Heart Disease: A Textbook of Cardiovascular Medicine*, 6th ed. Philadelphia, PA: W.B. Saunders, 2001.

Cameron JL (ed.). *Current Surgical Therapy*, 8th ed. St. Louis, MO: C.V. Mosby, 2004.

Cotran RS, Kumar V, Collins T. *Robbins Pathologic Basis of Disease*, 6th ed. Philadelphia, PA: W.B. Saunders, 1999.

Cunningham FG, et al. *Williams Obstetrics*, 21st ed. New York, NY: McGraw-Hill, 2001.

Hoffman R, et al. *Hematology: Basic Principles and Practice*, 3rd ed. New York, NY: Churchill Livingstone, 2000.

Jones KL (ed). *Smith's Recognizable Pattern of Human Malformations*, 5th ed. Philadelphia, PA: W.B. Saunders, 1997.

Jones KL (ed). *Smith's Recognizable Pattern of Human Malformations*, 5th ed. Philadelphia, PA: W.B. Saunders, 1997.

Kunimoto DY, et al. *The Wills Eye Manual: Office and Emergency Room Diagnosis and Treatment of Eye Disease*, 4th ed. Philadelphia, PA: Lippincott Williams & Wilkins, 2004.

Larsen PR, et al. *Williams Textbook of Endocrinology*, 10th ed. Philadelphia, PA: W.B. Saunders, 2003.

Ruddy S, et al. *Kelley's Textbook of Rheumatology*, 6th ed. Philadelphia, PA: W.B. Saunders, 2001.

Rudolph CD, Rudolph AM, Hostetter MK, Lister GE, Siegel NJ, et al. (eds.). *Rudolph's Pediatrics*, 21st ed. New York, NY: McGraw-Hill, 2003.

Sadock BJ, Sadock VA. *Kaplan and Sadock's Synopsis of Psychiatry*, 9th ed. Philadelphia, PA: Lippincott Williams & Wilkins, 2003.

Schwartz SI, Shires GT, Spencer FC, et al. (eds.). *Principles of Surgery*, 7th ed. New York, NY: McGraw-Hill, 1999.

Townsend CM, Beauchamp RD, Evers BM, et al. (eds.). *Sabiston Textbook of Surgery: The Biological Basis of Modern Surgical Practice*, 17th ed. Philadelphia, PA: W.B. Saunders, 2004.

CHAPTER 11

Practice Test 4
Questions

Read each question carefully and in the order in which it is presented. Then select the one best response option of the choices offered. More than one option may be partially correct. You must select ONE BEST answer.

Setting I: Office/Health Center

You see patients in two locations: at your office suite, which is adjacent to a hospital, and at a community-based health center. Your office practice is a primary care generalist group. Most of the patients you see are from your own practice and are appearing for regularly scheduled return visits. Occasionally you will encounter a patient whose primary care is managed by one of your associates. Reference may be made to the patient's medical records. Known patients may be managed by the telephone. You may have to respond to questions about information appearing in the public media, which will require interpretation of the medical literature. The laboratory and radiology departments have a full range of services available.

Questions 1 through 4

A 19-year-old Black male presents to your office for a precollege sports examination. He is planning to be on the college basketball team. He is playing basketball 5 days per week for 1–2 h each day. He has been healthy. He complains today of mild right flank discomfort which comes and goes. He denies any fever, chills, dysuria, or polyuria. He has no history of significant trauma or previous hematuria. He smokes one pack of cigarettes every 2–3 days, drinks 4–6 beers on weekends, and denies recreational drug abuse. His last diphtheria-tetanus (dT) shot was at age 14. His examination is normal. You order a urinalysis which shows 8 red blood cells (RBCs) per high-power field (HPF). Review of his chart shows that he had 6 RBCs/HPF in a urinalysis 6 months ago but he never returned for the requested follow-up examination.

1. What is the appropriate next step at this point?

    (A) observation
    (B) repeat urinalysis in 3 months
    (C) empiric antibiotic treatment of urinary tract infection (UTI)
    (D) intravenous pyelogram
    (E) plain abdominal x-ray

2. During this visit, you should

    (A) counsel patient regarding low back pain prevention
    (B) counsel patient regarding skin cancer prevention
    (C) provide alcohol abuse counseling
    (D) give dT booster
    (E) advise patient to do frequent testicular examination for testicular cancer screening

3. The number one cause of death in this patient's age group is

    (A) acquired immune deficiency syndrome (AIDS)
    (B) homicide
    (C) suicide
    (D) motor vehicle accident
    (E) cardiovascular disease

4. When you ask this patient why he smokes, the most likely answer will be

   (A) everyone around me smokes
   (B) I am addicted
   (C) it relaxes me
   (D) I have a habit
   (E) I am bored

Questions 5 and 6

A 42-year-old woman is referred to the clinic after recently moving to the area. She presents with numerous chief complaints, including severe headaches since childhood, arthritis pain, atypical chest pain, and chronic lower back pain. She also describes a history of intermittent diarrhea and unusual food intolerances. She has had irregular menstrual periods since menarche, and often becomes dizzy and unsteady on her feet. General review of her large medical chart documents frequent outpatient appointments, a number of hospitalizations, abundant tests and procedures, and multiple surgeries. Despite her extensive evaluations, there have not been definitive diagnoses or sufficient treatments to adequately address all of her difficulties. She clearly appears in significant distress regarding the amount of her suffering and perceived lack of attention she has received.

5. Which of the following is her most likely diagnosis?

   (A) conversion disorder
   (B) hypochondriasis
   (C) pain disorder
   (D) somatization disorder
   (E) undifferentiated somatoform disorder

6. Which of the following is the most useful approach in her management?

   (A) admission to the hospital for extensive workup
   (B) confrontation about the psychologic nature of her symptoms
   (C) reassurance that a diagnosis will eventually be found

   (D) referral to various outpatient specialists
   (E) regularly scheduled follow-up appointments

Questions 7 through 9

A 60-year-old White female presents to your office with the complaints of aching shoulders and sides of her hips. These symptoms have persisted for the past 4 weeks and have prompted her to avoid her water aerobics class at her local YMCA. She has lost 15 lbs in the past 4 weeks but denies any joint symptoms. Her physical examination demonstrates no loss of joint range or mobility, no synovitis in any joint, and tenderness of the neck and shoulders. Her motor strength in the upper and lower extremities is normal. Laboratory testing is significant only for an erythrocyte sedimentation rate (ESR) of 99 mm/h, a negative antinuclear antibody (ANA), and a normal creatine kinase (CPK).

7. Her clinical history and examination suggest which of the following diagnoses?

   (A) polymyositis
   (B) hypothyrodism
   (C) polymyalgia rheumatica
   (D) osteoarthritis of the neck and shoulders
   (E) fibromyalgia

8. What would be the most appropriate medical management for this patient?

   (A) thyroid hormone replacement
   (B) analgesic such as acetaminophen
   (C) prednisone in a dose of 20 mg daily
   (D) antidepressant medication (Amitriptyline 50 mg daily)
   (E) muscle relaxant (cyclobenzaprine 10 mg daily)

9. The patient returns to your clinic 5 days later saying that the symptoms are still present. In addition, the patient reports that she has been having headaches and blurriness of her vision. Laboratory studies demonstrate an ESR of 100 mm/h. These additional symptoms suggest which of the following diagnoses?

(A) rheumatoid arthritis

(B) giant cell arteritis

(C) systemic lupus erythematosus

(D) hypothyroidism

(E) the patient is depressed and is amplifying her symptoms

10. A 6-month-old female is brought to your clinic for a well child examination. Her height and weight are below the 50th percentile. The child has otherwise been healthy. On examination, the child has good color and is in no acute distress. During auscultation, you hear a loud, harsh, and blowing holosystolic murmur over the left sternal border. Which of the following would be the most likely cause of your clinical findings?

(A) ventricular septal defect

(B) tetralogy of Fallot

(C) transposition of the great vessels

(D) truncus arteriosis

(E) pulmonic atresia

Questions 11 through 13

A previously healthy 27-year-old female comes to your office with complaints of recurrent headaches over the past few days. She became alarmed when she recently visited a health fair and was told that she had elevated blood pressure (BP). She was started on oral contraceptives (OCPs) after the birth of her last child 1 year ago. In that year, she has gained 20 lbs and has developed bilateral ankle edema that worsens at night. She missed her last two menstrual periods and, this morning, she woke up with some vaginal bleeding. She wants to know what to do because at this point of her life "she just can't afford to get pregnant."

11. Which of the following would be the most appropriate next step?

(A) Advise that she stop the OCPs and get a urine pregnancy test.

(B) Obtain a urine pregnancy test but continue the OCPs.

(C) Reassure her that all of her symptoms are likely caused by the onset of menses.

(D) Emphasize to her that the headaches are likely due to social stressors and that her weight will likely stabilize in time.

(E) Recommend that she be started on diuretic medication to control her BP and reduce her edema.

12. Which of the following is an absolute contraindication to taking OCPs?

(A) a diagnosis of major depression

(B) a history of migraine headaches

(C) a history of oligomenorrhea

(D) smoking after the age of 35

(E) a history of any hemolytic anemia

13. Which of the following is considered an adverse effect of OCPs?

(A) thrombocytopenia

(B) ovarian cancer

(C) cholelithiasis

(D) irreversible infertility

(E) endometrial cancer

14. A 19-year-old college student is found to have an elevated serum calcium on routine physical examination. She has a family history of hypercalcemia that has not resulted in any known symptoms. Further workup reveals a slightly elevated serum parathyroid hormone with depressed levels of serum phosphate. A 24-h urine calcium excretion is obtained and is low. Which of the following is the correct diagnosis?

(A) familial hypocalciuric hypercalcemia (FHH)

(B) primary hyperparathyroidism

(C) secondary hyperparathyroidism

(D) tertiary hyperparathyroidism

(E) metastatic bone cancer

Questions 15 through 17

A 44-year-old divorced male is referred to the clinic for ongoing management of his hypertension and hypercholesterolemia. He begins the evaluation by remarking, "I came here because I heard you are the best. Those other doctors didn't like me very much. Besides, they don't know what they are doing." He subsequently admits to poor compliance with taking his medications or maintaining a low salt, low fat diet. He blames this on his boss, whom he calls a "task master . . . he works me to the bone, and I don't have time to eat properly." He denies pervasive depressive symptoms but claims to be "lonely and bored." He describes lifelong difficulties with his temper and he has frequently broken items of value when angry. He is not in a stable relationship but does admit to repeated promiscuity with women, where he will impulsively purchase expensive jewelry to curry favor with them in order to have sexual intercourse.

15. Which of the following is his most likely diagnosis?

(A) avoidant personality disorder
(B) borderline personality disorder
(C) dependent personality disorder
(D) paranoid personality disorder
(E) schizoid personality disorder

16. The above patient's comments demonstrate which prominent defense mechanism?

(A) denial
(B) displacement
(C) intellectualization
(D) splitting
(E) sublimation

17. Which of the following medications would be the most appropriate first-line treatment for his symptoms?

(A) clonazepam (Klonopin)
(B) haloperidol (Haldol)
(C) lithium
(D) sertraline (Zoloft)
(E) valproic acid (Depakene)

18. Which of the following patients with thyroid cancer has the best prognosis?

(A) a 16-year-old child with papillary carcinoma metastatic to three cervical lymph nodes
(B) a 42-year-old male with papillary carcinoma
(C) a 52-year-old female with follicular carcinoma confined to the thyroid capsule
(D) a 44-year-male with an occult focus of medullary carcinoma found incidentally after a subtotal thyroidectomy
(E) a 53-year-old female with a Hurthle cell carcinoma

19. A 36-year-old patient presents to her physician for a prescription for OCP. What medical history elicited from this patient would be an absolute contraindication to prescribing her OCP?

(A) hypertension
(B) type II diabetes mellitus
(C) epilepsy
(D) cigarette smoker
(E) menstrual migraines (without aura)

Questions 20 and 21

You are evaluating a 4-month-old girl for persistently poor weight gain. The mother relates that the child is "a very good eater" but cannot seem to keep weight on and that she has seemed to have an increase in her "spitting up." She was born at term with an uneventful perinatal history. On examination, she appears as a vigorous but wasted infant with decreased adiposity. Her weight and height are both below the 3rd percentile. Her examination is otherwise essentially normal. Laboratory studies include the following:

Na 135	K 5.2	Cl 111	Bicarbonate 16
BUN 15	Creatinine 0.9	Glucose	79
Urinalysis:	Specific gravity 1.010	pH 6.0	Blood and protein (−)

20. What is the most likely explanation for this child's poor weight gain?

(A) pyloric stenosis

(B) formula intolerance

(C) duodenal stenosis

(D) gastroesophageal reflux

(E) renal tubular acidosis

21. Which of the following would help confirm the diagnosis?

(A) an upper gastrointestinal (GI) contrast study

(B) an upper GI endoscopy

(C) a trial of sodium bicarbonate to assess urinary pH

(D) a trial of metoclopramide (Reglan)

(E) a trial of an elemental formula

22. A 55-year-old woman presents to her internist complaining of urinary frequency and irritation for the past 2 months. Last weekend your partner called her in a prescription for trimethoprim/sulfamethoxazole (Bactrim DS) for a presumed UTI. Her symptoms have persisted. In addition, she has noted increasing vaginal dryness and irritation during intercourse. These problems have been exacerbated since she discontinued her oral hormone replacement therapy last year. On examination, you would expect to find

(A) white, curdy vaginal discharge

(B) thin, pale vulvar skin and vaginal mucosa

(C) a fungating, friable lesion on her cervix

(D) a retained tampon

(E) a vesico-vaginal fistula

23. Regarding the Food and Drug Administration pregnancy categories for medication, which of the following statements is true?

(A) A higher category indicates a higher level of risk for congenital abnormalities.

(B) Category B drugs include those which have been shown to have teratogenic risk in animal studies but no such risk in human studies.

(C) Category C drugs show consistent evidence of risk in both animal and human pregnancy.

(D) Category D drugs are of high enough risk for causing congenital anomalies that women who take them should be advised not to become pregnant.

(E) Drugs in category X always cause birth defects.

24. A 25-year-old woman presents with bilateral galactorrhea, fatigue, and weight gain. She had menarche at age 12, had normal monthly periods until age 20, and then was placed on birth control pills for contraception until 18 months ago. She subsequently had a normal pregnancy with vaginal delivery 6 months ago. She nursed the child for 3 months and restarted her birth control pills. She also started a vigorous exercise program to lose weight. However, over the past 3 months, she has felt fatigued and has gained about 15 lbs. She has noticed muscle cramps while exercising, dry skin, and persistent hair loss. She also has felt depressed. On examination, her BP is 130/90, heart rate 60 bpm. There is a rough texture to her skin and her deep tendon reflexes are slow to relax.

Labs:		
	Total T4	4.5 (5–12 µg/dL)
	T3-resin uptake	20% (25–35%)
	Free thyroid index	0.9 (1.2–4.2)
	TSH	35 (0.4–5 uU/mL)
	Prolactin	40 (5–15 ng/mL)

Which of the following would be the most appropriate next step?

(A) MRI of pituitary

(B) nuclear thyroid scan

(C) stop OCP and repeat studies in 6 weeks

(D) initiate levothyroxine therapy

(E) thyroid replacement hormone (TRH) stimulation test

25. An 18-year-old primigravid woman had a complete hydatidiform mole evacuated by suction curettage. Her preevacuation serum human chorionic gonadotropin (hCG) level was 125,000 mIU/mL and her uterus was 22 weeks' gestational size. Postevacuation serum quantitative hCG levels were obtained every 2 weeks. Her hCG level decreased to 25,000 mIU/mL at 2 weeks, but then began to climb and is currently 32,000 mIU/mL after 4 weeks. Physical examination suggests a boggy uterus only. What is the most appropriate step in management at this point?

(A) repeat dilatation and curettage
(B) weekly hCG testing
(C) CT scan of the head, chest, abdomen, and pelvis
(D) hysterectomy
(E) pelvic ultrasound

Setting II: Inpatient Facilities

You have general admitting privileges to the hospital, including the children's and women's services. On occasion you will see patients in the critical care unit. Postoperative patients are usually seen in their rooms, unless the recovery room is specified. You may also be called to see patients in the psychiatric unit. There is a short-stay unit where you may see patients undergoing same-day operations or being held for observation. Also, you may visit patients in the adjacent nursing home/extended care facility and the detoxification unit.

26. A 74-year-old female, with a history of hypertension and hypothyroidism, is admitted with easy bruising, guaiac positive stools, and anemia (hemoglobin 8.1 g/dL). Screening coagulation tests reveal a prolonged activated partial thromboplastin time (aPTT) with a normal prothrombin time (PT) and platelet count. What is the next step in the diagnosis of this woman's problem?

(A) perform upper and lower endoscopy with biopsies
(B) check factors II, VII, IX, and X levels

(C) check factor VII level
(D) check FXI, VII, IX, and VIII levels
(E) check an aPTT 1:1 mix with normal plasma

27. A 42-year-old male with extensive Crohn's disease undergoes a near complete resection of the ileum. A deficiency of which of the following vitamin is likely to result?

(A) niacin
(B) thiamine
(C) vitamin B_{12}
(D) vitamin C
(E) vitamin B_6

Questions 28 through 30

A 55-year-old female presented with a 3-week history of feeling a lump in her breast on self-examination. The mass was painless and she did not notice skin changes, nipple discharge, or retraction. There was no family history of breast or ovarian cancer. The patient was otherwise healthy. On physical examination, a hard mass was found on the left upper quadrant of the breast measuring approximately 2 cm in diameter. After a mammography and clinical testing she underwent an excisional biopsy. The photomicrograph shown in Fig. 11-1 is a representative histologic section representing the tumor mass.

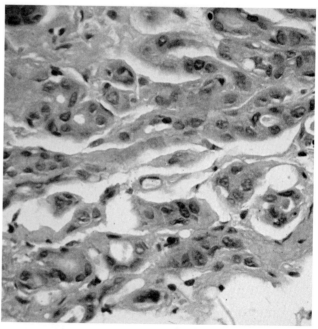

FIG. 11-1 (*Courtesy of Edison Catalano, MD.*)

28. What would be the diagnosis on the palpable tumor seen on the microphotograph?

   (A) infiltrating ductal carcinoma, poorly differentiated (grade III)
   (B) infiltrating ductal carcinoma low grade
   (C) microinvasive ductal carcinoma, papillary variant
   (D) atypical ductal hyperplasia
   (E) colloid carcinoma (mucinous secreting)

29. Indicate the most important prognostic finding in carcinoma of the breast.

   (A) presence of estrogen receptors
   (B) lymphatic invasion
   (C) cellular anaplasia
   (D) metastasis to the regional lymph nodes
   (E) nipple retraction

30. With which of the following breast tumors will you find axillary metastasis?

   (A) atypical lobular hyperplasia
   (B) lobular carcinoma in situ
   (C) atypical ductal hyperplasia
   (D) tubular adenoma
   (E) infiltrating ductal carcinoma

31. A patient with uncontrolled diabetes and chronic renal failure undergoes an uneventful debridement of a necrotic venous ulcer. On the second postoperative night, she is noted to have persistent bleeding and a prolonged bleeding time. Which of the following is the best intervention at this time?

   (A) compression dressing and subcutaneous injection of vitamin K
   (B) platelet transfusion
   (C) intravenous desmopressin (DDAVP)
   (D) transfuse fresh frozen plasma
   (E) correct hyperglycemic state

32. With pregnancy, physiologic alterations occur in nearly all organ systems. Regarding the hematologic system, which of the following is true?

   (A) The blood volume increases by 100% by the end of pregnancy.
   (B) The maternal red cell mass increases by 50% by the end of pregnancy.
   (C) The total iron demands for a term pregnancy to meet both maternal and fetal needs are 2500 mg.
   (D) Supplementation with 30 mg of elemental iron per day during pregnancy effectively prevents iron depletion.
   (E) Mean platelet counts in pregnant and nonpregnant women are the same.

33. Which of the following is an indication to resect a Meckel's diverticulum found incidentally during a laparoscopic appendectomy in a 52-year-old male?

   (A) any Meckel's diverticulum found incidentally should be removed
   (B) location within 12 in. of the ileocecal valve
   (C) history of rectal bleeding
   (D) presence of a wide neck
   (E) presence firm tissue at the base of the diverticulum

Questions 34 and 35

34. A 34-year-old male undergoes an uneventful excision of a parathyroid adenoma. The following postoperative day, he complains of numbness around his lips. Which of the following is the most likely cause of this symptom?

   (A) hypocalcemia secondary to hypomagnesemia
   (B) hypocalcemia due to acute renal failure
   (C) hypocalcemia due to hungry bone syndrome
   (D) hypocalcemia due to inadvertent injury to the recurrent laryngeal nerve
   (E) postoperative hematoma of the neck

35. Which of the following is the most appropriate intervention?

(A) oral calcium gluconate

(B) intravenous rehydration with normal saline

(C) intravenous magnesium sulfate infusion

(D) blood transfusion

(E) reassurance and close observation

Setting III: Emergency Department

Most patients in this setting are new to you, but occasionally you arrange to meet there with a known patient who has telephoned you. Generally, patients encountered here are seeking urgent care. Also available to you are a full range of social services, including rape crisis intervention, family support, and security assistance backed up by local police.

36. A CT scan in a patient with a temperature of 102.1°F and a history of an abdominal aortic graft reveals fluid around the graft. Which of the following is the most appropriate treatment?

(A) IV antibiotics and repeat CT scan in 24–48 h

(B) CT guided catheter drainage of fluid collection

(C) exploration with graft excision, irrigation, and replacement with fresh graft

(D) exploration with graft excision and construction of axillo-bifemoral graft

(E) open exploration with debridement and drainage of fluid collection

37. A 7-year-old girl presents to the emergency room (ER) with complaints of fatigue and pallor. She was treated by her primary care physician (PCP) earlier in the week for an upper respiratory infection. Your examination reveals splenomegaly and bruising on her upper extremities. You order laboratory work that shows a WBC of 11,000, hemoglobin of 6 g/dL, and a platelet count of 40,000. A Coombs test is also positive. What is the most likely cause?

(A) immune thrombocytopenic purpura

(B) Henoch-Schönlein purpura

(C) Evans syndrome

(D) meningococcemia

(E) hemolytic uremic syndrome

Questions 38 through 40

A 78-year-old female is transferred from the nursing home with nausea, vomiting, abdominal distention, and obstipation for the last 3 days. On examination, she is somnolent and tachycardic. Her abdomen is distended, tympanic, and diffusely tender. An abdominal x-ray is obtained and is shown in Fig. 11-2.

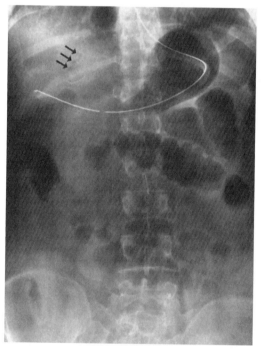

FIG. 11-2 (Reproduced, with permission, from Chen MYM, Pope TL Jr, Ott DJ. Basic Radiology. New York, NY: McGraw-Hill, 2004, p. 220.)

38. These findings are most consistent with

(A) gallstone ileus

(B) pancreatitis

(C) cholangitis

(D) small bowel neoplasm

(E) perforated appendicitis

39. The patient is at risk for

    (A) ascending cholangitis
    (B) small bowel perforation
    (C) colonic perforation
    (D) Ogilvie syndrome
    (E) massive lower GI bleed

40. The most appropriate intervention is

    (A) IV fluids, gastric decompression, antibiotics, and close observation
    (B) endoscopic retrograde cholangiopancreatography (ERCP) with decompression of the biliary tree
    (C) cholecystectomy
    (D) surgical exploration with enterotomy to relieve the obstruction
    (E) surgical exploration with enterotomy to relieve the obstruction and concomitant cholecystectomy

41. Which of the following conditions is the leading cause of death in the United States of infants between the ages of 1 and 12 months?

    (A) bacterial meningitis
    (B) congenital heart disease
    (C) congenital malformation syndromes
    (D) accidental poisonings
    (E) sudden infant death syndrome (SIDS)

Questions 42 and 43

An 84-year-old White female presents with acute vision loss that occurred several hours ago. She has a past history of hypertension and atrial fibrillation which are both controlled. She has been generally tired lately and is not eating well.

42. Which of the following tests should be ordered first?

    (A) MRI of brain and orbits with contrast
    (B) carotid Doppler
    (C) ESR
    (D) cardiac echo
    (E) complete blood count with differential and platelet count

43. Which of the following would you most likely find on fundoscopic examination?

    (A) retinal hemorrhages
    (B) lipid exudation
    (C) cherry red spot
    (D) AV nicking
    (E) cotton wool spots

44. A 62-year-old male presents to the ER with severe substernal pain following a prolonged episode of retching and vomiting. Work up, including a chest x-ray, reveals minimum air in the mediastinum. Which of the following is the most appropriate intervention at this time?

    (A) upper endoscopy
    (B) gastrografin swallow
    (C) place nasogastric and chest tubes, make NPO, and begin broad spectrum antibiotics
    (D) emergent left thoracotomy
    (E) emergent right thoracotomy

45. What is the most likely infectious agent in a 4-month-old with copious nasal secretions, wheezing, and cough in the winter?

    (A) group B *Streptococcus*
    (B) group A *Streptococcus*
    (C) respiratory syncytial virus
    (D) nonpolio enteroviru
    (E) *H. Influenzae*

46. A 35-year-old man presents to the ER with a third-degree flame burn of his right upper extremity, anterior trunk, and right lower extremity, sparing the genitalia. His estimated burn percentage is

    (A) 15%
    (B) 25%
    (C) 35%
    (D) 45%
    (E) 55%

Questions 47 through 50

A 50-year-old man presents to the ER following three episodes of massive hematemesis. The patient has never had prior similar episodes and is not currently bleeding. His vital signs are: temperature 98.8°F, BP 98/72 supine, 75/50 sitting up, pulse 110, respirations 17, oxygen saturation of 100% on room air. On examination, he is pale, dizzy, and weak. He has scleral icterus, spider angiomata on his chest, splenomegaly, and shifting dullness in his abdomen. His initial hematocrit is 30%. His prothrombin time is 31 s with an international normalized ratio (INR) of 3.1. The patient denies taking any anticoagulant medications. A GI consultation is requested.

47. Prior to upper endoscopy, the best initial step in the patient's management is

    (A) obtain hepatitis serologies
    (B) gastric lavage with nasogastric tube
    (C) CT scan to rule out hepatic disease
    (D) IV fluid resuscitation
    (E) correction of the patient's coagulopathy

48. Upper endoscopy reveals multiple grade 3 (out of 4) varices in the esophagus. One of the larger varices has a fibrin plug over what appears to be a break in the mucosa and is oozing fresh blood. What is the next best step in the patient's management?

    (A) endoscopic esophageal banding to treat the varices
    (B) endoscopic esophageal sclerotherapy to treat the varices
    (C) surgical therapy for definitive ligation of varices
    (D) institution of high-dose proton-pump inhibitor (PPI) therapy
    (E) placement of a transjugular intrahepatic portosystemic shunt (TIPS) via interventional radiology

49. The patient does well and does not rebleed while in hospital. Which additional therapy that can help prevent rebleeding in this patient should be provided as an outpatient?

    (A) endoscopic esophageal banding to treat the varices
    (B) endoscopic esophageal sclerotherapy to treat the varices
    (C) surgical therapy for definitive ligation of varices
    (D) institution of high-dose PPI therapy
    (E) placement of a TIPS via interventional radiology

50. Six months later the patient returns to the ER following another episode of massive hematemesis. Upper endoscopy performed in the hospital reveals actively bleeding gastric varices below the esophagogastric junction. The bleeding is torrential and the patient is hemodynamically unstable.

    What is the next best step in the patient's management?

    (A) endoscopic esophageal banding to treat the varices
    (B) endoscopic esophageal sclerotherapy to treat the varices
    (C) surgical therapy for definitive ligation of varices
    (D) institution of high-dose PPI therapy
    (E) placement of a TIPS via interventional radiology

Answers and Explanations

1. (D)

2. (C)

3. (D)

4. (C)

Explanations 1 through 4

Microscopic hematuria is defined as >3 RBCs/HPF on microscopic evaluation of the urinary sediment from two of three properly collected urinalysis specimens. Because the degree of hematuria bears no relation to the seriousness of the underling cause, hematuria should be considered a symptom of serious disease until proved otherwise (observation is incorrect). The initial step in evaluating microscopic hematuria is a thorough medical history and physical examination. Evaluation of the upper urinary tract is the next recommended step. Options for this include intravenous pyelography, ultrasonography, and CT scanning. *(Grossfeld GD, et al. Asymptomatic microscopic hematuria in adults: Summary of the AUA best practice policy recommendations. Am Fam Physician 2001;63: 1145–1154)*

During this visit you should provide alcohol abuse counseling. The U.S. Preventive Services Task Force (USPSTF) has a B recommendation (recommend routinely) for screening and behavioral counseling interventions to reduce alcohol misuse by adults in primary care settings. The USPSTF has an I recommendation (insufficient evidence) for skin cancer and low back pain prevention counseling and D recommendation (against) routine screening for testicular cancer in asymptomatic adolescent and adult males. The patient's last dT booster was at age 14, 5 years ago, so he does not need a dT booster at this time. *(USPSTF: www.preventiveservices.ahrq.gov)*

The number one cause of death in this patient's age group is motor vehicle-related injuries. The mortality rate for the 15–24 year age range due to unintentional injury is 38.7/100.000, most of it due to motor vehicle accidents. The next most common causes of death are other traumas, including homicide, suicide, and drowning. *(Maxcy-Rosenau-Last. Public Health and Preventive Medicine, 14th ed.)*

In a cross-sectional study of 354 inner city adolescents aged 12–21 were asked their reasons for continued smoking. The most common response was "it relaxes me," reported by 73%. This was followed by "I have a habit" (56%), "I am addicted (29%)," "I'm bored (22%)," and "Everyone around me smokes (17%)." In order to promote smoking cessation in this population, interventions need to focus on reduction in perceived stress, along with nicotine dependence *(Siqueira LM, Rolnitzky LM, Rickert VI. Smoking cessation in adolescents. Arch Pediatr Adolesc Med 2001;155:489–495)*

5. (D)

6. (E)

Explanations 5 and 6

Conversion disorder is diagnosed by the presence of neurologic symptoms or deficits associated with largely unconscious psychologic factors or conflicts, without the myriad of different symptoms seen in this case. Hypochondriasis is characterized by a preoccupation with fears of having a serious illness based on a misinterpretation of bodily sensations. Pain disorder involves significant distress or impairment in functioning as a result of pain. Psychologic factors are felt to play a role in the onset, severity, exacerbation, or maintenance of the pain. Nonpain-related symptomatology, as demonstrated in this patient, is not a feature.

Undifferentiated somatoform disorder is diagnosed when there are unexplained physical complaints which do not meet full criteria for somatization disorder. This case represents somatization disorder, characterized by a pattern of recurring, multiple somatic complaints, beginning before the age of 30, which are not fully explained by any known medical condition (DSM IV).

If a patient is diagnosed with somatization disorder, admission to the hospital for an extensive workup and multiple referrals may reinforce the process of somatization and worsen symptoms. Confronting the individual will likely anger the patient and lead to an increase in somatic complaints. Reassurance that a diagnosis will be discovered is inaccurate, misleading, and can eventually result in a lawsuit. The most appropriate management for these individuals is to schedule regular, brief appointments addressing any new physical complaints. Laboratory tests, studies, and procedures should be limited in nature. An abbreviated physical examination will reassure the patient that they are cared for and taken seriously. After a therapeutic alliance is better established, eventual referral to a psychiatrist may help to decrease health care utilization and to treat any comorbid psychopathology. (*Synopsis, p. 647*)

7. (C)

8. (C)

9. (B)

Explanations 7 through 9

Polymyalgia rheumatica is an inflammatory syndrome of older individuals characterized by pain and stiffness in the shoulder and pelvic girdles. Patients are typically >50 years old, have bilateral symptoms, and the ESR is frequently elevated above 40 mm/h. The absence of muscle weakness and normal CPK argue against polymyositis. Although hypothyroidism can cause musculoskeletal pain, it is not associated with an ESR of 99 or weight loss (typically weight gain). Osteoarthritis of the

neck and shoulders would demonstrate abnormalities in the range of motion associated with pain—this patient has muscle tenderness only. Fibromyalgia is a chronic noninflammatory and nonautoimmune diffuse pain syndrome of unknown etiology, with an average age of onset of between 35 and 40 years of age and characteristic tender points (11 of the 18 tender points need to be present for at least 3 months and exist both above and below the waist). Given the advanced age of this patient (60-year-old), the presence of symptoms for only 1 month and evidence for systemic inflammation (ESR = 99), the diagnosis of fibromyalgia is highly unlikely.

Prednisone in a dose of 10–20 mg daily usually results in a dramatic and rapid response in polymyalgia rheumatica. Most patients are significantly better in 1–2 days and the ESR should steadily decline. The use of TRH would be appropriate if this patient's symptoms were due to hypothyroidism. Analgesics will not help the inflammation (indicated by the elevated ESR) in polymyalgia rheumatica. Although this patient could have depression, the elevated ESR argues against this and the use of a muscle relaxant for a systemic inflammatory disease is unlikely to be helpful.

Giant cell (or temporal) arteritis occurs synchronously or sequentially in patients with PMR. Symptoms include headache, jaw claudication, visual disturbance, and scalp tenderness. The failure of prednisone to significantly improve symptoms (at doses of 20 mg daily) or normalize the ESR should suggest the presence of temporal arteritis and prompt temporal artery biopsy. Rheumatoid arthritis is unlikely, as there is no evidence of synovitis of any of the joints. Systemic lupus erythematous is possible, but highly unlikely, in a patient of this age who is ANA negative. This patient's symptoms are not typical for hypothyroidism (absence of muscle weakness, weight loss instead of weight gain, and an elevated ESR ~ 100 mm/h). To assume that the patient is depressed and is amplifying her symptoms despite laboratory evidence of systemic inflammation (ESR ~ 100 mm/h) would not be prudent. (*Ruddy, pp. 1155–1162*)

10. (A) Cyanotic congenital heart lesions are usually the result of right-to-left shunting. This results in the shunting of blood past the pulmonary system and the absence of gas exchange. Tetralogy of Fallot, transposition of the great vessels, truncus arteriosus, and pulmonic atresia are all causes of cyanotic congenital heart disease. The child in the case presented, however, does not have a cyanotic lesion. Of the listed heart lesions, only the ventricular septal defect (VSD) results in left-to-right shunting. *(Fleisher and Ludwig, pp. 187–191)*

11. (A)

12. (D)

13. (C)

Explanations 11 through 13

The patient likely has elevated BP secondary to OCP medication. This is the most common cause of secondary hypertension in the patient and, at its onset, the medication should be stopped. In addition, she has developed other side effects from OCPs, including weight gain and edema. Given her current symptoms, it is reasonable to assume that her BP may be elevated and hence should be checked during this visit. The vaginal bleeding and missed menses may signify that she is currently pregnant. Therefore, a urine pregnancy test should be obtained and the OCP stopped immediately until pregnancy is ruled out.

The only absolute contraindication listed is smoking after the age of 35, although heavy smoking at any age is also considered a relative contraindication. With the exception of hemolytic anemia, the rest of the choices are all considered relative contraindications to prescribing OCPs. The only hemolytic anemia which is considered an absolute contraindication is sickle cell disease, due to an increased risk of thrombosis.

Cholelithiasis is a well-established potential side effect of OCPs. Others include thromboembolic disease, hypertension, weight gain, fluid retention, edema, glucose intolerance, headaches, melasma, and nausea. The risk of developing endometrial cancer and ovarian cancer may, in fact, be reduced with the use of OCPs. The temporary infertility induced by OCPs should be reversible on discontinuation. Prolonged infertility following the cessation of OCPs should prompt a workup for other causes. Thrombocytopenia is not considered to be an expected side effect of OCPs. *(Larsen, pp. 672–691)*

14. (A) FHH, or familial benign hypercalcemia, is a rare condition characterized by asymptomatic or mildly symptomatic hypercalcemia. It is inherited as an autosomal dominant trait and the parathyroid glands are usually normal in size. The basis for the development of FHH appears to be mutations in the calcium-sensing receptor gene which regulates the parathyroid gland set point and modulates the extracellular calcium concentration. The condition may be mistaken for primary hyperparathyroidism because, in both conditions, the serum calcium and parathyroid hormone levels are elevated with a concomitant low serum phosphate. The distinction is made by obtaining a 24-h urine calcium excretion level. In patients with FHH, the urine calcium level is low, whereas in primary hyperparathyroidism the level is high. The distinction is important, as patients with primary hyperparathyroidism benefit from surgery and those with FHH do not. *(Cameron, p. 602)*

15. (B)

16. (D)

17. (D)

Explanations 15 through 17

Avoidant personality disorder is characterized by a pattern of inhibition in social situations and feelings of inadequacy. These individuals are more likely to blame themselves for their difficulties rather than criticize others, as illustrated in the above case. Patients with dependent personality disorder display a pervasive need to be taken care of that leads to submissive behavior. They are not likely to be hostile or as labile as in the above example. Paranoid individuals maintain chronic mistrust and suspiciousness of others. They assume that others will or have harmed them. They are not liable to enter into numerous relationships or admit to feelings of loneliness in the way that the above patient demonstrates. Schizoid personality disorder is diagnosed in patients with a pervasive pattern of detachment and restricted range of expression in interpersonal relationships. Schizoid individuals do not seek out relationships, preferring solitary activities. They are not as explosive as the patient in the case. The above example represents a man with borderline personality disorder, characterized by instability of relationships, affects and sense of self, as well as impulsivity, anger control problems, and chronic feelings of emptiness (DSM IV).

Denial is classified as a primitive or psychotic defense mechanism, where an individual avoids awareness of an external reality by negating sensory data. Displacement is considered a neurotic defense, characterized by shifting feeling from one person or situation to another that will evoke less distress. Intellectualization is another neurotic defense, utilizing intellectual processes in order to avoid affective experience. Sublimation is classified as a mature defense, where a person will direct an impulse toward a socially acceptable goal. The above patient demonstrates the defense mechanism of splitting. Splitting is considered a primitive defense and is commonly seen in severe personality disorders, especially borderline personality disorder. In splitting, patients divide feelings, people, and behavior into separate good and bad categories rather than deal with their ambivalence. (Synopsis, pp. 207–208, 802)

While benzodiazepines, such as clonazepam, may help with anxiety and agitation in individuals with borderline personality disorder, they are not considered first-line medications due to the paucity of data, risk of abuse, and the possibility of worsening behavioral dyscontrol. Antipsychotics, like haloperidol, may be beneficial for anger control and self-mutilation, but the effects are nonspecific. Given the significant side effects, especially the risk of tardive dyskinesia, they are not considered to be used as solo agents. Mood stabilizers, such as lithium and valproic acid, are sometimes used to treat the impulsive aggression and mood lability common in borderline patients. However, there is legitimate concern in using lithium in these impulsive, often suicidal patients, given its toxicity in overdose. While valproate is safer in overdose, there are less data to support its efficacy in this patient population. Antidepressants in general, especially serotonin-specific reuptake inhibitors (SSRIs) like sertraline, have been shown to be efficacious in treating the symptoms of mood lability, impulsivity, aggression, hostility, and self-mutilation seen in borderline personality disorder. SSRIs have been the most widely studied medications and are very safe in the event of an overdose. These factors favor their use as a first-line pharmacotherapy in these patients, although no agents are currently FDA approved for this illness. (Practice Guideline for the Treatment of Patients with Borderline Personality Disorder, 2001, APA)

18. **(A)** Thyroid cancer is classified as papillary, follicular, Hurthle cell, medullarly, or anaplastic. Of all subtypes, papillary carries the best overall prognosis. In addition to the subtype of cancer, there are several important prognostic indicators, referred to as the AGES scale. The AGES scale includes the **A**ge of the patient, pathologic tumor **G**rade, **E**xtent of disease, and **S**ize of tumor. Other important factors include the presence of distant metastases, the extent of original surgical resection, and the presence of extrathyroidal invasion. Of all factors, age is the most important (age < 40). For instance, a 16-year-old male with thyroid cancer and metastasis to regional lymph nodes has a 90% chance of survival. (Schwartz, pp. 1682–1683)

19. **(D)** Absolute contraindications to the use of combined OCPs include history of thrombotic disorders, vascular disease (e.g., cerebral, coronary), impaired liver function (or liver tumor), history of hormone-dependent cancer (e.g., breast), smoker over the age of 35, known or suspected pregnancy, undiagnosed vaginal bleeding, and congenital hyperlipidemia. (Beckmann, p. 335)

20. (E)

21. (C)

Explanations 20 and 21

This child has a "narrow-gap" metabolic acidosis. Given her history, this would be most consistent with renal tubular acidosis (RTA). In her case, this represents the presence of a proximal renal bicarbonate threshold (proximal RTA). She is unable to retain bicarbonate enough to raise her serum level. Persistent vomiting (pyloric stenosis, duodenal stenosis, or gastroesophageal reflux) would result in the loss of bicarbonate and thus a serum alkalosis, not acidosis.

In proximal RTA (type II RTA), there is a failure to reabsorb bicarbonate. There is a "threshold" level of serum bicarbonate above which the kidney will "spill" the bicarbonate into the urine. For example, if the "threshold" is a serum level of 15, the addition of bicarbonate to the serum will result in the bicarbonate spilling into the urine, with a resulting increase in the urinary pH. The addition of bicarbonate into the serum would result in a transient increase in the serum level, with a gradual decrease back to the "threshold" level. When the serum bicarbonate level reaches 15, the threshold level, the urinary pH will return to normal (slightly acidic, pH of approximately 5–7). In distal RTA (type I RTA), there is an inability to maintain a proton "gradient." This results in an abnormally high urinary pH in the face of acidemia (the inability to lower urinary pH). Distal RTA will also have hypokalemia, as a result of maintaining electroneutrality. In evaluation of a proximal RTA, the diagnostic work-up includes a trial of bicarbonate. This trial will demonstrate the transient rising of the urinary pH and serum bicarbonate. (*Rudolph, pp. 1710–1712*)

22. (B) This patient has symptoms and physical findings of vulvovaginal atrophy due to the hypoestrogenic state of menopause. Irritative bladder symptoms are common with this condition as the lower GU tract has estrogen receptors like the vagina and vulva. A white, curdy discharge of a yeast infection is possible, and would be more common following a course of antibiotic. It would not be consistent with the time course of her symptoms, however. A retained tampon would tend to cause a malodorous vaginal discharge. The likelihood of this woman using a tampon would also be low, as she is postmenopausal. A vesico-vaginal fistula would tend to cause a leakage of urine from the vagina rather than irritative bladder symptoms. A fungating cervical mass (i.e., advanced cervical carcinoma) would be a rare occurrence. (*Hendrix SL. Long-term use of hormone therapy for urogenital complaints. Med Clin North Am 2003;87(5):1029–1037*)

23. (B) The FDA drug categories provide a very basic guideline as to the safety of prescribing a medication during pregnancy. However, being a member of a higher category does not automatically confer a higher risk. While, in fact, a number of category X drugs are associated with a higher risk of congenital abnormalities, some are simply listed as category X because there is no conceivable use for these agents during pregnancy and not because they are teratogenic. A good example is OCP tablets. Drugs in category D have been shown to have at least some risk for congenital abnormalities, such as valproate with a 10-fold increase for neural tube defects; however, the risk to the fetus of taking the medication may be outweighed by controlling the underlying medical problem. Many drugs in FDA category C suffer from a relative lack of data in either animal or human studies. Drugs in category B fall into two groups. They either have not been shown to be teratogenic in animals, with no human data available, or have been shown to have risk in animals but controlled studies have not shown evidence of risk. This is consistent with the wide variation in teratogenesis between species. (*Briggs, Freeman, Yaffe (eds.). Drugs in Pregnancy and Lactation, 6th ed. Baltimore, MD: Lippincott Williams & Wilkins, 2001*)

24. (D) The diagnosis is primary hypothyroidism, most likely due to postpartum thyroiditis. The essential laboratory finding is the elevated TSH and low free thyroid hormone levels in the setting of weight gain and fatigue. The low T3-resin uptake indicates increased thyroid binding globulin (TBG) from either hypothyroidism or estrogen effect. The free thyroid index is derived by multiplying T3-uptake times the total T4. As both levels are low, the free thyroid index will also be low. The galactorrhea and the elevated prolactin are not uncommon in patients with hypothyroidism and relate to the increased levels of TRH, a potent stimulant for prolactin. The prolactin should no longer be elevated from nursing, but OCPs also increase prolactin levels. As the baseline TSH is elevated, there is no indication for a TRH stimulation test. Nuclear thyroid scans give useful information in the differential diagnosis of hyperthyroidism but are not helpful in the diagnosis of hypothyroidism. (*Larsen, pp. 423–428, 440*)

25. **(C)** Follow-up of patients with hydatidiform mole indicates evacuation is curative in 80% of cases. In roughly 20% of cases, however, trophoblastic tissue will persist and the diagnosis of gestational trophoblastic neoplasia (GTN) will be made. This diagnosis includes a spectrum of disease including invasive mole, choriocarcinoma, and placental site trophoblastic tumor.

Following evacuation of a molar gestation, appropriate surveillance followup should include serial hCG values obtained q 1–2 weeks until normal times three and then monthly thereafter, to complete 1 year of surveillance. Birth control is recommended during this period, preferably with OCPs. In the setting of stable or rising hCG levels, as in the case noted above, metastatic workup is indicated with a CT scan of the head, chest, abdomen, and pelvis.

Patients at risk for the development of postevacuation GTN include those with (1) preevacuation uterus >16 weeks size; (2) preevacuation bilateral ovarian enlargement (theca-lutein cysts); (3) age greater than 40; (4) preevacuation hCG levels greater than 100,000 mIU/mL; (5) prior hydatidiform mole; (6) medical complications of molar pregnancy including toxemia, hyperthyroidism, and trophoblastic embolization.

Indications for treatment of postmolar trophoblastic tumor include: (1) plateauing hCG levels for three consecutive determinations, (2) rising hCG levels for two consecutive determi-

nations, (3) hCG levels greater than 20,000 mIU/mL 4 or more weeks postevacuation, (4) detection of metastases, or (5) histopathologic diagnosis of choriocarcinoma.

A repeat D&C is rarely indicated following evacuation of a molar gestation; it is not curative in the setting of GTN and may be associated with an increased risk of uterine perforation. (*Diagnosis and management of gestational trophoblastic neoplasia. Best Pract Res Clin Obstet Gynaecol 2003;17(6):893–903*)

26. **(E)** The initial step in identification of the cause of a prolonged PT or aPTT is to establish if the addition of normal plasma can correct the deficit. Failure to correct the prolonged PT or aPTT by addition of 50% normal plasma is indicative of the presence of a specific (against one of the coagulation factors) or nonspecific inhibitor (e.g., lupus anticoagulant). If, after the 1:1 mix, the PT or aPTT tests correct, a plasma factor(s) deficiency is the most likely cause. The most common inhibitor in a non-hemophilia individual is against factor VIII, as is this woman's case. (*Hoffman, p. 1843*)

27. **(C)** The distal small bowel (ileum) is the site of absorption of fat-soluble vitamins (vitamins A, D, E, and K) as well as vitamin B_{12}. Vitamin B_{12} binds with intrinsic factor, a glycoprotein secreted from parietal cells of the gastric fundus and body. Specific receptors in the terminal ileum take up the B_{12} intrinsic factor complex. Vitamin B_{12} deficiency leads to megaloblastic anemia. The patient will require monthly vitamin B_{12} injections. (*Schwartz, p. 1255*)

28. **(A)**

29. **(D)**

30. **(E)**

Explanations 28 through 30

The photomicrograph shows malignant tumor cells infiltrating between the collagen bundles and in some focal areas, growing as a solid nest. The tumor shows high degree of anaplasia with prominent nucleoli and scant cytoplasm. Formation of ductal structures is minimal and, for all of these reasons, it is a poorly differentiated tumor (grade III). Carcinoma of the breast affects one out of nine women in the United States and one-third of these patients will die of the disease. Cancer of the breast is rarely found before the age of 25, except when there is a familial predisposition. Family history is a risk factor for the development of breast cancer in 5–10% of the cases. Two genes have been implicated in the genetic inheritance of cancer of the breast those are, BRCA-1 and BRCA-2; however, less than 20% of women with a family history of breast cancer carry these genes. A proliferative breast disease (atypical ductal hyperplasia) is also associated with an increase in risks for developing breast cancer. Also associated with the increased risk of developing carcinoma of the breast is increasing age, carcinoma of the contralateral breast or endometrium, radiation exposure, length of reproductive life, parity, obesity, and estrogen (although questionable). Invasive or infiltrating ductal carcinomas are the major variety of the carcinomas (70–80%). Most of these cancers exhibit a marked increase in fibrous tissue stroma, which gives the stony hard consistency. On histologic examination, the tumor consists of malignant cells forming cords, solid nests, and tubules. The cytologic appearance of these tumor cells varies from low to high grade. *(Cotran, 6th ed., pp 1104–1111)*

The prognosis of breast cancer is directly related to its staging using the TNM system. In the absence of distant metastasis, the stage of the tumor is determined by the size of the primary tumor and the presence or absence of regional lymphadenopathy. Other prognostic factors, such as the presence of lymphatic invasion or hormone receptor status, may influence survival, but it is not clear whether they add to the information from pathologic staging.

Atypical lobular hyperplasia, atypical ductal hyperplasia, and tubular adenoma are benign breast diseases and would not cause adenopathy. Lobular carcinoma in situ, by definition, is not an invasive cancer and, therefore, would not cause the presence of axillary adenopathy. However, approximately 30% of patients who undergo excision of lobular neoplasia may develop invasive carcinoma in the following 15–20 years, usually infiltrating ductal carcinoma. Of the options listed, only infiltrating ductal carcinoma would be expected to cause axillary metastasis. *(Harrison's Principles of Internal Medicine, 15th ed., pp. 574–577)*

31. **(C)** Prolonged bleeding time is the hallmark of platelet pathology. Impaired platelet adhesion is seen in both acute and chronic renal insufficiency. The mechanism is unclear, although data imply that uremic toxins in plasma result in disaggregation of factor VIII, which is required for proper platelet function. DDAVP (1-desamino-8-D-arginine vasopressin) is a synthetic derivative of vasopressin and administration results in a dose-dependent increase of factor VIII from endothelial cells. It is therefore used to help control postoperative bleeding in uremic patients. Alternatively, transfusion with cryoprecipitate is useful because it contains high levels of factor VIII. Ultimately, correction of the uremic state with dialysis may be indicated. Transfused platelets will not correct the condition, as they will be deactivated by the circulating toxins. Vitamin K is used to correct bleeding caused by a defective extrinsic pathway of the coagulation cascade. Fresh frozen plasma does not contain high levels of factor VIII. Hyperglycemia is not related to bleeding tendency. *(Jarrell BE, et al. National Medical Series for Independent Study, Surgery, 4th ed. Philadelphia, PA: Lippincott Williams & Wilkins, 2000, pp. 130–131; Schwartz, p. 82)*

32. **(D)** Physiologic changes in the cardiovascular and circulatory systems are significant and may affect underlying maternal illness. Blood volume increases by 40–50% by term pregnancy, with red cell mass lagging behind and increasing by only 20–25%; this differential has been referred to as the physiologic anemia of pregnancy. The total requirement for term pregnancy to meet maternal, fetal, and placental needs is 1000 mg of iron. This need can be met by preexisting iron stores in iron-replete women, but at the risk of depleting their iron stores, resulting in postpartum anemia. Iron depletion can be prevented by the administration

of 30 mg of elemental iron per day, which can be obtained by taking one ferrous gluconate 325 mg tablet per day. *(Romslo I, Haram K, Sagan N, et al. Iron requirement in normal pregnancy is assessed by serum ferritin, serum transfer and saturation and erythrocyte protoporphyrin determinations. Br J Obstet Gynecol 1983;90:101)*

33. **(E)** Meckel's diverticulum, the most common true diverticulum of the GI tract, is a congenital diverticulum that results from incomplete closure of the omphalomesenteric, or vitelline, duct. It is characteristically found within 2 ft of the ileocecal junction and along the antimesenteric border of the ileum. A Meckel's may be asymptomatic and found incidentally during surgical exploration. In this scenario, resection is indicated only if there are signs of potential complications. Such findings include the presence of palpable firm tissue at the base. This represents heterotrophic gastric or pancreatic tissue, which may result in an adjacent ulcer and bleeding. If a connection or adhesion from the Meckel's to the umbilicus is present, resection would be indicated to prevent the risk of future intestinal rotation, volvulus, and obstruction around the adhesion. Finally resection should be contemplated if the neck of the Meckel's is narrow, as this may result in future obstruction by a fecalith with resulting diverticulitis and perforation. The morbidity from incidental removal can be as high as 12% and is therefore limited to these indications. *(Schwartz, p. 1249)*

34. **(C)**

35. **(A)**

Explanations 34 and 35

Hungry bone syndrome refers to hypocalcemia following surgical correction of hyperparathyroidism in patients with severe, prolonged disease, as serum calcium is rapidly taken from the circulation and deposited into the bone. Symptoms usually occur within 24–48 h following parathyroidectomy, when calcium levels reach a nadir. Early symptoms include numbness and tingling in the perioral area, fingers, or toes. Advanced symptoms include

nervousness, anxiety, and increased neuromuscular transmission evidenced by positive Chvostek's and Trousseau's signs, carpal pedal spasm, and hyperactive tendon reflexes. In severe cases, one may develop a prolonged QT interval on ECG.

Patients who manifest any signs or symptoms of hypocalcemia always require intervention. In severely symptomatic patients, treatment should begin with intravenous calcium gluconate. Mildly symptomatic patients may be given oral calcium in the form of calcium lactate, calcium carbonate, or calcium gluconate. If hypocalcemia remains despite calcium supplementation, additional therapy with vitamin D may be needed. Supplemental calcium and vitamin D therapy should be continued until serum calcium levels return to normal. *(Schwartz, p. 1701)*

36. **(D)** The triad of fever, abdominal fluid collection, and history of abdominal graft surgery indicates the development of a graft infection. The most common organism isolated is *Staphylococcus aureus*. It is a rare, but morbid, complication, with mortality rates as high as 36%. The infection may rapidly result in sepsis, hemorrhagic shock, and septic embolization.

The standard treatment is early detection and surgical removal of the infected graft, with primary closure of the aorta and creation of an extraanatomical reconstruction—most commonly an axillo-femoral bypass. Such a bypass carries its own morbidities, including risk of limb loss, aortic stump blowout, and pelvic ischemia. *(Am J Surg 1999;178(2):136–140)*

37. **(C)** Evans syndrome is the combination of immune thrombocytopenic purpura (ITP) and autoimmune hemolytic anemia. The triggers of these events remain speculative. Children with Evans syndrome will have a Coombs positive anemia with various levels of thrombocytopenia. Corticosteroids may be warranted to control acute hemolysis or thrombocytopenia. *(Rudolph, p. 1546)*

38. **(A)**

39. **(B)**

40. (D)

Explanations 38 through 40

Gallstone ileus causes 1–2% of mechanical small-intestine obstructions. It results from erosion of an impacted gallstone through the wall of the gallbladder into the wall of the adjacent duodenum. The gallstone then passes through the small intestine. The size of the stone is important, since stones smaller that 2 cm usually pass, while larger stones may cause an obstruction. When obstruction occurs, the site is usually at the terminal ileum, which is the narrowest portion of the small intestine. The resulting obstruction results in large fluid losses and electrolyte abnormalities. Edema, ulceration and, ultimately, necrosis of the bowel may occur, resulting in perforation.

The correct preoperative diagnosis is infrequently made. However, radiographic examination is diagnostic if gas is demonstrated within the biliary tree in the presence of a small intestine obstruction. In 20% of cases a radiopaque stone is also visualized.

Definitive therapy requires urgent surgical intervention. The patient is explored and the small bowel is opened (enterotomy) just proximal to the lodged stone. The stone is extracted and the small bowel is primarily closed. Prolonging the operation to perform a cholecystectomy in an ill, elderly patient adds to potential operative morbidity and is generally not warranted. (*Schwartz, pp. 1450–1452*)

41. (E) SIDS is the most common cause of death in children between 1 and 12 months of age. In the first month of life, perinatal complications (i.e., prematurity) are the most common cause of death. The diagnosis of SIDS requires a review of the medical history, a death scene investigation, as well as a full postmortem examination. The rate of SIDS has decreased dramatically with the onset of the "Back to Sleep" campaign, which recommends placing infants on their back or side—not abdomen—to sleep. While bacterial meningitis can be a devastating disease, it is rarely fatal when treated. Death from congenital malformations will usually occur within the first month of a neonate's life. (*Rudolph, pp. 1935–1936*)

42. (C)

43. (C)

Explanations 42 through 43

This patient is presenting with symptoms most consistent with central retinal artery occlusion. This typically causes painless, acute, unilateral vision loss. Sometimes there will be an associated history of amaurosis fugax. Characteristic diagnostic signs of this are a cherry red spot in the center of the macula and superficial opacification or whitening of the retina in the posterior pole. Common etiologies of this include embolus from the heart or carotid artery, thrombosis, giant cell arteritis, other collagen vascular disease, and hypercoagulable states.

For this patient, who has atrial fibrillation, which would put her at an increased risk of embolic disease, the most important test to order emergently would be an ESR. This would help to determine whether the etiology of the event is more likely embolic or related to giant cell arteritis. If the ESR were markedly elevated then high-dose steroids should be immediately started. The other tests listed may be part of the later work-up but would not be as important immediately to determine the urgent treatment required. (*Wills Eye Manual, Section 11.5*)

44. (B) Esophageal perforation has a poor survival rate, especially if the diagnosis is delayed. When suspected, urgent posterior-to-anterior (PA) and lateral chest x-rays should be obtained. Positive findings include mediastinal emphysema, mediastinal-widening secondary to edema, pneumothorax, and pleural effusion; however, these findings may take over an hour to appear. The diagnosis is confirmed with a water-soluble contrast (gastrografin) esophagogram. If the gastrografin study is negative, a thin-barium swallow should be performed. Barium extravasation may result in a severe mediastinitis. (*Cameron, p. 8*)

45. **(C)** In the wintertime, greater than 90% of children younger than 3 years of age will become infected with respiratory syncitial virus (RSV). It can cause a bronchiolitis in infants which occasionally results in hypoxia. Most otherwise healthy infants will not require hospitalization. Risk factors for complications from RSV bronchiolitis include bronchopulmonary dysplasia, congenital heart disease, and prematurity. *(Red Book, pp. 523–528)*

46. **(D)** There are two methods commonly utilized to estimate the total burn surface area: the palm method and the rule of nine. The palm method is based on the fact that patient's palm approximates 1% of his/her total body surface area. This method is particularly useful in those with a patchy pattern of burn injury. Rule of nine divides the body surface into several areas, each of which represents 9% or an interval of 9%. The head and neck represents 9% and each of the upper extremity equals 9% of the total body surface area. The anterior and posterior trunk each accounts for 18% as does each lower extremity. The genital area is 1%. In the above scenario, the patient has a burn involving his right upper extremity (9%), anterior trunk (18%), and right lower extremity (18%), a total of 45%. *(Schwartz, p. 228)*

47. **(D)**

48. **(A)**

49. **(A)**

50. **(E)**

Explanations 47 through 50

The patient is symptomatically orthostatic when switching from a supine to sitting position following massive hematemesis and needs urgent IV volume repletion to help prevent end-organ damage from hypovolemia. Hepatitis serology data, gastric lavage, correction of coagulopathy, and radiologic studies, while all important, should be deferred until after the patient has been hemodynamically stabilized.

Endoscopic esophageal banding would be the procedure of choice for this patient. Banding is superior to sclerotherapy in terms of efficacy for stopping variceal bleeding, although sclerotherapy might be a second option if banding fails or causes more bleeding. Surgery in patients with bleeding esophageal varices involves a very high risk due to portal hypertension and concomitant coagulopathy. PPI therapy would do little to help this patient as his illness is not due to acid reflux. A TIPS is not first-line therapy for acute variceal bleeding.

The patient had bleeding esophageal varices that have been successfully treated via banding. Banding rarely completely ablates varices in a single session. Multiple sessions are often required to completely thrombose and scar the varices to the point where they cannot rebleed. Sclerotherapy is not usually performed in patients who have responded to banding. High-dose PPI therapy would not help to prevent rebleeding from esophageal varices. A TIPS is not required in patients who have had bleeding controlled endoscopically and are doing well. Endoscopic therapy is preferable to surgery as an outpatient management strategy in patients with portal hypertension.

Gastric varices, often seen in patients with portal hypertension, respond poorly to endoscopic banding or sclerotherapy. A PPI would not help to stop the bleeding. Surgery in this patient is possible but highly risky given his hemodynamic instability. A TIPS could be performed in an emergent fashion and would decompress his portal system and would have the best chance of stopping the bleeding from the gastric varices. *(Harrison's Principles of Internal Medicine, pp. 252–253, 1760–1761)*

BIBLIOGRAPHY

American Academy of Pediatrics. *The Red Book, 2003 Report of the Committee on Infectious Diseases*, 26th ed. Elk Grove Village, IL: American Academy of Pediatrics, 2003.

American Psychiatric Association. *Diagnostic and Statistical Manual of Mental Disorders*, 4th ed., Text Revision. Washington, DC: American Psychiatric Association, 2000.

American Psychiatric Association. *Practice Guideline for the Treatment of Patients with Borderline Personality Disorder.* Washington, DC: American Psychiatric Association, 2001.

Beckmann CRB, Ling FW, Laube DW, et al. *Obstetrics and Gynecology*, 4th ed. Baltimore, MD: Lippincot Williams & Wilkins, 2002.

Braunwald E, et al. *Harrison's Principles of Internal Medicine*, 15th ed. New York, NY: McGraw-Hill, 2001.

Cameron JL (ed.). *Current Surgical Therapy*, 8th ed. St. Louis, MO: C.V. Mosby, 2004.

Cameron JL (ed.). *Current Surgical Therapy*, 8th ed. St. Louis, MO: C.V. Mosby, 2004.

Cotran RS, Kumar V, Collins T. *Robbins Pathologic Basis of Disease*, 6th ed. Philadelphia, PA: W.B. Saunders, 1999.

Fleisher GR, Ludwig S (eds.). *Textbook of Pediatric Emergency Medicine*, 4th ed. Baltimore, MD: Lippincott Williams & Wilkins, 2000.

Hoffman R, et al. *Hematology: Basic Principles and Practice*, 3rd ed. New York, NY: Churchill Livingstone, 2000.

Kunimoto DY, et al. *The Wills Eye Manual: Office and Emergency Room Diagnosis and Treatment of Eye Disease*, 4th ed. Philadelphia, PA: Lippincott Williams & Wilkins, 2004.

Larsen PR, et al. *Williams Textbook of Endocrinology*, 10th ed. Philadelphia, PA: W.B. Saunders, 2003.

Ruddy S, et al. *Kelley's Textbook of Rheumatology*, 6th ed. Philadelphia, PA: W.B. Saunders, 2001.

Rudolph CD, Rudolph AM, Hostetter MK, Lister GE, Siegel NJ, et al. (eds.). *Rudolph's Pediatrics*, 21st ed. New York, NY: McGraw-Hill, 2003.

Sadock BJ, Sadock VA. *Kaplan and Sadock's Synopsis of Psychiatry*, 9th ed. Philadelphia, PA: Lippincott Williams & Wilkins, 2003.

Schwartz SI, Shires GT, Spencer FC, et al. (eds.). *Principles of Surgery*, 7th ed. New York, NY: McGraw-Hill, 1999.

Index

Page numbers followed by italic *f* or *t* denote figures or tables, respectively.